Ambulance Care Essentials

Disclaimer

Class Professional Publishing have made every effort to ensure that the information, tables, drawings and diagrams contained in this book are accurate at the time of publication. The book cannot always contain all the information necessary for determining appropriate care and cannot address all individual situations; therefore, individuals using the book must ensure they have the appropriate knowledge and skills to enable suitable interpretation. Class Professional Publishing does not guarantee, and accepts no legal liability of whatever nature arising from or connected to, the accuracy, reliability, currency or completeness of the content of Ambulance Care Essentials. Users must always be aware that such innovations or alterations after the date of publication may not be incorporated in the content. Please note, however, that Class Professional Publishing assumes no responsibility whatsoever for the content of external resources in the text or accompanying online materials.

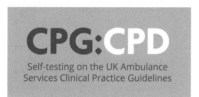
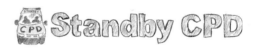

Ambulance Care Essentials

Richard Pilbery
and
Kris Lethbridge

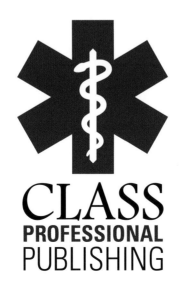

CLASS
PROFESSIONAL
PUBLISHING

Printing history

Preliminary edition published 2015

This edition first published 2015. Reprinted 2015, 2016 and 2017

The accompanying online resource published 2015

The authors and publisher welcome feedback from the users of this book.

Please contact the publisher:

Class Professional Publishing,

The Exchange, Express Park, Bristol Road, Bridgwater TA6 4RR

Telephone: 01278 427800

Email: post@class.co.uk

Website: classprofessional.co.uk

Class Professional Publishing is an imprint of Class Publishing Ltd

A CIP catalogue record for this book is available from the British Library

Paperback ISBN: 978-1-85959-582-4

eBook ISBN: 978-1-85959-583-1

Line illustrations by David Woodroffe with additional drawings by Nigel Downing

Cover design by Hybert Design Limited, UK

Designed and typeset by David Lewis XML Associates Ltd

Printed in Slovenia by KINT

Contents

Chapter 21: Cardiac Arrest

Acronyms

ABC	airway, breathing, circulation
ABG	arterial blood gas
ACP	advance care plan
ACS	acute coronary syndrome
ADRT	advanced decision to refuse treatment ('living will')
AED	automated external defibrillator
AF	atrial fibrillation
AMHP	approved mental health professional
AMI	acute myocardial infarction
ANF	autonomic failure
ANS	autonomic nervous system
APGAR	appearance, pulse, grimace, activity, respiration [test on newborns]
ASM	airway smooth muscle
ATMIST	age, time of incident, mechanism of injury, injuries, signs and symptoms, treatment given/immediate needs
ATP	adenosine triphosphate
AVPU	alert, voice, pain, unresponsive
BLS	basic life support
BURP	backwards, upwards, right pressure [manoeuvre]
BVM	bag-valve-mask
CES	cauda equina syndrome
CHALETS	casualties, hazards, access, location, emergency services, type, start a log
CNS	central nervous system
CO/COHb	Carbon monoxide/carboxyhaemoglobin
COPD	chronic obstructive pulmonary disease
CPR	cardiopulmonary resuscitation
CRT	capillary refill time
CSF	cerebral spinal fluid
CT	computerised tomography
CVP	central venous pressure
DIC	disseminated intravascular coagulopathy
DNA	deoxyribonucleic acid
DNACPR	do not attempt cardiopulmonary resuscitation
DOPES	displacement, obstruction, pneumothorax, equipment failure, stomach
DSH	deliberate self harm
ECA	emergency care assistant
ECG	electrocardiogram
ECSW	emergency care support worker
ED	emergency department
EOC	emergency operations centre
EOLC	end-of-life care
ET	endotracheal
EtCO2	end-tidal carbon dioxide [monitor]
GCS	Glasgow Coma Scale
HART	hazardous area response team
HCAI	healthcare-associated infection
HCPC	Health and Care Professions Council
HIN	Hazard Identification Number
HPV	hypoxic pulmonary vasoconstriction
ICP	intracranial pressure
ICU	intensive care unit
ICV	immediate care vehicle
IR	infrared
IV	intravenous
JVD	jugular venous distension
kPa	kilopascal
LAD	left anterior descending artery
LAFB	left anterior fascicular block
LBBB	left bundle branch block
LCA	left coronary artery
LMA	laryngeal mask airway
LOC	level of consciousness
MDT	Mobile Data Terminal
METHANE	major incident, exact location, type of incident, hazards, access, number of casualties, emergency services
MHA	Mental Health Act
MI	myocardial infarction
MILS	manual in-line stabilisation
MIU	minor injuries unit
MOI	mechanism of injury
MSC	motor, sensory, circulation [function]
MTC	major trauma centre
NAI	non-accidental injury
NIBP	non-invasive blood pressure measurement
NOI	nature of illness
NSAIDs	non-steroidal anti-inflammatory drugs
NSR	normal sinus rhythm
NSTEMI	non-ST-segment elevation myocardial infarction
OH	orthostatic hypotension
OPA	oropharyngeal airway
PDA	posterior descending artery
PEA	pulseless electrical activity
PICU	paediatric intensive care unit
pPCI	primary percutaneous coronary intervention
PND	paroxysmal nocturnal dyspnoea
PPE	personal protective equipment
PPH	primary postpartum haemorrhage
PPV	positive pressure ventilation
RCA	right coronary artery
RCT	randomised controlled trial
RINDs	reversible ischaemic neurological deficits
RNA	ribonucleic acid
ROLE	recognition of life extinct
ROM	range of movement
ROS	reactive oxygen species [free radicals]
ROSC	return of spontaneous circulation
RRV	rapid response vehicle
RTC	road traffic collision
RVI	right ventricular infarction

SA	sino-atrial	SOBOE	shortness of breath on exertion
SAD	supraglottic airway device	SpO2	blood oxygen saturation
SAMPLE	signs and symptoms of presenting complaint, allergies, medications, past medical history, last oral intake, events leading to current illness/injury	STEMI	ST-segment elevation myocardial infarction
		SUDICA	sudden unexpected death in infants, children and adolescents
SARS	severe acute respiratory syndrome	SVC	superior vena cava
SC	subcutaneous	SW	support worker
SCENE	safety, cause including NOI/MOI, environment, number of patients, extra resources needed	TBI	traumatic brain injury
		TBSA	total body surface area
		TXA	tranexamic acid
SCI	spinal cord injury	UA	unstable angina
SIDS	sudden infant death syndrome	URTI	upper respiratory tract infection
SIRS	systemic inflammatory response syndrome	UTI	urinary tract infection
SNS	sympathetic nervous system	WHO	World Health Organization

Acknowledgements

Class Professional Publishing would like to thank the following for their co-operation in the production of this book:

- Iris Murch, Mervyn Murch, Sarah Petter, Steven Petter, Karina Pilbery, Megan Pilbery, Vicky Pilbery and the team at SWAST for modelling
- Daniels for the loan of patslide equipment
- Ken Wenman and Claire Warner at SWAST for the loan of the ambulance
- Mangar for the loan of the Mangar ELK
- Mike Page for consulting
- Nigel Wilson for photography work
- Rose Teanby, for photographic editing
- SP Services for first aid and medical devices
- University of the West of England for the loan of the Lifepak and introductions to the students

The authors and publisher would like to thank the following for their invaluable feedback on earlier drafts of this book:

- Victoria Burnham, Head of Professional Practice, Scottish Ambulance Service
- Anne-Marie Chatwin, PA / OT, Clinical Education Manager, East Midlands Ambulance Service NHS Trust
- Jon Ellis, MAEd, FHEA, FIfL, MCPara, Advanced Paramedic Practitioner, Head of Education, Peritorum Ltd
- Steve Evans, MCPara, Paramedic Training Manager, Training, Education & Development, North West Ambulance Service
- Gary Heaps, M/c Para, BSc, ADI, Paramedic Training Manager, Training, Education and Development, North West Ambulance Service
- Frederick Lawrence, FASI, Educational and Training Consultant, North West Ambulance Service
- Sid Marshall, Education Manager, South Central Ambulance Service NHS Foundation Trust
- Neil Monery, Senior Learning and Development Manager, South East Coast Ambulance Service NHS Foundation Trust
- Ian Mullineaux, BSc, CertED, PGCODE, ELearning Coordinator, North West Ambulance Service
- Boyd Murdoch, S.R.P. Tutor, Paramedic Training Manager, Training and Education, North West Ambulance Service
- Jim Petter, Head of Education and Professional Development, South Western Ambulance Service NHSFT
- Dawn Stevenson, HDip EMT, Senior Training Officer, Education & Competency Assurance, National Ambulance Service College
- Ian Teague, Assistant Director of Education, South Central Ambulance Service NHS Foundation Trust
- Hannah Turner, SR Para, MCPara, MIFL, BSc (Hons), Clinical Tutor/Practice Placement Educator, South Western Ambulance Service NHSFT
- John Walker, Learning and Development Lead, South East Coast Ambulance Service NHS Foundation Trust HQ
- Kenny Weir, Practice Placement Lead (IQA), Scottish Ambulance Service

The following images are © Richard Pilbery 2015:

- Chapter 5 Figure 3.2 Non-latex disposable gloves
- Chapter 5 Figure 3.3 Surgical face mask and FFP3 mask
- Chapter 10 Figure 2.1 Oxygen cylinders – CD (portable) and HX (fitted to ambulance)

We would like to thank the following for their kind permission to publish material:

- Chapter 4 Figure 1.1 The health and care system. © Crown copyright. Available at: https://www.gov.uk/government/publications/the-health-and-care-system-explained/the-health-and-care-system-explained
- Chapter 5 Alcohol Handrub Procedure. Based on the 'How to Handrub' poster © World Health Organization 2009. All rights reserved
- Chapter 5 Handwashing Procedure. Based on the 'How to Handwash' poster © World Health Organization 2009. All rights reserved
- Chapter 7 Figure 2.1 An incident command structure showing examples of the additional support roles that may be required. Reproduced by the kind permission of the National Ambulance Resilience Unit (NARU)
- Chapter 7 Figure 2.2 The triage sieve. Copyright National Ambulance Resilience Unit, 2014
- Chapter 9 Figure 2.2 Mechanical suction device. Image reproduced by the kind permission of Laerdal Medical
- Chapter 9 Figure 2.3 Hand-operated suction device. Image reproduced by the kind permission of Ambu A/S
- Chapter 9 Figure 3.2, 3.3 and 3.4 Tracheostomy tubes. Images reproduced by the kind permission of Kapitex Healthcare Ltd
- Chapter 9 Figure 4.3 The choking algorithm. Reproduced with the kind permission of the Resuscitation Council (UK)
- Chapter 9 Figure 5.1 Management of choking in the paediatric patient. Reproduced with the kind permission of the Resuscitation Council (UK)
- Chapter 10 Figure 2.6 A firesafe. Image reproduced by the kind permission of BPR Medical
- Chapter 10 Figure 2.8 Bag-valve-mask with oxygen reservoir bag attached and inflated. Image reproduced by the kind permission of Ambu A/S
- Chapter 10 Instructions for use of oxygen images. © BOC Ltd 2014. Image reproduced by the kind permission of BOC healthcare
- Chapter 10 Figure 2.11 The Pneupac paraPac 200DProcedure. Image property of Smiths Medical and reprinted with permission from Smiths Medical, ASD, Inc

- Chapter 10 Figure 3.2 A patient providing a peak flow reading. Images reproduced with the kind permission of East of England Ambulance Service
- Chapter 10 Figure 3.3 Normal adult peak flow values. Image reproduced by the kind permission of Clement Clarke International
- Chapter 11 Figure 2.6 An aneroid sphygmomanometer. Image reproduced by the kind permission of Welch Allyn
- Chapter 12 Figure 3.2 Petechial non-blanching rash. Courtesy Meningitis Research Foundation www.meningitis.org
- Chapter 12 Figure 3.3 Maculopapular rash with scanty petechiae. Courtesy Meningitis Research Foundation www.meningitis.org
- Chapter 14 Procedure for Jext autoinjector. Images reproduced with the kind permission of ALK
- Chapter 15 Procedure – Prometheus pelvic splint equipment. Image reproduced courtesy of Prometheus Medical Ltd
- Chapter 15 Procedure – Extrication in a time-critical situation. Images reproduced with the kind permission of East of England Ambulance Service
- Chapter 15 Figure 5.1 Orthopaedic stretcher. Image reproduced by the kind permission of Ferno (UK) LTD
- Chapter 15 Table 3.1: Visual guide to estimating blood loss. Republished with permission of Wiley Blackwell. Source: Bose, P., Regan, F. and Paterson-Brown, S. (2006), Improving the accuracy of estimated blood loss at obstetric haemorrhage using clinical reconstructions. BJOG: An International Journal of Obstetrics & Gynaecology, 113: 919–924
- Chapter 17 Figure 4.1 Newborn life support algorithm. Reproduced with the kind permission of the Resuscitation Council (UK)
- Chapter 21 Figure 1.1 The chain of survival. Image reproduced by the kind permission of Laerdal Medical
- Chapter 21 Figure 3.4 A LIFEPAK 15 monitor/defibrillator commonly used by ambulance services. Image reproduced by the kind permission of Physio-Control

Every effort has been made to secure permission to reproduce copyright images. If any have been inadvertently overlooked, the copyright holders are invited to contact Class Professional Publishing and the omission will be rectified in the next printing as well as all further editions.

Foreword

Welcome to the first edition of *Ambulance Care Essentials*, which has been written by Richard Pilbery and Kris Lethbridge and peer reviewed by the National Education Network for Ambulance Services (NENAS). The textbook supports the UK Ambulance Services Level 3 Diploma in Clinical Healthcare Support: Ambulance (QCF).

Over the last few years, the emergency and urgent care landscape has changed dramatically. In response to this, the Association of Ambulance Chief Executives (AACE) asked NENAS to undertake an education transformation project to ensure we can meet the developing skills of our future workforce. NENAS are pleased to be working with Class Professional Publishing and others to help deliver the required change. We trust that this textbook will be of the upmost use and will promote pleasure and satisfaction in its readers.

Julian Rhodes, National Education Network for Ambulance Services and Head of Education & Training, West Midlands Ambulance Service NHS Foundation Trust

The Association of Ambulance Chief Executives welcomes the addition of *Ambulance Care Essentials* to its portfolio of endorsed publications. This innovative textbook will assist many in learning essential ambulance skills at the start of their careers and provides a solid foundation for those who later undertake paramedic studies. The progressive manner of introducing new concepts, skills and knowledge gives the reader a complete understanding of what is required of today's multi-skilled ambulance staff. AACE also welcomes the publication of the online course which supports the book. We look forward to future editions.

Steve Irving, Executive Officer, the Association of Ambulance Chief Executives

Chapter 1: **Introduction**

1 **Course guide**

1.1 **Introduction**

This is the companion workbook to the online learning resource, Ambulance Care Essentials. This course is designed to help prepare you to work as an ambulance service support worker (SW). The content is based on the curriculum for the Level 3 Diploma in Clinical Healthcare Support: Ambulance (QCF).

Each chapter comprises a number of topics centred by a theme, such as Health and Safety, or the Airway. The learning objectives for each chapter are mapped to modules within the Diploma, enabling you to claim credit for these if your service supports the Diploma. However, the content is relevant to all those working in supporting roles on ambulances.

Access the online materials through your Trust or visit http://ambulancecareessentials.co.uk

1.2 **Online course**

The online materials are run within the Moodle open-source learning platform, which is widely used by universities, colleges and ambulance services throughout the UK and beyond, to deliver education via distance learning, in a mature online learning environment.

The workbook mirrors the static content of the online materials, but omits the interactive components including:

- Animations
- Videos
- Quizzes.

In addition, the grade report within Moodle has been configured to allow for instructors to monitor the progress of their students through the course and, if required, record evidence of their achievement of clinical competencies, which are required by vocational qualifications such as the level 3 Diploma in Clinical Healthcare Support: Ambulance (QCF).

1.3 **Workbook**

This workbook, like the online materials, is designed to be read from start to finish on the first reading. This is because concepts introduced later on in the book assume that you already have knowledge of the content that has been covered in earlier chapters. However, once the course has been completed, this workbook will be a useful reference which you can return to again and again, reflecting on the learning points which are highlighted.

1.4 **Getting started**

To help get you orientated to the course and the relevance of the various chapters to clinical practice, the next lesson, ANATOMY OF AN EMERGENCY CALL, will take you step by step through an emergency attended by an ambulance crew, highlighting the variety of knowledge and skills that you will require in order to be an effective SW.

Each chapter is split into lessons, which are typically laid out in the following way:

- Learning objectives: To clearly highlight what you are expected to learn in the chapter
- Introduction: Setting the scene for the theme of the chapter
- Content: The content!

2 **Anatomy of an emergency call**

2.1 **Introduction**

This course consists of a number of modules that are completed in sequence and all contribute an essential part of your role as an emergency care support worker. It can be helpful to find out WHY you need to learn something. In order to see these in context, let's review a typical clinical scenario that you may be faced with when working on an emergency ambulance (Figure 2.1).

2.2 **The emergency operations centre**

When Mrs. Brown makes a 999 call, she speaks to a telephone operator who asks her which service she requires. She asks for the ambulance

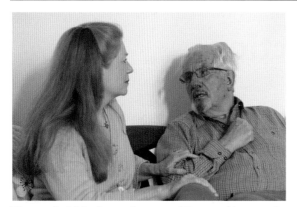

Figure 2.1 Mr. James Brown, a 59-year-old man who has chest pain, with his wife, Patricia

service and is put through to her local ambulance service's emergency operations centre (EOC, Figure 2.2).

While she talks to the call taker, the dispatcher allocates the ambulance that you are working on to the emergency call. Since it has been categorised as a Red call by the medical priority dispatch system, you need to arrive as soon as possible. National targets require an ambulance service response within 8 minutes for 75% of Red calls.

You will learn more about the ambulance service, including the roles and responsibilities of its staff, and ambulance and clinical quality indicators in THE AMBULANCE SERVICE chapter.

2.3 **Arriving on scene**

You will have been conducting a scene assessment, even before arriving at the address. This will include the location, time of day, and type of incident, and it is a dynamic process, i.e. should be constantly reviewed as the scene can change rapidly. You will learn about SCENE ASSESSMENT AND SAFETY later in the course.

In addition to scene safety, you will consider the need for personal protective equipment. At a residential address, this may be limited to a pair of disposable gloves, but at the scene of a road traffic collision, you will need a helmet, and high-visibility jacket as well.

With the help of your paramedic colleague, you carry the immediate aid kit, oxygen, drugs bag and monitor/defibrillator to the front door, where Mrs. Brown is anxiously waiting (Figure 2.3).

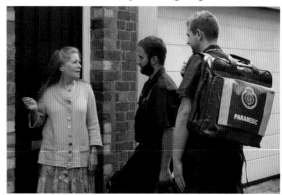

Figure 2.3 The crew arrive at the address

2.4 **Principles of communication**

You are shown into the living room where Mr. Brown is sitting on the sofa, clutching his chest and looking rather grey and sweaty. Your paramedic colleague introduces himself and you to Mr. and Mrs. Brown and clarifies what Mr. Brown prefers to be called. He tells you to call him Jim (Figure 2.4).

Communication is a fundamental aspect of all ambulance work and your role as an SW. It is

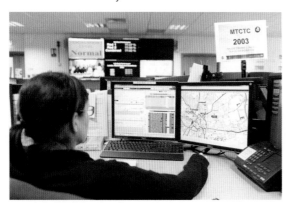

Figure 2.2 A dispatcher in the EOC

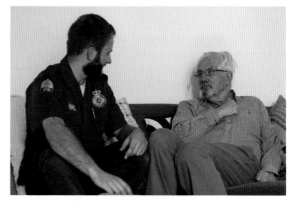

Figure 2.4 The paramedic talking to Jim

not always easy as you will have to communicate with patients, friends and family members, and other healthcare professionals, and adapt your approach and style appropriately. In addition, you cannot communicate the same way with an elderly person as you would a 2-year-old child. Some patients will not, or cannot, communicate with you, because they are depressed or don't speak English, for example. The lesson on the PRINCIPLES OF COMMUNICATION in chapter 3 will cover this in more detail.

2.5 **Patient assessment**

Your paramedic colleague completes an initial airway, breathing, circulation, disability, exposure/environment (ABCDE) assessment of Jim and asks you to obtain a set of baseline observations to support this. Jim's Airway is patent; he is Breathing at a rate of 16 breaths per minute, which is in the normal range. After obtaining permission (actually, consent, an important legal concept, covered in the CONSENT AND CAPACITY lesson in chapter 4) from Jim, you apply a pulse oximeter to one of his fingers. His oxygen saturations are 93% on air and, having excluded the presence of chronic obstructive pulmonary disease (COPD, which you will learn about in the COMMON RESPIRATORY CONDITIONS lesson in chapter 10), the paramedic asks you to administer low-flow oxygen via a simple face mask.

Continuing with the assessment of Jim's Circulation, you measure his blood pressure and apply electrodes to each of his limbs in order to record a 3-lead electrocardiogram (ECG), apply your disposable gloves to check his blood sugar (covered in the ASSESSMENT OF DISABILITY lesson in chapter 12) and finally, check his temperature.

2.6 **Patient history**

Jim tells the paramedic that he experienced a sudden onset of central chest pain radiating to his jaw, back and both arms an hour prior to his wife's 999 call. It feels like a heavy pressure, which he scores a 7 out of 10, and is associated with shortness of breath, nausea and sweating. His wife states that he has been very pale since the onset of pain. You are asked by the paramedic to prepare the entonox administration set for Jim to use (covered in the USING MEDICAL GASES SAFELY lesson in chapter 10).

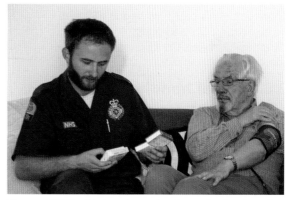

Figure 2.5 Reviewing the patient's medication is an important part of the history

The paramedic asks about Jim's past medical history and is told that he has high cholesterol and hypertension, both of which he is medicated for (Figure 2.5). He has never suffered from a heart attack (myocardial infarction, MI), but does admit to suffering from occasional chest pain on exertion over the past month or so.

2.7 **The 12-lead ECG**

The paramedic asks you to record a 12-lead ECG (Figure 2.6), while he administers aspirin and GTN to Jim, having checked that there are no contra-indications to administration (criteria when the drugs should not be given to the patient).

After obtaining consent, you open Jim's shirt and prepare his chest for the electrodes, which is not easy as his skin is greasy with sweat. Having prepared the skin (covered in the ASSESSMENT OF CIRCULATION lesson in chapter 11), you identify the anatomical landmarks to ensure you place the electrodes in the correct location. Once completed, you connect up the ECG leads to the monitor/defibrillator, enter the patient's age and gender and press the 12-lead ECG button.

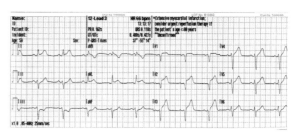

Figure 2.6 A 12-lead ECG showing signs of a heart attack

There is a short pause while the machine acquires the ECG and prints it out for you. The paramedic reviews the ECG and asks you to fetch the carry chair.

2.8 **Manual handling**

You return with the carry chair, complete a Task, Individual, Load, Environment, Equipment (TILEE) assessment and explain to Jim how you would like him to transfer onto the carry chair. Ensuring that you have a hand on the back of the chair at all times, you assist Jim onto the chair and fasten the safety strap across his chest. Before tipping the chair back onto the wheels, you warn Jim, and then proceed out of the house, stopping to allow your colleague to exit first to lift the chair over the lip of the doorframe and outside step.

You wheel Jim onto the ambulance tail-lift and remain with him while your colleague raises it (Figure 2.7). Once at ambulance level, you carefully wheel Jim alongside the ambulance stretcher so that he can transfer onto it.

The TILEE manual handling assessment tool and the equipment used for manual handling are covered in the lessons: PRINCIPLES OF MANUAL HANDLING and MOVING AND HANDLING EQUIPMENT AND TECHNIQUES in chapter 6.

2.9 **Assist the paramedic**

With the patient safely aboard the ambulance, you reconnect the monitor/defibrillator so that the paramedic can observe changes in Jim's condition en route to hospital. However, the paramedic would like to cannulate before leaving and asks you to help.

Assisting the paramedic is part of the SW role, so you quickly gather the equipment he requires,

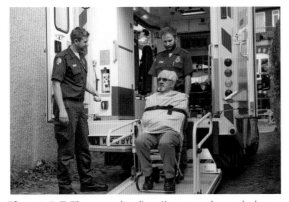

Figure 2.7 The crew loading Jim onto the ambulance

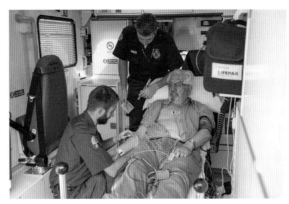

Figure 2.8 Assisting the paramedic with cannulation

including a selection of cannulas, a dressing pack, alcohol wipes, syringes and a saline flush (Figure 2.8). Having identified a vein and prepared the site, the paramedic inserts the cannula and advances it, releasing the tourniquet and removing the needle, which is safely deposited in a sharps bin that you have already placed close to him.

With this completed, and due to the fact that Jim is having a heart attack, the paramedic requests that you drive on blue lights and sirens to the local heart attack centre and not the local emergency department (ED). Thanks to your knowledge of the ambulance service, you are aware of this pathway and know which hospital is the regional centre capable of performing primary percutaneous coronary intervention (pPCI). You pass the paramedic the mobile phone to pre-alert the hospital and head for the driver's seat.

2.10 **Hospital arrival**

Traffic is light and you make good progress, arriving at the heart attack centre within 30 minutes. Just as you are pulling up outside the doors to the hospital, the paramedic shouts through that Jim has suffered a cardiac arrest.

You park up and leap into the back of the ambulance to assist. The paramedic is already performing chest compressions and asks you to connect the defibrillator pads.

You apply the pads as you have been taught, removing the chest leads that are obstructing the placement of one of the pads. The paramedic pauses chest compressions to check the rhythm and recognises it at once as ventricular fibrillation (VF), one of the shockable rhythms. You are

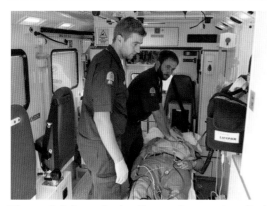

Figure 2.9 Resuscitating Jim requires good quality basic life support and early defibrillation

asked to charge the defibrillator as the paramedic resumes chest compressions (Figure 2.9).

The constant tone of the defibrillator tells you it is ready to deliver the shock and, after checking that no-one is touching the patient, the paramedic instructs you to press the shock button. Jim jolts upwards slightly as his chest muscles contract, and you take over chest compressions while the paramedic inserts an oropharyngeal airway (OPA) and connects the bag-valve-mask (BVM) to high-flow oxygen.

After two minutes of cardiopulmonary resuscitation (CPR), the paramedic asks you to stop chest compressions to assess the rhythm. The ECG shows an organised rhythm and a pulse check reveals that Jim's heart is beating again. His breathing is not adequate, however, and en route to the cardiac catheter lab, the paramedic

ventilates Jim with the BVM and by the time you arrive, Jim is making some respiratory effort.

The paramedic provides a hand-over to the waiting staff, explaining Jim's history, findings on examination, treatment you have administered and the cardiac arrest which you have just successfully resuscitated.

2.11 Clean up and prepare for the next call

With Jim safely in the hands of the cardiac catheter lab staff, you return with the paramedic to the ambulance to clean up, restock and get ready for the next emergency call (Figure 2.10).

You find out later that Jim had an occluded left anterior descending coronary artery, which was cleared and reopened by the cardiac catheter lab staff. He is recovering well and due to be discharged from hospital soon.

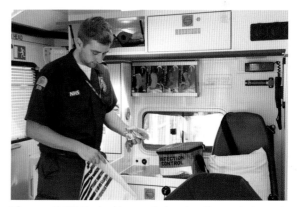

Figure 2.10 Restocking and cleaning the ambulance is a less glamorous, but still important, part of the SW role

Chapter 2: **The Ambulance Service**

1 **Response to a 999 call**

1.1 **Learning objectives**

By the end of this lesson you will be able to:

- Explain how the ambulance service manages an emergency call
- State some of the alternative services callers may be directed to when an emergency ambulance is not required.

1.2 **Introduction**

The response to a 999 call can be complex and varies between each incident depending on the degree of need. The three main stages of a response are:

- Call for help and triage
- Ambulance service response
- Onward care of patient.

1.3 **Call for help and triage**

When someone calls 999 (or 112) in the UK, they are connected to an operator from the national telephone network. Once the nature of the emergency has been established, the call will be forwarded to the police, fire or ambulance services or coastguard, depending on the most appropriate response(s) required.

Once the call is connected to the ambulance service emergency operations centre, a qualified call handler will ask a series of questions. These questions usually come from a package of software called 'NHS Pathways', a system designed to triage calls and identify those that need an ambulance most urgently. Pathways can also identify those callers who do not need an ambulance and for whom an alternative care pathway, such as visiting the GP or self-presenting at a Minor Injuries Unit (MIU), would be more appropriate [HSCIC, 2014a].

As the call handler works through the questioning, the triage system will identify how urgently an ambulance is required and arrive at a triage code and a response category (Table 1.1) [NEAS, 2011].

During this triage, a clinician is often available to assist in 'enhanced triage'. This is particularly useful when dealing with patients who have complex needs which the standard pathways system may not be set up to deal with.

Also during triage, the call handler will identify if there is a need for other emergency services, or whether there may be any dangers to the responding ambulance clinicians present (such as an assailant still at scene). Where required, other services will be contacted and ambulance crews can be advised of the risks.

1.4 **Ambulance service response**

Based on the information gathered during the triage process, the most appropriate response can be determined. There are two main types of response, which are:

- Hear and treat
- Physical response.

Hear and treat

Hear and treat is where the patient is advised how to look after themselves, or recommended to self-present to a more appropriate care provider, such as a GP or MIU. In late 2014, the number of patients being managed in England through this route was around 8% of all 999 calls [NHS England, 2015].

Physical response

For the majority of 999 calls, the ambulance service will send a physical response. Depending on the need of the patient and the scale of the incident, this may include:

- Community responder
- Rapid response car
- Response motorcycle
- Emergency ambulance
- Air ambulance
- Specialist practitioner in urgent care
- Hazardous area response team (HART)
- Ambulance service officer/commander
- Specialist operations response team
- Medical support such as British Association for Immediate Care (BASICS).

Table 1.1: Ambulance response categories

Category	Description	Example	Response
Red 1	Most severe life-threatening emergencies	Cardiac or respiratory arrest	Emergency: Within 8 minutes
Red 2	Life-threatening emergencies	Stroke or breathing emergency	Emergency: Within 8 minutes
Green 1	Serious but not life-threatening	Diabetic problems	Emergency: Within 20 minutes
Green 2	Serious but not life-threatening	Suspected fracture	Emergency: Within 30 minutes
Green 3	Non-emergency call	Non-serious assault injuries	Enhanced telephone triage within 20 minutes. Physical response within 60 minutes, if required
Green 4	Non-emergency call	Fall with no apparent injuries	Enhanced telephone triage within 60 minutes. Physical response within 90 minutes if required.

1.5 Onward care

Where necessary, patients will be transported to hospital for emergency care and treatment. This is frequently to emergency departments (EDs) but now also includes an increasing number of specialist emergency care departments, such as stroke units or cardiac wards.

In addition to this, ambulance clinicians now have a range of alternative care pathways available to them, in order to avoid hospital admission where appropriate. During late 2014 in England, in 37% of incidents where patients had a response from the ambulance service they were not transported to an ED, but were either managed at scene ('see and treat') or taken to an alternative care provider [NHS England, 2015].

Alternative care providers may include:

- Specialist paramedics in urgent care: paramedics with additional training who can manage a range of minor injury and illness within the community
- GPs
- GP drop-in centres
- Out-of-hours services

- Mental health teams
- Minor Injury Units
- Pharmacies
- 111
- Social services
- 'Hospital at home' teams
- Emergency residential care
- Community hospitals.

Given the current pressure being faced by urgent care services within the UK, it is likely that more routes for referral and additional training in managing more patients in the community will feature prominently in ambulance service development over the coming years [NHS England, 2014a].

2 Roles within the ambulance service

2.1 Learning objectives

By the end of this lesson you will be able to:

- Identify a number of clinical and leadership roles within the ambulance service and briefly explain what the role entails.

2.2 Introduction

There are 11 NHS ambulance trusts in England, as well as NHS ambulance services in Scotland, Wales and Northern Ireland, who are statutory providers of ambulance services for the Government within the UK [NHS Choices, 2011].There are also a range of voluntary services, including St John Ambulance and the British Red Cross, and a variety of independent sector services, ranging from the very small to national scale organisations.

Each service is structured differently, so it is not possible to give a definitive list of the different roles. However, over the following pages are descriptions of some of the roles you may find, which could be broadly divided into:

- Clinical
- Clinical leadership
- Command and control.

2.3 Clinical roles

Community responder

Community responders come from a variety of backgrounds and volunteer their time to the ambulance service. They respond to incidents close to where they live or work, often in remote settings, which can take longer for an ambulance to get to. Responders carry basic life-saving equipment including an automated external defibrillator (AED) and devices for managing a patient's airway. In some places the fire service and other similar agencies may also act as first responders for the ambulance service [SWAST, 2014b].

Support worker (SW)

SWs work alongside paramedics on front line ambulances. They are trained in providing emergency care, basic emergency interventions and life support, and are qualified emergency drivers. SWs normally work under the supervision of a qualified clinical colleague. SWs may also work on support vehicles that are used to transport patients to hospital when they have been assessed by another healthcare professional and are deemed as needing a less urgent admission to hospital.

Technician

Technicians are non-registered clinicians who normally work alongside a paramedic, but may also work on their own. They have a range of skills relevant to emergency and urgent care and can undertake a number of pre-hospital procedures and administer a range of medications. There is national variation in the skill sets of technicians and the way in which they are deployed by different services.

Paramedic

Paramedics are qualified and registered clinicians who specialise in working in the urgent and emergency care setting. They are trained in the examination and treatment of emergency conditions, have a wide range of skills and treatment options and are considered as specialists in emergency care. Registered with the Health and Care Professions Council (HCPC), paramedics have a degree of autonomy in their practice and can be held accountable to the HCPC for their actions and omissions that arise from providing clinical care to patients.

Specialist paramedic – urgent care

Specialist paramedics have been known by a range of titles including emergency care practitioner and paramedic practitioner. They have undertaken an enhanced course of learning, usually at degree level, along with a range of placements that equip them with the skills and knowledge to treat urgent care patients. These patients include those with acute illnesses such as respiratory tract and urinary tract infections or minor injuries and wounds. Specialist paramedics have a broad range of skills in the management of urgent patients and can administer a greater variety of medications [CoP, 2014].

Specialist paramedic – critical care

Also known as Critical Care Paramedics (CCP), these clinicians have also undertaken enhanced study, but with a focus on dealing with the most critically ill or injured. Specialist paramedics in critical care will often work as part of a multidisciplinary team alongside a doctor who specialises in emergency pre-hospital care [CoP, 2014].

Hazardous area response team (HART)

HART are groups of paramedics, and sometimes technicians, who have been specially trained to work in difficult situations and alongside the police and fire service at large and dangerous incidents. They have a special set of skills and equipment, which can include swift water rescues, working at heights, and use of breathing apparatus. This allows them to safely access patients in remote and difficult settings. There is a network of HART bases around the country and their help can normally be requested through the emergency operations centre.

2.4 Clinical leadership roles

Running any ambulance service requires a large range of clinical leaders. Some of the common roles include:

- Paramedic consultant
- Clinical development manager
- Pharmaceutical adviser
- Medical director.

Paramedic consultant

The paramedic consultant is a relatively new role in some ambulance trusts throughout the UK. The role of the consultant is to act as a senior clinical leader involved in service development; clinical leadership; research and evaluation; and education and professional development. Consultants will normally work in a mixed role providing advanced clinical support to operational staff while also undertaking their other responsibilities. After the medical director, a consultant paramedic is normally the most senior clinical leader in an ambulance trust.

Clinical development manager (CDM)

Normally a specialist paramedic, the CDM is responsible for ensuring that clinical policies and procedures are up to date. They also consider what new procedures and medication may be beneficial for patients.

Pharmaceutical adviser

Most organisations will have a pharmacist working for them at least part time. This is to ensure that the use of medications by the service

is safe and appropriate and that the relevant laws are being followed.

Medical director

The medical director, normally a doctor with a background in emergency and/or critical care, is the ultimate person responsible for the clinical care inside an organisation. They are a very senior clinical leader and answerable for clinical errors and omissions within an organisation.

2.5 Command and control roles

Inside every large organisation is a command and control structure. This structure is required to co-ordinate and effectively deliver the functions of the organisation, but it becomes particularly relevant in emergency services at times of complex or major incidents. All commanders receive specific training relevant to their role. Different command roles do not necessarily indicate rank or seniority within an organisation, but are instead allocated so that those involved understand their role in managing an incident. Following criticism of emergency services not communicating effectively at previous major incidents, the national Joint Emergency Services Interoperability Principles programme (JESIP) has been launched in the UK so commanders from all the emergency services know better how to work together and communicate at complex and major incident scenes [JESIP, 2013].

Operational commanders

Operational commanders, broadly equivalent to what were formerly known as 'bronze commanders', are present at the scene of an incident and are responsible for organising the delivery of care and the safety of those working at a scene. They have to assess what resources are available to them, or have been made available to them by tactical and strategic commanders, and utilise those resources in the most effective way possible.

Depending on the size of the incident, operational commanders work alongside a number of other officers from both the ambulance and other emergency services to ensure services are being provided in an effective and co-ordinated manner.

Operational commanders receive direction from tactical commanders, with whom they have to constantly liaise closely to ensure they have the resources they require to manage an incident.

Tactical commanders

Formally known as 'silver' commanders, the tactical commander is responsible for ensuring that all the tactical resources a bronze commander requires for the management of the incident are in place. They will communicate closely with other emergency services and agencies and may or may not be present at the actual incident, depending on the scale and nature of the incident as well as the amount of time it goes on for. At some incidents there may be multiple operational commanders, each dealing with different sections of the incident, in which case, the tactical commander will be responsible for co-ordinating their actions.

The tactical commander achieves a level of oversight for an incident that cannot normally be achieved by an operational commander on the ground. From this position, the tactical commander can ensure there is effective joint working of agencies and that the deployment of resources and the tactics being used to manage an incident are appropriate.

Strategic commanders

Formally known as 'gold' commanders, strategic commanders are responsible for devising and making available the resources to implement a strategy for managing an incident. The strategic commander usually has control over all of the organisation's resources and is responsible for making these resources available to the tactical and operational commanders.

Strategic commanders, like tactical commanders, get an oversight of the management of an incident and are responsible for ensuring the tactics being used are appropriate, that all services are working effectively together and that clear lines of communication are in place. Where necessary, strategic commanders are responsible for national level communication to make available further resources if they are required.

National inter-agency liaison officer (NILO)

The NILO is a nominated person who has had specific training and experience to ensure that agencies such as fire, police and ambulance services can communicate effectively during a major or serious incident. They will normally work remotely from the scene of an incident to ensure that all agencies are communicating effectively [NARU, 2012].

Chapter 3: **Communication**

1 Principles of communication

1.1 Learning objectives

By the end of this lesson you will be able to:

- Identify the different reasons people communicate
- Explain how communication affects relationships in the work setting
- Describe the factors to consider when promoting effective communication
- Explain how people from different backgrounds may use and/or interpret communication methods in different ways
- Identify barriers to effective communication
- Explain how to access extra support or services to enable individuals to communicate effectively.

1.2 Introduction

Communication will be at the core of your role in your day-to-day management of patients and when attending incidents. As inter-personal communication forms such a fundamental aspect of our daily lives we rarely stop to think about how we do it. But, as will be discussed throughout this lesson, effective communication, especially in a high-stress environment, is a skill that requires development and practice in order to be effective.

Poor communication is one of the most frequently received complaints for healthcare organisations, including the NHS [HSCIC, 2013]. The World Health Organization (WHO) recognises that communication is a key aspect of improving medical safety; poor communication has previously been responsible for disastrous medical and surgical errors, including the removal of incorrect organs and limbs [WHO, 2009a].

As a health professional, effective communication will be a key standard against which your employer will expect you to perform. For registered professionals, including paramedics, being able to communicate effectively is one of the fundamental standards of registration [HCPC, 2014].

1.3 Basics of communication

Traditionally, communication has been regarded as the sending of a message from one person to another (Figure 1.1) [Corcoran, 2013].The sender (person A) has a message they wish to pass to the receiver (person B). The message exists within the consciousness of the sender initially, and then they decide on a method of passing that message. Before it can be passed it must be 'encoded'. This encoding may be the selecting of certain words, certain emphasis during part of the sentence, or other verbal or non-verbal features. The receiver must then 'decode' the message as they receive it and try to interpret the original message from all the verbal and non-verbal information they have received. Clearly, this model is not sufficient in healthcare, as it implies a one-way communication, not the two-way communication that is essential for providing best care to patients.

A modified model has been suggested, which includes the variables of understanding and feedback, and is a cyclic process (Figure 1.2). This inclusion of checking the understanding of the message given, and receiving feedback, is fundamental to ensure that messages have been understood in the way in which they were intended [Corcoran, 2013].

This is particularly important in high-stress situations or when communicating information a person may not understand well (such as a medical complaint), to ensure that the correct message has been received and understood. In these situations it is very easy for a message to be misinterpreted, with potentially disastrous consequences.

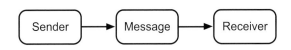

Figure 1.1 Basic model of communication

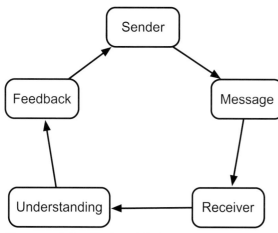

Figure 1.2 Modified model of communication

1.3.1 **Verbal skills**

Verbal communication can be divided into two broad areas [Blaber, 2008]:

- Language and vocabulary
- Paralinguistic features of communication.

Language and vocabulary

Working in healthcare you must be able to adjust your language and vocabulary so that it is suited to the person you are communicating with. When communicating with colleagues and other health professionals you will need to use more complex and professional language. However, there will be times when you need to adjust to communicate with those who have a narrower range of language skills, which may include children or those with cognitive impairment.

Paralinguistic features

'Paralinguistic' refers to the modification of the way in which we speak and place emphasis in communication. This includes:

- Volume
- Rhythm
- Pitch
- Pace
- Intonation
- Tone.

1.3.2 **Non-verbal communication**

Non-verbal communication can have a dramatic impact on the message you are sending and the way that it is then interpreted. It can be possible to communicate entirely by non-verbal means,

especially if you know the person well [Blaber, 2008].

Examples of non-verbal communication include:

- Eye contact
- Facial expression
- Gesture and posture
- Personal space and touch.

All of these should be used in a manner that is appropriate to the situation. For example, when gathering a history from a patient, if you are head down and writing as they speak then the patient may get the impression you are not paying attention to them and might leave out key details. In contrast, if you are making eye contact, nodding your head and acknowledging their communication with small verbal cues, such as 'OK' and 'yes' as they are speaking, then they are more likely to continue communicating and reveal all the information you need in order to assess them properly.

1.4 **Social context**

Communication relies heavily on the social context in which it takes place. Consider the two following scenarios and how the changing social context may influence how you communicate [Hartley, 1999]:

- Scenario A: You attend a small child who has fallen and injured their wrist. As part of your assessment you need to look at the wrist, but the child is wary of letting you get close, due to fear of you causing more pain
- Scenario B: You are called to give evidence in court at the case of a serious assault you attended. You are placed in the witness box and asked a series of questions by the prosecution, prior to cross-examination by the defence.

In both these scenarios, effective communication is critical to ensure that others receive the message you intended to send: however, the way in which you communicate these messages will be vastly different. Your role is to ensure you encode the message, using both verbal and non-verbal features of communication, in such a way that it is likely it will be decoded in the manner you intended.

This concept extends well beyond the extreme examples cited above and into your daily role as an SW. You will, every day, meet people from a wide range of social and cultural backgrounds. Every one of these people will have a different social context in which they exist, and you will need to be mindful of modifying your communication, based on the needs of the individual, to ensure that accurate messages are passed and misunderstanding does not occur.

1.5 **Barriers to communication**

Barriers to communication are anything that influences your ability to effectively pass on and receive back the message you need. You will frequently encounter difficult-to-manage barriers to communication and will need to think of ways of dealing with them. Here are some examples of barriers to communication and how they can be overcome:

- Physical obstacles: Such as distance or your patient being stuck the other side of a closed door. The clear answer here is to remove the obstacle, but in some situations this may not be possible, so you will need to think of novel solutions. Examples may include: establish contact via a phone; use an intermediary to relay messages; signal with your hands or other props

- Language: You will inevitably meet people with whom you cannot communicate in their native language. The use of a family member as a translator can be helpful; alternatively, your service may have provided you with other tools such as phrase books or access to Language Line, a telephone service that provides translators for a wide range of languages over the phone

- Emotions: You will frequently encounter patients and situations where those involved are experiencing extreme emotions. At these times people are less able to understand what is being said to them or asked of them. Use of your verbal and non-verbal skills of communication will be key here to ensure clarity of message

- Age: Young patients in particular will need to be communicated with in a way that is suitable to them and that they can understand. Using pictures, drawings and other props can be an effective means of overcoming barriers to communication.

This is just a short list of examples of barriers that you may experience in communicating. It is worth noting that whenever you adapt your communication to overcome such difficulties there is an increased risk of your message being misinterpreted, so you should make doubly sure that what you wanted to communicate is the message the person has received.

1.6 **Summary**

Communication is a natural skill that we all use on a daily basis; however, in your front line role you will routinely be faced with challenging and demanding communication scenarios. To help overcome these, having an understanding of the theory of communication and a strong working knowledge of what resources are available to you locally will be helpful. You will also need to be adaptive, creative, responsive and innovative in overcoming barriers to communication on a daily basis. Only when you can overcome barriers can you be sure of providing the right care to your patient.

Long after your patients have forgotten what you did for them, they will remember the way in which you went about doing it. Communication may be one of the most frequently received complaints for healthcare services, but being treated with care and compassion, and effectively communicated with, is also one of the most frequently praised attributes of individual health professionals.

2 **Practical communication**

2.1 **Learning objectives**

By the end of this lesson you will be able to:

- Explain the importance of clear, concise reporting of findings to the clinician

- Explain the importance of recording patient observations

- Describe the procedure for clinical handover to medical professionals

- Explain the procedure for communicating via radio.

2.2 **Introduction**

This lesson will consider the importance of communication in your role as a support worker.

2.3 **Recording and passing on information**

In your role you will normally be working alongside a clinician who will be responsible for patient care. It is likely that you will frequently be asked to undertake examinations and record observations.

Keeping accurate records and gaining accurate observations is critical to safe patient care as it forms a part of the continuity of their care. Changes in observations can indicate a deteriorating or improving patient, so if there are errors in the recorded observations it can create a false perception of the patient's changing state of health.

The following tips will help to ensure patient safety when undertaking this part of your role:

• Pass on, or record, all the information you obtain. If you are not sure of its relevance, pass it on to the clinician responsible for their care

• If you are asked to undertake procedures, observations or interventions that are outside your skill set, politely inform the responsible clinician that you are not able to do this

• If you are struggling or unsure, make your supervising clinician aware

• Never fabricate, estimate or make up observations. Doing so not only exposes the patient to risk but would also be considered as unprofessional conduct when discovered.

2.4 **Handover**

The process of a handover is passing on the care of your patient to another healthcare provider(s). During handover, all information relevant to the care of the patient should be provided in a concise and effective manner.

You may, on occasion, be required to undertake a handover, whether it be to hospital staff, GPs, or any of the other vast range of clinicians or other services involved in the provision of care to your patients. It is well recognised that handovers are a high-risk aspect of a patient's care, where important information can be forgotten or missed out [BMA, 2014]. This can lead to errors or omissions on the part of the receiving clinician and then harm to the patient as a result.

This risk of error is increased in high-stress situations, for example where patients are critically ill or injured: just the time when that information needs to be passed on in the most effective manner.

There are many models to help facilitate clinical handover and thereby reduce the risk of key information being forgotten. The UK Ambulance Services Clinical Practice Guidelines recommend the use of the 'ATMIST' model as a quick and easy way of conducting a handover [AACE, 2013]:

• A: Age of patient

• T: Time of incident

• M: Mechanism of injury

• I: Injuries sustained

• S: Signs and symptoms

• T: Treatment given/immediate needs

Other principles to consider when conducting a handover include:

• Make sure the person you are handing over to is the person responsible for the patient's care

• Have your handover ready: Make notes in advance to help if necessary

• Make it concise: Especially for the critically ill and injured patient you will have a very limited period of time (often less than 60 seconds) in which to provide a handover

• Make sure you have everyone's attention prior to beginning your hand over

• Provide written copies of all information as well as a verbal account whenever you hand over the care of your patient.

2.5 **Radio communication**

Most ambulance services use radios in one form or another as a means of communication (Figure 2.1). Your service should introduce you to the technical aspects of how your radio system works, but below are some general guidelines and etiquette on using a radio as a form of communication:

• Unlike on a mobile phone, only one person at a time can talk on a radio, so check frequently with the person you are talking to that they are receiving your message

- Be concise: Often several people will share the same radio channel or be trying to talk to the same person (the emergency operations centre, for example) so keep your messages as concise as possible so as not to jam up the line
- Be clear: Radios often distort sounds, especially if the receiving party has a poor signal. Speak slightly more slowly than usual, in a normal tone of voice
- Consider security: Think about who could be listening to your broadcast. Do not pass sensitive or confidential information over the radio unless you are authorised to do so
- Know your call sign and the call sign of the person you are speaking to: When making a call you should use the call sign of the person you are calling, followed by your call sign. For example: 'Control, this is Alpha two six, come in, over.'

Certain phrases that have specific meanings may be used when talking via the radio (Table 2.1).

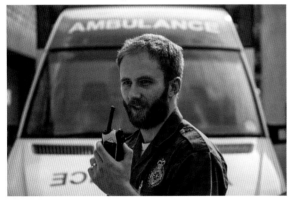

Figure 2.1 Communicating by radio

Table 2.1: Phrases to use when talking via the radio

Phrase	Meaning
Go ahead	Indicates you are ready to receive a message
Wait one	I need to pause for a few seconds
Stand-by	Acknowledge the other party, but you are not able to reply immediately
Negative	No
Affirmative	Yes
Say again	Repeat last message
Over	You have finished your message and are ready for the other party to reply
Out	The conversation between you and the other party has finished and others can now use the same channel
Copy	You have understood the message
Wilco	You 'will comply' with the broadcast message
Priority	You are requesting priority over other radio traffic as you have an urgent message
Come in	Asking another party to acknowledge that they can hear your broadcast
So far?	When broadcasting a longer message you should stop periodically and check if the person is receiving the message clearly

When spelling out words, use the phonetic alphabet to avoid confusion of letter sounds:

- A: Alpha
- B: Bravo
- C: Charlie
- D: Delta
- E: Echo
- F: Foxtrot
- G: Golf
- H: Hotel
- I: India
- J: Juliet
- K: Kilo
- L: Lima
- M: Mike
- N: November
- O: Oscar
- P: Papa
- Q: Quebec
- R: Romeo
- S: Sierra
- T: Tango
- U: Uniform
- V: Victor
- W: Whiskey
- X: X-Ray
- Y: Yankee
- Z: Zulu

Chapter 4: **Legal, Ethical and Professional Issues**

1 Being a healthcare professional

1.1 Learning objectives

By the end of this lesson you will be able to:

- Explain what it means to have a duty of care
- Explain how duty of care contributes to the safeguarding or protection of individuals
- Describe potential conflicts or dilemmas that may arise between the duty of care and an individual's rights
- Describe how to manage risks associated with conflicts or dilemmas between an individual's rights and the duty of care
- Explain where to get additional support and advice about conflicts and dilemmas
- Describe how to respond to complaints
- Explain the main points of agreed procedures for handling complaints
- Explain expectations about your work role as expressed in relevant standards
- Explain the importance of reflective practice in continuously improving the quality of service provided
- Describe how your values, belief systems and experiences may affect working practice
- Explain how a working relationship is different from a personal relationship
- Describe different working relationships in health and social care settings
- Describe why it is important to adhere to the agreed scope of the job role
- Explain how and why person-centred values must influence all aspects of health and social care work
- Explain why it is important to work in partnership with others.

1.2 Introduction

This lesson will describe what it means to be a healthcare professional, with a focus on:

- Values-based healthcare
- Duty of care
- Scope of practice
- Standards
- Complaints
- Reflection.

1.3 Values-based healthcare

Working as a healthcare professional is an extraordinarily privileged role. As an ambulance clinician you will often be caring for people when they are at their most vulnerable. The majority of people have less than a handful of contacts with the ambulance service throughout their lifetime, so when they do call during extreme life events, patients will look to you for help, guidance and support in whatever situation they find themselves in. Being in this privileged role, it is important to recognise that you should be patient focused and the attitudes and beliefs that you hold can influence the care you provide to your patient.

Staffordshire Hospital

Stafford hospital was an acute hospital that became the focus of a national outcry about standards of care. Following concerns raised by the families of patients around poor standards of care and further concerns around unusually high mortality rates, especially for emergency admission patients [Cure the NHS, 2014], the Healthcare Commission conducted an investigation in 2008 looking into care at the hospital. This uncovered deficiencies at virtually every stage of the pathway of emergency care [HC, 2009].

The resulting public inquiry and report, widely known as the Francis report, painted a damning picture of a place where there were fundamental failures of care. These included [Francis, 2013]:

- Patients were left in excrement-soiled bedclothes for lengthy periods
- Assistance was not provided with feeding patients who could not eat without help
- Water was left out of reach
- Staff treated patients and those close to them with what appeared to be callous indifference.

Although a definitive number has never been released, it is suspected that hundreds of patients died unnecessarily and thousands more suffered at the hands of poor care.

The final report made 290 recommendations in total, many of which have been or are being adopted nationally. There have been a number of other reports published since into improving care within the NHS, but perhaps the most influential is the one conducted by the National Advisory Group on the Safety of Patients in England [DoH, 2013b]. This review made a number of key recommendations including:

- The NHS should continually and forever reduce patient harm by embracing wholeheartedly an ethic of learning
- Patients and their carers should be present, powerful and involved at all levels of healthcare organisations from 'wards to the boards'.

Not only does this philosophy make the NHS an organisation that learns from and builds on its errors, but it puts the patient at the core of all activities. Health professionals must always apply a culture of compassionate care when looking after patients, a culture that is best summarised by the 6 Cs:

1. Care
2. Compassion
3. Competence
4. Communication
5. Courage
6. Commitment.

1.3.1 What influences your values and attitudes?

There are multiple aspects that influence our own attitudes, but understanding this and understanding how our attitudes impact on the management of our patients is an important distinction to make. Everyone harbours

prejudgements about certain people or groups of people. These can be positive or negative and these stereotypes are used as a form of mental shortcut [Paul, 1998]. However, this can also be dangerous, as it can lead to judgements being made about people based on limited information. These judgements can even influence the way in which a patient is treated, which in turn can lead to errors.

Consider the following scenario:

- You are working a Friday night shift in a busy urban setting. It's 03:00 and for the last 3 hours you've attended 4 different patients all of whom are worse for wear through the consumption of alcohol. You're overdue your meal break and are beginning to run low on fuel, but the emergency operations centre have just allocated you to attend a 20-year-old male who is lying on the pavement outside a city-centre night-club. On arrival you are greeted by a crowd of his friends, who tell you that it is his birthday, he (and they) have been drinking excessively during the evening and he is known for being a 'lightweight'. It appears the alcohol has got the better of him. The senior clinician quickly checks him out; there are no signs of injury, so he advises the man's friends to call a taxi and take him home.

Is there a risk of stereotyping influencing your practice in this scenario? The answer is almost certainly yes, particularly if you approach the incident thinking 'here we go again', wondering how long it will be until you get your meal break, and whether you will make it to the fuel station before running out of diesel. If you think in this way, you are not focused on how best to care for your patient.

Alcohol consumption can mask a range of conditions which, if not carefully examined for, can easily go unnoticed. If you attend multiple, drink-related incidents in the course of one shift, your brain will naturally want to shortcut or apply a stereotype ('they're just drunk'), especially if you are hungry, tired and late for a rest period.

1.3.2 Patient-centred NHS

Take a moment to review the Department of Health's graphic that demonstrates how the NHS links together (Figure 1.1) [DoH, 2013c]. The NHS is a huge organisation and requires many different components to come together and form

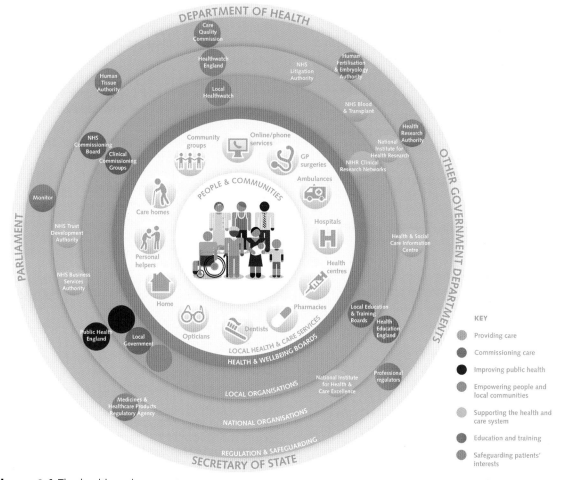

Figure 1.1 The health and care system
© Crown copyright. Available at: https://www.gov.uk/government/publications/the-health-and-care-system-explained

it. Note that people and communities, including patients, are at the very centre of the organisation.

1.4 Duty of care

Duty of care is a civil law concept within the UK and exists to ensure that one party does not allow unreasonable harm or loss to occur to another [Dimond, 2011]. As a healthcare professional, you owe a duty of care to your patient from the point at which they are accepted as a service user [HCPC, 2012]. From that point onwards you must act in a way to prevent harm where a reasonable person could see that harm might occur. If you breach this duty of care and someone suffers as a result, then this can lead to the civil wrong of negligence.

Negligence

Negligence occurs when duty of care is breached and reasonably foreseeable harm occurs as a result. If a party is guilty of negligence, they can be pursued through the civil courts for damages. There are four stages for negligence to be proven [Pilbery, 2013]:

- Establish a duty of care
- Breach of duty
- Harm occurred
- Causation.

Establishing a duty is usually straightforward, since as a healthcare professional you owe a duty to any patient you encounter.

Breach of duty occurs when a reasonably foreseeable consequence of a person's action leads to harm. The difficult part to measure in this section is what counts as 'reasonably foreseeable' and this is a point that the courts may have to decide upon. Special legal tests based on the Bolam and Bolitho cases can be used to determine what is or is not reasonable. In these tests, a body of professional opinion will be consulted to determine whether the actions of a practitioner were reasonable, but they must also stand up to logical analysis [Dimond, 2011].

A claimant must be harmed or suffer a loss in order for a claim to be successful. Normally this will be physical harm, but may also include:

- Emotional distress
- Loss of income, future earnings or enjoyment of life.

For each harm the claimant alleges they suffered, they must be able to prove it was due to the actions or omissions of the practitioner.

Causation is the final step in proving negligence. It is not enough for a duty of care to exist and for that duty to be breached. That breach of duty has to go on to cause harm and it should be evident that this breach was the cause. Also sometimes referred to as the 'but for' principle, it is applied by asking 'But for the (action or omission) would harm have occurred?' If the answer to this is 'yes', then negligence is not proven; if the answer is 'no', then it is likely that negligence exists.

As a health professional you need to bear in mind the principle of duty of care and always consider whether you are providing care in the best interests of your patient.

1.5 Scope of practice and standards

Your scope of practice as a support worker will most likely be established by your employer through a series of standards. Such standards are treated as the benchmark for determining whether or not a person is working within their scope of practice and also whether or not they are fit to be a health professional for other reasons.

Standards can cover a wide range of topics, not just clinical skills. It is not possible to list the standards for emergency care assistants here, as they will vary from organisation to organisation, but for paramedic colleagues, standards are set nationally by the Health and Care Professions

Council (HCPC) [HCPC, 2014]. These standards include:

- Standards of proficiency: The skills required to do the job
- Standards of conduct, performance and ethics: Ensuring that registered health professionals conduct themselves and their business in an ethical and moral fashion
- Standards of education and training: To ensure that each registrant receives, and the educational institution provides, a satisfactory level of education and training.

You should be aware of the standards expected of you from your organisation and make sure you practise within those standards. You should not attempt to undertake any activity outside your scope of practice as you are not likely to have the knowledge, skill or experience to do so safely and would therefore be putting the patient and yourself at risk.

What constitutes negligence was outlined earlier, and it should be noted that any activity undertaken outside of your scope of practice, and which leads to harm, is likely to be grounds for a claim of negligence.

If at any point it becomes unavoidable for you to step outside your scope of practice, you should report this through the usual reporting mechanisms within your organisation. This is not just to protect yourself, but so that the organisation as a whole can learn from the experience.

1.6 When things go wrong

All ambulance services strive to be a 'no harm' organisation, but it is probably an unavoidable fact that systems as large and complex as modern ambulance services will always have adverse incidents. However, these errors should not lead to patient harm, and lessons should be learnt from mistakes when they occur.

The National Advisory Group on the Safety of Patients in England has made recommendations in the light of the Francis report discussed above, advising that the NHS needs to become a learning organisation and that a blame culture should be abandoned in preference for a just and reporting culture, which in turn leads to a learning culture. It is also noted that many failings in the NHS are not down to staff; instead they are caused by poor processes and systems, which in turn lead to errors [DoH, 2013b].

All health organisations should learn from mistakes. They should also be promoting a learning culture where staff are not unnecessarily blamed for mistakes, and where people feel safe in reporting incidents so that the larger organisation can learn from those incidents, even small ones.

1.6.1 Failure to achieve standards

This concept of reporting extends to yourself and your own practice as well. If you recognise that in the course of your duty you have failed to achieve the expected standards for someone in your role, then you should make this known. Different organisations will have different methods of reporting, but most now have a central system for reporting incidents and a dedicated team that deals with those reports.

1.6.2 Complaints

During the course of your duty it may be the case that someone wishes to make a complaint about you, your colleagues, your organisation or another organisation. This can be challenging, as the natural response is to be defensive, but remember that the principles of a learning organisation together with opportunities to reflect should be seen as a way of improving our services and should be welcomed as such.

It is likely that your service will have specific guidelines or a policy on handling complaints, which you should be familiar with, but good general guidelines include:

- Record facts and pass them on to appropriate people: do not undertake the investigation yourself
- If someone wishes to make a complaint, take the details and pass them on to relevant parties, or give the person the contact details of the relevant people inside your organisation
- Do not challenge facts about a complaint; if necessary this can be done later on, once all the facts have been established
- Provide contact details so that patients know how to get in touch should they wish to.

If you become involved in an investigation or complaint then you should do all you can to support the investigation. Withholding key information may be seen as a misconduct

offence, which is likely to be handled very differently from learning from a genuine error.

Additional sources of support

You may find that you need other sources of support should you be made aware of a complaint. Such sources may include:

- Organisational policy
- Your line manager
- Making Experiences Count (or similar) investigation team within your organisation [DoH, 2007a].

1.6.3 Whistleblowing

Improving patient safety relies on staff identifying when things are not right, or when mistakes have been made, so organisations can learn and prevent similar circumstances from arising again in the future. Whistleblowing is the act of reporting suspected wrongdoing at work. Whistleblowers should be supported and congratulated for speaking up and so providing an opportunity to remedy the problem. However, whistleblowers are not always treated fairly by their employers, with instances of bullying and dismissal occurring [Francis, 2015].

Changing an organisation's culture takes time, but all organisations should be committed to embracing a learning culture and taking staff concerns seriously, whilst treating the staff involved fairly. A report into NHS whistleblowers recommends that all NHS organisations should appoint a 'Freedom to Speak Guardian' who will be responsible for ensuring that all staff that raise concerns are treated fairly [Francis, 2015].

1.7 Reflection

Everyone reflects on a near-constant basis throughout their life, but lending structure to reflection can make it a powerful tool for learning and developing. The ability to reflect critically on one's own performance should be seen as a key skill for any health professional and for many, including paramedics, it is a standard of their ongoing registration that they undertake regular reflection [HCPC, 2014].

Gibbs' reflective cycle

Gibbs' reflective cycle is probably one of the most commonly used models in healthcare reflection (Figure 1.2). This is a simple-to-follow model that invites you to look back on an experience and then consider the different

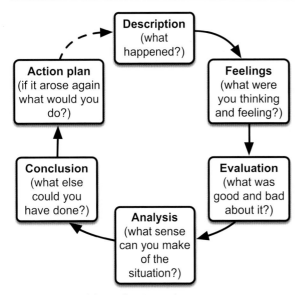

Figure 1.2 Gibbs' reflective cycle
Source: Gibbs G (1988) Learning by Doing: A guide to teaching and learning methods. Further Education Unit, Oxford Polytechnic: Oxford
Available at: http://www.brookes.ac.uk/students/upgrade/study-skill/reflective-writing-gibbs

elements in specific stages [Gibbs, 1988]. If applied correctly, you should analyse your actions, in detail, before deciding on what could have been done differently and action-planning how to implement those changes to your practice.

When undertaking reflection, it is tempting to focus on mistakes exclusively. Although reflecting on errors is a helpful process and provides insight into how to avoid similar mistakes in the future, you should do this not only when things have not gone as you would like, but also when things have gone well. It is just as important to identify the good things, so they can become a part of ongoing practice, as well as those things you may wish to change.

Reflective models such as Gibbs' reflective cycle are primarily intended for formal, written reflections, but this is not always required. A brief chat with your colleagues following a challenging incident may be all that is necessary [Jasper, 2003].

1.7.1 **Description**

This should provide a brief overview of what happened. It needs to be an objective account, i.e. just the facts. Although you need to cover the incident from start to finish, you do not need

to elaborate on aspects that you will not discuss further in your reflection. For example, if the journey to hospital was uneventful, then that is all you need to say about it. On the other hand, if the journey to the emergency department was the most important part of the incident, then you will need to say more. If this reflection is going to be read by someone else, you need to pre-alert your reader to the aspects of the incident you intend to discuss (i.e. flag important points). It may help to use some of the following questions [Jasper, 2003]:

- Where were you?
- Who else was there?
- Why were you there?
- What were you doing?
- What were other people doing?
- What was the context of the event?
- What happened?
- What was your part in this?
- What parts did other people play?
- What was the result?

1.7.2 **Feelings**

Recall and explore the things that were going through your mind:

- How were you feeling when the event started?
- What were you thinking about at the time?
- How did it make you feel?
- What did other people's actions/words make you think?
- How did you feel about the outcome?
- What do you think about it now?

1.7.3 **Evaluation**

Evaluation involves valuing or measuring something against some sort of standard. This might be ambulance clinical practice guidelines if you intend to discuss a method of treating a patient or an advanced intervention that you assisted a senior colleague with. You might also want to rate your performance against the legal, ethical and professional frameworks that govern practice. Relevant questions in this section include:

- What was good about the experience?
- What was bad about the experience, or didn't go so well?

1.7.4 Analysis

Analysis involves breaking things down into their component parts, so that they can be explored separately. Questions that you might want to answer in this section include:

- What went well?
- What did I do well?
- What did others do well?
- What went wrong, or did not turn out the way I thought it should?
- In what ways did I contribute to this?
- Why might these things have happened?

1.7.5 Conclusion

Now you have successfully taken the incident apart, you need to make sense of what you have found out in order to prepare for the next section – the action plan. In addition, you will need to show that you have developed some insight into your own and other people's behaviour in terms of how they contributed to the event.

1.7.6 Action plan

Now you have reassembled the incident, you are in a position to plan for next time. Factors you might like to consider are:

- What do you want to achieve as a result of your action?
- How will you do it?
- When will you do it?
- Where will you do it?
- Who will be part of the action?

1.8 End of Lesson

You've reached the end of the lesson. Why not test your knowledge by taking the BEING A HEALTHCARE PROFESSIONAL QUIZ?

2 Consent and capacity

2.1 Learning objectives

By the end of this lesson you will be able to:

- Assess capacity
- Gain consent
- Maintain consent
- Analyse factors that influence the capacity of an individual to express consent

- Describe different ways of applying active participation to meet individual needs
- Describe how to support an individual to question or challenge decisions concerning them that are made by others.

2.2 Introduction

As a support worker employed in a front line role, you will regularly have to apply the concepts of consent and mental capacity to your work, often in challenging and confusing situations where a rapid assessment and fast action may be required to determine a defendable and lawful decision.

Having a good understanding of the basic principles will make this easier and help to remove doubt when tackling challenging and potentially confusing scenarios.

2.3 Consent

In the United Kingdom, case law has determined that adult patients with mental capacity (or competence) must give consent before they are touched. Failure to do this leaves the ambulance crew open to civil claims for trespass against the person, which includes assault and battery [Dimond, 2008].

Valid consent

In order for consent to be valid, it must be given voluntarily, i.e. free from pressure exerted by relatives, partners, ambulance staff or police officers. In addition, patients need to be appropriately informed about the nature and purpose of any intervention or plan of action that they are consenting to. Finally, the person consenting needs to have the mental capacity to consent. This is usually the patient, but includes someone with parental responsibility in patients less than 18 years of age, or a person who has been given a Lasting Power of Attorney or authority by a court to make treatment decisions [DoH, 2009a].

Implied consent

As a rule, if your patient is over 18 years of age, only they can consent to any intervention. Lying unconscious in the street covered in vomit after consuming a litre of vodka and Red Bull® does not imply consent. Prior to the Mental Capacity Act 2005, you would have cared for this individual in the absence of consent as part of your duty of care for the patient and out of necessity in an emergency. Now, this is covered by the Mental Capacity Act [Dimond, 2011].

Implied consent is more appropriate for situations where non-verbal communications by the patient make it clear that they are giving consent, for example rolling up a sleeve for a blood pressure recording (you don't record blood pressures over clothes, do you?). However, it is best to obtain at least a verbal consent in this situation so that the patient knows what you are about to do. This should avoid confusion and surprise when your patient expects a blood pressure recording and gets an intramuscular injection, for example!

2.4 **Mental capacity**

Case law has clearly laid out the right of a mentally competent adult to refuse any treatment, including life-saving interventions, regardless of the reason, or for no reason at all. This has now been incorporated into several statutory frameworks. In England and Wales, this framework is the Mental Capacity Act 2005 (MCA), and in Scotland, the Adults with Incapacity (Scotland) Act 2000.

Central to all of these is the concept of personal autonomy, that is, the right of an individual to 'govern themselves' according to their own set of personal values, preferences, commitments and character traits [Freyenhagen, 2009]. This can come into conflict with an ambulance crew's tendency towards beneficence (i.e. serving the best interests of patients [Moye, 2007]) and wanting to safeguard their job.

Mental capacity is the ability to make a decision, and covers everything from when to get up to how much alcohol to drink and whether to go to hospital as advised by the ambulance crew. A lack of capacity is defined as an inability of your patient to make a specific decision at the time they are required to make it, due to an impairment of, or disturbance in the functioning of, the mind or brain. It does not matter if this impairment or disturbance is temporary or permanent. Examples of impairment include:

- Temporary:
  - Post-ictal following a convulsion
  - A diabetic suffering a hypoglycaemic event
  - Ingestion of alcohol or drugs

- Permanent:
  - Dementia
  - Significant learning disabilities
  - Long-term effects of brain damage.

2.4.1 **MCA code of practice**

All patients have the right of autonomy over decisions relating to their healthcare (in all but a few specific circumstances) if they have the 'capacity' to make those decisions and these decisions are made voluntarily.

The MCA code of practice explains the five statutory principles that need to be foremost in your mind when making capacity decisions [DCA, 2014]:

1. A person must be assumed to have capacity unless it is established that they lack capacity

2. A person is not to be treated as unable to make a decision unless all practicable steps to help them to do so have been taken without success

3. A person is not to be treated as unable to make a decision merely because they make an unwise decision

4. An act done, or decision made, under this Act for or on behalf of a person who lacks capacity must be done, or made, in that person's best interests

5. Before the act is done, or the decision is made, regard must be had to whether the purpose for which it is needed can be as effectively achieved in a way that is less restrictive to the person's rights and freedom of action.

It is important to note that a person cannot be said to generally have capacity or to lack capacity; instead, capacity relates to a specific decision needing to be made. For example: a person may have capacity to make simple decisions such as day-to-day control of finance for purchasing essential items, but they may lack the capacity to make more complex long-term investment decisions.

Another important consideration is whether a decision can be delayed. If a person is experiencing a temporary disturbance or impairment, it may be reasonably foreseeable that they will regain capacity and can then make the decision for themselves in the future. There are several situations in the emergency setting where this will not be the case, for example patients suffering from stroke or severe breathing difficulties, but if the decision is not urgent and the patient is not likely to come to harm as a result of not making the decision immediately then it should be delayed where possible, pending the return of normal capacity [DCA, 2014].

2.4.2 Assessing capacity

The MCA describes a two-stage test to determine whether your patient has mental capacity. Stage 1 requires you to identify whether the patient has an impairment of, or a disturbance in the functioning of, their mind or brain. If they do not, then you cannot say that the patient lacks capacity under the Act. Stage 2 requires you to determine whether this impairment or disturbance means that the person cannot make the specific decision currently required of them.

Stage 1

Evidence of impairment is required for stage 1 to be positive. Impairments may be temporary or permanent, as discussed above, but impairment must be present before moving on to the next stage. If no such impairment is present, the person will not lack capacity under the Act. If the patient does have such impairment, this does not in itself mean that they lack capacity, but instead the healthcare person undertaking the assessment should progress to stage 2 of the test. Otherwise, you should assume that the patient does have capacity and it is not necessary to undertake stage 2 of the test.

Stage 2

To help define whether a person is unable to make a specific decision there are four aspects to test during stage 2:

1. Is the person able to understand relevant information about the decision to be made? Relevant information includes:
   - The nature of the decision to be made
   - The reason why the decision is needed
   - The likely effects of deciding one way or another, or of making no decision at all.
2. All the information required to cover these three points should be conveyed, in a suitable manner for the person receiving the information to understand. The healthcare person undertaking the capacity assessment should then check, by whatever means is most suitable, that the patient understands the relevant information.
3. Is the person able to retain the information in their mind for the period of time required to make the decision? The patient must be able to hold the information in their mind long enough to make an effective decision. The Act makes it clear that being able to retain information for only a short period does not in itself mean a person lacks capacity: it depends on the complexity of the decision needing to be made.
4. Is the person able to use or weigh information as part of the decision-making process? To have capacity a person must have the ability to weigh up information and use it to arrive at a decision. That decision does not have to be the right one in the view of the person undertaking the assessment, but instead the person being assessed must show they have used the information to arrive at their decision. Some patients with brain damage may understand the information, but not be able to use it to arrive at a decision and may make impulsive decisions regardless of the information they have been given.
5. Is the person able to communicate their decision? A person must be able to communicate their decision, although this does not have to be in verbal or written form.

If the answer to any of these questions in stage 2 is 'No' then it is likely the person lacks capacity. If the answer to all is 'Yes' then it is presumed the patient has mental capacity.

2.4.3 Supporting patients with capacity assessments

A person can only be said to lack capacity if all reasonable steps to help them to reach the decision themselves have been made. These may include:

- Presenting information in a way that is easy for them to understand
- Using illustrations to help describe certain procedures
- Exploring alternative methods of communication where possible

- Taking time to give the patient the best opportunity to make a decision for themselves
- Utilising a relative or carer who understands a particular barrier and how to overcome it.

Capacity in emergency situations

In certain time-critical situations, such as a stroke affecting a patient's speech or understanding for example, it may not be possible to take the additional time to help the person to make their own decisions, as to do so may lead to the patient suffering harm due to delaying treatment.

In these circumstances healthcare staff should work on the basis of a patient lacking capacity and should act in their best interests. However, staff should still communicate with the patient and keep them informed of what is happening. They should work to the principle that only those actions which must be immediately taken are taken, and that other decisions, which can be safely delayed, should be.

2.4.4 Patients who lack capacity

All acts undertaken and decisions made on behalf of a person who lacks capacity should be done in the 'best interests' of that person. Establishing what is in a person's best interests for the management of emergency conditions is usually simple, but there may be occasions where more complex decisions are required. We all have our own attitudes and beliefs, and therefore what we believe to be in someone's best interests may differ from someone else's idea.

When considering what is in the best interests of a person lacking capacity you should try to:

- Encourage participation: Do whatever is possible to encourage the person to take part in the decision-making process
- Identify all relevant circumstances: Try to identify all the things that the person who lacks capacity would take into account if they were making the decision or acting for themselves
- Find out the persons views, such as:
  - Past and present wishes and feelings
  - Beliefs and values that would be likely to influence the decision in question
  - Any other factors the person themselves would be likely to consider if they were making the decision

- Avoid discrimination: Do not make any decisions based purely on discriminating factors such as age, gender, appearance or behaviour
- If the decision concerns life-sustaining treatment: Do not be motivated in any way by a desire to bring about the person's death. You should not make assumptions about the person's quality of life.

If one is present, you should also follow any information available in an advanced directive (living will), or if a Lasting Power of Attorney has been appointed, that person should be consulted.

2.5 Summary

Decisions relating to capacity and consent can be difficult and often present themselves at the least opportune moment, frequently out-of-hours when other advice and support is limited. These decisions can also be emotive and charged with ethical dilemmas.

Having a good understanding of the law and the principles that accompany these laws is vital and will give you a strong base from which to practise. Remember these key concepts:

- The Mental Capacity Act applies to anyone aged 16 or over
- All persons are assumed to have capacity unless shown otherwise
- A person with capacity has the right to make their own decisions, even if unwise
- When a person lacks capacity you should act in their best interests
- For a person with capacity, you must seek consent before giving treatment.

3 Confidentiality

3.1 Learning objectives

By the end of this lesson, you will be able to:

- Explain the meaning of the term 'confidentiality'
- Demonstrate ways to maintain confidentiality in day-to-day communication
- Describe the potential tension between maintaining an individual's confidentiality and disclosing concerns.

3.2 Introduction

All health professionals have a duty of confidentiality to their patients, whereby they must protect all patient information and handle it in an approved manner. This is emphasised in the professional standards for all registered professions, including paramedics [HCPC, 2014], but equally applies to other ROLES WITHIN THE AMBULANCE SERVICE (see chapter 2). Failure to follow strict organisation polices and, where relevant, codes of conduct in relation to handling information can be a source of distress for patients and embarrassment for organisations. It can also result in legal or disciplinary action for both organisations and individuals [NHS England, 2014].

Within your role, you will routinely have access to confidential, patient-identifiable information. This information should not be shared without the consent of the patient or unless there is some other compelling reason to do so, as discussed later in this lesson.

What should be considered as patient-identifiable information?

Patient-identifiable information is anything that may enable a patient to be identified, either directly or indirectly [AACE, 2013]. This includes obvious personal information, such as name, address, date of birth etc. However, it also includes less commonly considered things, such as:

• Clinical record numbers
• Images or voice recordings of a patient
• Rare disease information.

Consider the following scenario:

'You work in a small town with a population of around 25,000 people. In this town lives a patient who suffers with Addison's disease: a rare endocrine disorder. The patient frequently suffers from crisis due to their Addison's, and when this happens family members call for an ambulance. You attend this patient suffering a crisis one day; as this is not a condition you are familiar with, on returning to the ambulance station you decide to ask colleagues for some information about the condition. You are mindful not to disclose the name or location of the patient (to prevent a breach of confidentiality), but instead describe the incident and ask for advice.'

Considering that Addison's is a rare disease and this one person, in a small community, frequently requires ambulance assistance, is it reasonable that on the balance of probabilities your colleagues would be able to identify whom you are talking about, just by describing the condition?

Any information that has the potential to identify the patient, however remotely, should be considered as identifiable and managed in such a way as to help avoid a breach of confidentiality from occurring [AACE, 2013].

3.3 Maintaining confidentiality

Organisations should have policies in place to describe how they handle information and protect confidentiality. As a healthcare worker, you have a legal obligation to maintain confidentiality so should have a good working knowledge of these policies [NHS England, 2014].

During the course of a working day, it may be necessary to discuss or share patient-identifiable information on a number of occasions. Such occasions may include:

• Discussing the care of your patient with another healthcare professional
• Handing over the care of your patient to another professional
• Requesting support in clinical decision-making for your patient
• Contacting other organisations or services to help provide care or support.

These communications can take many forms including:

• Face to face
• Written
• Telephone
• Mobile data systems
• E-mail.

Throughout all of these, you should consider how best to maintain confidentiality. Your employing organisation should make a copy of its policy available, but some good practice guidelines include [NHS England, 2014]:

- **Seek consent before sharing information**: Before you share patient information you should seek consent from the patient to do so. However, in a limited range of situations it may be appropriate to share information without the patient's consent, for example:
  - It is not possible to gain consent
  - There is a legal requirement to make certain disclosures
  - It is in 'the public interest' to make a disclosure.

- **Share only that information which is necessary**: If you phone a GP to discuss the care of your patient then it may be necessary to discuss all aspects of the patient and their medical history and current episode in order to reach an appropriate management plan. In contrast, when you initially phone the surgery and speak to a receptionist, it would not normally be necessary to provide more than a name and address of your patient (so that their notes can be identified) and a brief description of the reasons for your call (so that it can be triaged for priority)

- **Maintain physical security of information**: Patient information is collected and held in a range of physical and electronic devices, including: written records, mobile data terminals, mobile phones, e-mail inboxes and a range of clinical monitoring equipment, such as ECG machines. At all times consider how the safety of this equipment and the data it contains is being managed. If clinical records are completed on paper, where are these stored? If you are working in an ambulance setting, these records should be safely stored, out of view from those looking into the vehicle and in such a manner that they could not accidentally fall out when a door to the ambulance is opened. Other security measures include:
  - Keep the environment secure: lock doors and close windows when a building or vehicle is unattended
  - Log off or 'lock' computers when leaving your desk
  - Delete electronic records on insecure monitoring equipment, in line with local

policy, once relevant information has been collected and recorded
  - If it is necessary to share identifiable information via e-mail then you should do so via a secure system
  - When speaking on the phone, have you taken all reasonable steps to ensure you are speaking to the correct person?
  - When discussing the care of a patient either over the phone or face to face, could you be overheard? If so, move to a private place where this could not happen.

- **Access only the information that you need**: During the working day, you may have access to a wide range of information about a large number of individuals. This access should be used only when you have reasonable grounds to do so. You should not access records or information about incidents or individuals that are not of relevance to you. Most electronic systems have means for monitoring those who access personal information and any unauthorised access will not only likely breach local policy but may also constitute an offence under the Data Protection Act (1998).

Further sources of information

Issues relating to confidentiality can be complex and you should know where to turn in order to find further information or support if required. Sources of support in different organisations vary, but may include:

- All organisations should have a policy detailing how they handle information and maintain confidentiality
- The NHS has a published code of conduct in respect to confidentiality [DoH, 2003]
- All organisations should have a lead of confidentiality, normally an 'information governance manager' or 'data protection officer'. They can be approached with any queries in relation to confidentiality and the handling of data
- All NHS organisations have a Caldicott Guardian – this person is responsible for ensuring that standards of confidentiality are maintained and that appropriate information-sharing arrangements are in place [HSCIC, 2014].

3.3.1 **Making a disclosure**

In the course of your role, you may be faced with the need to disclose information to other bodies or organisations. The primary principle here is that, wherever possible, consent should be gained prior to sharing information. However, in certain circumstances it may be necessary to make a disclosure without that consent [DoH, 2003].

Below is an outline of some scenarios where it may be necessary to share information without patient consent [AACE, 2013; GMC, 2009; DoH, 2010]:

- **Police**: The police have the right to personal information (name, address, contact details etc.) in the detection and prevention of a crime; however, this does not extend to personal health information unless it is in the investigation or prevention of a serious crime (rape, arson, murder etc.) or related to terrorism offences. On most occasions this information can be requested by the police through locally agreed channels and only information required immediately in the prevention and detection of crime should be shared by ambulance crews.
- **Local authorities**: A local authority officer who believes a person to be at risk is allowed access to health, financial and other records in order to determine whether any action needs to be taken to protect them.
- **Coroner**: An ethical duty of confidentiality continues after a patient has died, but relevant information should be disclosed to a coroner or similar officer in the investigation of an inquest or fatal accident inquiry.
- **Notifiable diseases**: If a patient suffers from a notifiable disease then there is a legal requirement to disclose this, even without patient consent. However, patients should still be informed that this has happened.
- **Risk of well-being**: In certain situations there may be a risk to a patient's well-being by not informing other professionals and/or the relevant authorities: for example, safeguarding concerns relating to vulnerable adults and children.
- **Unable to gain consent**: If a person lacks the capacity to consent to their information

being shared, it is possible to share that information which is relevant to the situation. However, information should be shared cautiously, and if one exists then a proxy, guardian or parent should be consulted first, if available.

- **Public interest**: It may be permissible to share information if it is in the public interest. This may be to prevent or detect a serious crime or in cases where others are placed at risk. Examples include:
  - Reporting a patient to the Driver & Vehicle Licensing Agency when they reject medical advice not to drive (although health professionals should inform the patient of their intention to report it)
  - Releasing relevant confidential information to social services where there is a risk of significant harm to children. In all cases consent should be sought prior to disclosure unless it is not practical to do so, or it would be inappropriate because, for example, they lack capacity to consent, or they are suspects who should not be informed that they are under criminal investigation.

Services should have policies in place that cover the majority of the above circumstances and these policies should be studied and followed when making a disclosure. In the absence of a specific policy, wherever possible, the organisation's data protection officer/information governance manager/Caldicott Guardian should be consulted prior to releasing information, but this should not be at the cost of endangering patient care due to the delay in passing on information.

3.4 **Key points**

Remember these key points relating to confidentiality:

- Patients are the owners of information or data relating to them
- Patient-identifiable information comes in many forms and is communicated in a range of ways
- Patient-identifiable information should not be shared without consent except in specific circumstances
- Only share information that is necessary
- Consider how to maintain security of data in order to prevent accidental disclosures

- In certain circumstances it may be permissible to share information without patient consent: you should be aware of these
- Organisations should have policies in place for protecting information and you should be familiar with these
- If you require further information, speak to your information governance manager, data protection officer or Caldicott Guardian.

4 Equality and diversity

4.1 Learning objectives

By the end of this lesson you will be able to:
- Explain what is meant by
  - Diversity
  - Equality
  - Inclusion
- Explain the links between identity, self-image and self-esteem
- Analyse factors that contribute to the well-being of individuals
- Describe the potential effects of discrimination
- Explain how inclusive practice promotes equality and supports diversity
- Explain how legislation and codes of practice relating to equality, diversity and discrimination apply to your own work role
- Describe how to challenge discrimination in a way that promotes change.

4.2 Introduction

Promoting equality should be at the heart of a healthcare organisation's values. It ensures that organisations work in a way that is fair, so that no community, group or individual is left behind [NHS England, 2015a].

It is helpful to understand what the terms 'diversity', 'equality' and 'inclusion' mean:
- Diversity: This involves recognising and valuing the difference between individuals across groups. Such difference should be seen as 'assets to be valued and affirmed, rather than as problems to be solved' [Thompson, 2006a]
- Equality: In its simplest form, equality is about being treated fairly. Equality recognises that people are different (diversity) but that those differences do not mean that a person should be discriminated against, as everyone should be treated fairly and equally. Equality also recognises that inequality exists and needs to be overcome for a truly fair society
- Inclusion: Positively striving to meet the needs of different people and taking deliberate action to create environments where everyone feels respected and able to achieve their full potential [NIHR, 2012].

4.3 Discrimination

Discrimination occurs when someone treats one person less favourably than they would another, because of a personal characteristic. This is often due to stereotyping.

Under the Equality Act 2010, it is unlawful for a person to discriminate against another with respect to their:
- Age
- Disability
- Gender
- Gender reassignment
- Marriage and civil partnership
- Pregnancy and maternity
- Race
- Religion and belief
- Sexual orientation.

Discrimination in your role

Classifying people or objects into broad groups makes it easier to make sense of society; this is known as typification. When these typifications become broad and rigid, stereotypes are formed [Blaber, 2008].

Using these stereotypes is a natural process as it allows us to 'shortcut' our thinking, but often they are not accurate. Making such shortcuts in healthcare can be dangerous as we will make incorrect assumptions about our patients and fail to challenge our own thought processes.

Applying such stereotypes is probably unavoidable, but we must be prepared to challenge our own thinking and the assumptions made on the basis of that thinking. For example, elderly patients have very varied life expectancies. Some patients may suffer a multitude of medical conditions in their early seventies and therefore have a relatively limited life expectancy, whereas many people will live late into their nineties and beyond with very few medical concerns.

Applying the same thought process to all patients is clearly inappropriate and could lead to your making unreasonable, unjustifiable and unethical decisions. You must actively practise treating all patients equally and base your care on their specific circumstances, rather than on those of a group they may fit into.

Challenging discrimination

When you see signs of discrimination in practice it should be challenged, not least because, in healthcare, discrimination based on stereotypes, whether it be on purpose or unthinking, can lead to patient harm.

Challenging discrimination can be difficult, and if not done in an appropriate manner could lead to conflict. Each situation will be unique, so there is no single solution that can be described here. However, some general guidance includes:

- Promoting discussion, rather than telling someone they have got it wrong: during discussion most people will realise their mistakes
- Encouraging an open environment, where people can feel safe to discuss a wide range of difficult and complex issues
- Providing sources of further information
- If you feel that you are not able to manage the issue yourself, or it is too serious for that, then you should discuss the matter with a line manager for advice and support.

4.4 Identity, self-image and self-esteem

The way in which we see others is, in part, based on the way in which we see ourselves.

Identity

Your identity is 'what makes you the person you are'. It is normally a collection of characteristics that, when brought together, make you a unique individual. It may include things like:

- Your beliefs and values
- Outstanding personal attributes
- Life goals
- Political, social and ethical beliefs
- Life experiences that have moulded you.

Self-image

Self-image is similar to identity, but rather than consisting of what goes together to make you, it is about how you see yourself. It may include:

- How you think you look
- What your place is in society
- How you believe others see you and think of you
- What job you have.

Self-esteem

Self-esteem is about how you feel about yourself and your self-image. For example, you may not have the physical attributes you would like to, or you may not be in a job you enjoy or that you feel gives you sufficient status. Although we all have times where we lack confidence, prolonged periods of low self-esteem can have harmful effects on our mental health and our lives [NHS Choices, 2014a].

Being aware of what influences our self-esteem means we can, with time, change it and also support those around us who wish to change their own image or identity.

When dealing with patients, you should bear in mind a person's self-image and be careful not to do anything that may offend or cause unnecessary upset to that image, as to do so may have a harmful effect on that person's psychological well-being and also on your relationship with them.

5 Safeguarding adults and children

5.1 Learning objectives

By the end of this lesson you will be able to:

- Define the various types of abuse
- Identify the signs and/or symptoms associated with each type of abuse
- Describe factors that may contribute to an individual being more vulnerable to abuse
- Explain the actions to take if there are suspicions that an individual is being abused
- Explain the actions to take if an individual alleges that they are being abused
- Identify ways to ensure that evidence of abuse is preserved

- Identify national policies and local systems that relate to safeguarding and protection from abuse
- Explain the roles of different agencies in safeguarding and protecting individuals from abuse
- Identify reports into serious failures to protect individuals from abuse
- Identify sources of information and advice about your own role in safeguarding and protecting individuals from abuse
- Explain how the likelihood of abuse may be reduced
- Describe unsafe practices that may affect the well-being of individuals
- Explain the actions to take if unsafe practices have been identified
- Describe the action to take if suspected abuse or unsafe practices have been reported but nothing has been done in response.

5.2 **Introduction**

Abuse or neglect is a commonly encountered scenario for those working in healthcare. You are likely to be in a key position to identify and assist victims of abuse or neglect. In order to do this, you will need to have a good understanding of the forms abuse can take, the signs and symptoms of those suffering, what increases a person's risk of being a victim of abuse, and also how to get help and support for victims.

5.3 **Learning from previous cases**

The vast majority of abuse and neglect happens behind closed doors and rarely reaches the attention of the public. However, over recent years there have been a number of notable cases, including:

- Winterbourne View: In 2011 a BBC Panorama programme showed staff at Winterbourne View, a private hospital caring for patients with disabilities, abusing their patients in a range of both physical and psychological manners. A national outcry followed, and in the subsequent investigation 11 staff were convicted of criminal offences and the hospital was shut. The investigation also identified that there were serious warning signs evident at the hospital for a long time prior to the discovery

of abuse, which had not been properly looked into [DoH, 2013d]

- Daniel Pelka: Daniel died aged 4 years and 8 months following a period of sustained abuse and neglect by his mother and her partner. His death was caused by a serious head injury, but he had been physically beaten and starved for a prolonged period prior to his death. In the serious case review following his death, it was identified that although the family and Daniel were well known to police, social services, healthcare services and his school, the warning signs had not been correctly picked up on or appropriate action taken. The report said that Daniel was 'invisible against the backdrop of his mother's controlling behaviour' and that professionals involved in his case had failed to 'think the unthinkable' [CSCB, 2014].

Sadly, this failure to notice warning signs is not unique and other equally tragic cases, such as the murders of Victoria Climbie and baby Peter Connelly (baby P), had very similar findings in their investigations.

Abusers can be skilled at explaining away injuries or unusual behaviour and making professionals feel relaxed about the situation they find. In your front line role, you may be the only person that comes into contact with a vulnerable person over a prolonged period of time, so you must be prepared to identify and raise concerns where necessary, in order to help prevent further similar cases to those above. You must be prepared to 'think the unthinkable'.

5.4 **Vulnerability**

People are considered to be vulnerable when they are at a greater than normal risk of abuse. For vulnerable adults, this can include [NHS Choices, 2015]:

- Those with learning difficulties
- Older people who are isolated
- Those with memory problems
- Those who are dependent on others for support
- Those whose carer is addicted to alcohol or drugs
- Those who live with a carer.

Abusers of vulnerable adults

Vulnerable adults may be abused by a wide range of people, including: relatives and family, professional staff, paid care workers, volunteers, other service users, neighbours, friends and those who deliberately target and exploit the vulnerable [DoH, 2000].

Risk factors for child abuse

All children are vulnerable to abuse, but those who may be more so include those in the following situations [NICE, 2009]:

- Parental or carer drug or alcohol misuse
- Parental or carer mental health problems
- Intra-familial violence or history of violent offending
- Previous child maltreatment in members of the family
- Known maltreatment of an animal by the carer or parent
- Vulnerable and unsupported parents or carers
- Pre-existing disability in the child.

5.5 Forms of abuse

There are four types of abuse common to both adults and children [DfE, 2013; DoH, 2011a]:

- Physical abuse
- Psychological/emotional abuse
- Sexual abuse
- Neglect.

For vulnerable adults there is also [Age UK, 2014b]:

- Financial abuse
- Discriminatory abuse.

5.5.1 Physical abuse

Physical abuse, also known as non-accidental injury (NAI), involves contact intended to cause, or resulting in, pain, injury or other physical harm. It may including striking someone (with or without an object), kicking, grabbing, biting or inappropriate restraint. For older patients in particular, it may also include being handled roughly, or moved in a way that causes pain without the appropriate lifting or moving aids [DfE, 2013; Age UK, 2014b].

Physical harm can also be caused when a carer or parent fabricates illness, or induces symptoms of an illness, in an adult or child (Munchausen's syndrome by proxy).

Signs may include:

- Bruising at multiple stages of repair
- Bruises on children who are not yet crawling
- Injuries inconsistent with age of patient
- Frequent attendance at hospital
- Inappropriate history for injury demonstrated
- Specific injuries, such as cigarette burns and 'hand-grip' bruises
- Fear of those around them
- Fear of making mistakes
- Being very withdrawn and quiet
- Delays in seeking help for illness or injury.

5.5.2 Psychological/emotional abuse

Psychological, also known as emotional, abuse is a form of abuse characterised by damaging a person's psychological well-being. This is often seen in situations of power imbalance, such as abusive relationships. It may include conveying a feeling of unworthiness, unimportance or being unvalued. It may also include making a person feel ashamed or humiliated through the words or actions of another person.

Over a prolonged period, this form of abuse can allow the abuser to mentally control the abused person and can seriously damage emotional and psychological development. All forms of abuse usually contain an element of psychological abuse, as abusers will try to control the actions and behaviour of their victim [DfE, 2013; Age UK, 2014b].

Signs may include:

- Lack of social skills
- Low self-worth
- Depression
- Self-harm
- Poor relationships with others
- Helplessness
- Excessive fear or anxiety.

5.5.3 Sexual abuse

Sexual abuse involves forcing or enticing a person to take part in sexual activity against their wishes, or for which they are not able to consent. Activities may involve physical assault, including penetration (for example rape or oral sex), or they can be non-penetrative, such as kissing, masturbation or touching the outside of clothing. Sexual abuse can also include non-contact activities such as indecent exposure, or forcing a person to watch, or to be involved in the production of, explicit sexual material. Grooming a person in preparation for abuse is also a form of sexual abuse [DfE, 2013; Age UK, 2014b].

Signs may include:

- Physical signs such as anal or vaginal soreness
- Sexually transmitted infection
- Unusual discharge
- Inappropriate use of sexual language for age
- A child being sexually active at a young age
- Guilt or shame
- Appearing frightened by or avoiding being near to certain people.

5.5.4 Neglect

Neglect is the persistent failure to meet a person's physical and/or psychological needs. A carer or parent should take reasonable steps to prevent harm from occurring to a dependant, and failure to do so may be neglect. Neglect can be deliberate or accidental, due to not fully understanding the needs of a dependent person.

Neglect may include:

- Failure to provide adequate food, warmth or shelter for a dependant
- Failure to ensure adequate access to appropriate medical care.

Signs of neglect include:

- Poor appearance and hygiene
- Untreated injuries or dental issues
- Poor physical development for age
- Poor language or communication skills for age
- Pressure sores
- Signs of malnourishment or dehydration
- Dirt, urine or faecal smell in person's environment.

5.5.5 Financial abuse

This is the unlawful use of a person's property, money or other valuables. It may include an individual being pressured into lending or giving money or other belongings to another person. A carer could start to take control of personal

finance and then use that control to gain profitably without consent. It may also include charging excessive amounts of money for simple services or goods. Relatives are often perpetrators of this kind of abuse and may move into a patient's house in order to be able to exert the influence required to take financial control [Age UK, 2014b].

Signs of financial abuse can include:

- Unexplained loss of money
- Unusual bank account activity
- Rapid deterioration in a person's standard of living as they can no longer afford essential goods and services
- A relative or carer moving into the home and taking control.

5.5.6 Discriminatory abuse

A person can be discriminated against based on their age, gender, race, ethnicity, religion, culture, beliefs or some other aspect or value of their life. It could include a failure to take into account personal or religious beliefs in the provision of care, and could impact on the spiritual welfare of a person. Age-related discrimination is an offence under the Equality Act 2010 [Age UK, 2014b].

5.6 Managing abuse or disclosures of abuse

The primary goal in the management of a patient who has suffered abuse should be their long-term safety. The situation may be highly emotionally charged, not least for you as a responder, but your actions in the immediate moments on scene may influence the entire course of protecting a vulnerable person.

You should remain calm and professional, and not judge those around you. Situations are rarely as simple as they may initially appear, and in the amount of time you will be in contact with a person it is unlikely that you will discover the full truth.

When managing an incident where a safeguarding concern is evident [AACE, 2013]:

- Consider not just the patient, but also others present. For example, you may be called to manage an adult with chest pain initially, but if you are concerned about the welfare of a child living in the same house you have the same duty to report and raise concerns as if that child was the original patient

- Your first priority should be to manage the presenting condition and ensure medical well-being: i.e. provide the usual clinical management for the presenting complaint and transport anyone with significant illness or injury to further care without delay

- Limit your questioning to that which is relevant: stop questioning if your suspicions are confirmed, as unnecessary questioning or probing may affect the credibility of subsequent evidence

- Accept any given explanation. Even if you do not believe the answer, do not make suggestions to the patient on how an incident may have occurred

- Do not directly accuse parents or carers of abuse, as to do so may result in refusal of further care or transport, thereby increasing the risk a patient faces

- Wherever possible you should work in partnership with the parents or carers, and inform them of your concerns and the need to share these concerns with other agencies. The only exemption to this rule is when you believe that doing so may put the patient at greater risk of harm. You will have to exercise professional judgement on this point and should record in detail your justification for not informing, if that is the option you choose

- Take any and all accusations seriously: it is not your role to decide on their validity or to investigate further, but instead you should refer your concerns to the appropriate authorities

- If a person makes a disclosure make sure you treat them with respect and dignity, and act in a manner which suggests you believe them. Body language and your words can have a massive influence on a patient's behaviour and confidence in you, and if they feel you do not believe them then they may not disclose what they were going to

- Complete full and accurate records of events. Where possible try to record word-for-word what the patient has disclosed

- If transporting your patient, make sure you fully hand over to the receiving staff all details, your concerns and reasons for those concerns, and details of any further action you are going to take.

Reporting an urgent concern

An urgent concern exists where you believe a person may be at immediate risk of further harm. In those circumstances you should work to ensure the immediate safety of the patient. This can often be best achieved by transporting the patient to hospital where they can be monitored and assessed while awaiting the support of other services.

In the most serious circumstances it may be necessary for you to contact the police via the emergency operations centre with your concerns to ensure immediate patient safety.

Follow local policy on deciding the urgency of the situation, and where necessary seek further advice from your organisation's safeguarding team, named professional for safeguarding, on-call social worker, or ambulance service officer.

In all cases, a safeguarding referral should be completed as soon as possible after the incident, in line with appropriate policies and procedures.

5.7 Safeguarding referrals

Whenever you believe a person is being abused or neglected, or is at risk of either, you should raise your concerns through a safeguarding referral. Different organisations will have different policies based on the local arrangement of who is responsible for the delivery of social care. You should be familiar with arrangements and policies in your local area, but some common guidelines normally include:

- Report all concerns: Any concerns you have, however small, should be reported through your safeguarding referral pathways. Experienced and qualified safeguarding professionals can judge for themselves whether further investigation or action is required. They will also know whether the patient, place of care, or family is known for previous safeguarding concerns, information that may not be available to you

- Additional sources of help: All services should have safeguarding teams including named professionals responsible for safeguarding. These teams are experienced in the management of safeguarding issues and have established relationships with the multidisciplinary teams that work around those issues

- Role of social services: In most areas, social services are the main organisation around which safeguarding concerns articulate. Social workers are experienced in dealing with vulnerable people and with cases of abuse and neglect, and can be a great source of support and advice. In some circumstances, social services may want to get in touch with you for more information following a safeguarding referral. You should work fully with social workers to provide whatever information you can in order to ensure the best available support and protection for individuals

- Escalating concerns: All care organisations should be well prepared for managing safeguarding concerns, but in the unlikely event that you do not believe that your concerns are being managed in an appropriate manner, you have a duty to escalate your concern [AACE, 2013]. To do this you should speak to a senior manager, colleague or a named professional. Ensure you make records of all concerns that you pass on.

5.8 **Summary**

Safeguarding can be a highly emotive topic for all concerned, and this should be at the front of your mind when managing a situation where safeguarding is a concern. Try to remain calm, impartial and factual and keep the immediate safety of patients as your primary goal.

Remember the cases of Winterbourne View and Daniel Pelka, where key signs were missed and professionals failed to 'think the unthinkable'.

Be aware of the signs of abuse or neglect and immediately raise any concerns you have through local policy for doing so. Also be mindful that dealing with safeguarding incidents can be emotionally traumatic for responders, and following such incidents you may need to make use of your organisation's counselling or support services.

Chapter 5: **Health and Safety**

1 **Health and safety policies and legislation**

1.1 **Learning objectives**

By the end of this lesson you will be able to:

- Identify legislation relating to health and safety in the ambulance service
- Explain the main points of health and safety policies and procedures
- Analyse the main health and safety responsibilities for:
  - Yourself
  - Your employer or manager
  - Others in the work setting
- Describe types of hazardous substances that may be found in the work setting.

1.2 **Introduction**

A variety of the legislation that relates to the ambulance service has been reviewed in the LEGAL, ETHICAL AND PROFESSIONAL ISSUES chapter, but it is also important that you are aware of the legislation relating to health and safety, and in particular, that you know your and your employer's legal responsibilities.

This lesson will provide an overview of the following legislation that directly applies to health and safety, including manual handling:

- Health and Safety at Work etc. Act 1974 (HSWA)
- Management of Health and Safety at Work Regulations 1999 (MHSWR)
- The Manual Handling Operations Regulations 1992 (MHOR) (as amended 2002)
- The Provision and Use of Work Equipment Regulations 1998 (PUWER)
- The Lifting Operations and Lifting Equipment Regulations 1998 (LOLER)
- The Personal Protective Equipment at Work Regulations 1992
- The Control of Substances Hazardous to Health Regulations 2002.

1.3 **Health and Safety at Work Act**

All workers have a right to work in places where risks to their health and safety are properly controlled. Health and safety is about stopping you getting hurt at work or ill through work. Your employer is responsible for health and safety, but you must help [HSE, 2009].

Employers must do the following in order to comply with the Act [HSE, 2009]:

- Decide what could harm you in your job and what precautions could prevent it. This is part of RISK ASSESSMENT
- In a way you can understand, explain how risk will be controlled and tell you who is responsible for this
- Consult and work with staff and the health and safety representatives, to protect everyone from harm in the workplace
- Provide (free of charge) health and safety training and provide equipment and protective clothing that you need to do your job
- Provide toilets, washing facilities, drinking water and adequate first-aid facilities
- Notify the Health and Safety Executive in the event of any major injuries and fatalities at work
- Have insurance that covers staff in the event of injury at work
- Display a physical or electronic copy of the current insurance certificate where you can easily read it
- Work with other employers or contractors sharing the workplace to ensure that everyone's health and safety is protected.

You have a number of responsibilities as an employee too [HSE, 2009]:

- Follow the training you have received when using any work item your employer has provided
- Take reasonable care of your own and other people's health and safety
- Co-operate with your employer on health and safety

- Tell someone (for example your employer, line manager or safety representative) if you think that a method of working or inadequate precautions are putting anyone's health and safety at serious risk.

1.4 Management of Health and Safety at Work Regulations

The Management of Health and Safety at Work Regulations 1999 require employers to put in place arrangements to control health and safety risks. These include [HSE, 2013a]:

- A written health and safety policy
- Assessments of the risks to employees, contractors, customers, partners, and any other people who could be affected by work-related activities, and record significant findings in writing
- Arrangements for the effective planning, organisation, control, monitoring and review of the preventive and protective measures that come from risk assessment
- Access to competent health and safety advice
- Providing employees with information about the risks in the workplace and how those employees are protected
- Instruction and training for employees in how to deal with the risks
- Ensuring there is adequate and appropriate supervision in place
- Consulting with employees about their risks at work and current preventive and protective measures.

1.5 Manual Handling Operations Regulations

Any transporting or supporting of a load (including the lifting, putting down, pushing, pulling, carrying or moving thereof) by hand or by bodily force is considered to be a manual handling operation by the Manual Handling Operations Regulations 1992.

Employers are required to make a suitable and sufficient assessment of the risks to the health and safety of their employees while at work. Where this assessment indicates the possibility of risks to employees from the manual handling of loads, the Regulations require a hierarchy of measures that must be adhered to. These include

avoiding hazardous manual handling operations so far as is reasonably practicable and assessing any hazardous manual handling operations that cannot be avoided so as to reduce the risk of injury, as far as is reasonably practicable.

No doubt you have noticed the term 'reasonably practicable' appearing a couple of times. This means that the employer's duty to avoid manual handling or to reduce the risk of injury can be limited, if the employer can show that the cost of any further preventive steps would be grossly disproportionate to their perceived benefit. Employees are also expected to play their part by following appropriate systems of work laid down by their employer to promote safety during the handling of loads [HSE, 2004a].

Emergency services

Preventing all potentially hazardous emergency service manual handling operations would result in an inability to provide the general public with an adequate rescue service. As an employee of an ambulance service, you may be asked to accept a greater risk of injury than someone employed to move inanimate objects (like boxes). In this case, additional relevant factors may include:

- The seriousness of the need for the lifting operation
- The ambulance service's duty to the public overall and the patient who requires assistance.

Taking these factors into account, the level of risk which an employer may ask an employee to accept may, in appropriate circumstances, be higher when considering the health and safety of those in danger, although this does not mean that employees can be exposed to unacceptable risk of injury [HSE, 2004a].

1.6 Provision and Use of Work Equipment Regulations

Work equipment as defined by the Provision and Use of Work Equipment Regulations 1998 is any machinery, appliance, apparatus, tool or installation for use at work. This includes equipment which employees provide for their own use at work. The scope of work equipment is therefore extremely wide. The use of work equipment is also very widely interpreted: it covers any activity involving work equipment and includes starting, stopping, programming, setting, transporting, repairing, modifying, maintaining, servicing and cleaning.

Employers must manage the risks from that equipment, including [HSE, 2014c]:

- Ensuring equipment is constructed or adapted to be suitable for the purpose it is used or provided for
- Taking account of the working conditions and health and safety risks in the workplace when selecting work equipment
- Ensuring work equipment is only used for suitable purposes
- Ensuring work equipment is maintained in an efficient state, in efficient working order and in good repair.

1.7 Lifting Operations and Lifting Equipment Regulations

Lifting equipment includes any equipment used at work for lifting or lowering loads, along with attachments used for anchoring, fixing or supporting it, including hoists and ambulance trolleys.

Employers are required to ensure that all lifting equipment is [LOLER, 1998]:

- Sufficiently strong, stable and suitable for the proposed use. Similarly, the load and anything attached must be suitable
- Positioned or installed to prevent the risk of injury, e.g. from the equipment or the load falling or striking people
- Visibly marked with any appropriate information to be taken into account for its safe use, e.g. safe working loads. Accessories, e.g. slings, clamps etc., should be similarly marked.

Additionally, employers must ensure that [LOLER, 1998]:

- Lifting operations are planned, supervised and carried out in a safe manner by people who are competent
- Where equipment is used for lifting people it is marked accordingly, and it should be safe for such a purpose, i.e. all necessary precautions have been taken to eliminate or reduce any risk
- Where appropriate, before lifting equipment (including accessories) is used for the first time, it is thoroughly examined. Lifting equipment may need to be thoroughly examined in use at

periods specified in the Regulations (i.e. at least six-monthly for accessories and equipment used for lifting people and, at a minimum, annually for all other equipment) or at intervals laid down in an examination scheme drawn up by a competent person. All examination work should be performed by a competent person (someone with the necessary skills, knowledge and experience)

- Following a thorough examination or inspection of any lifting equipment, a report is submitted by the competent person to the employer to take any appropriate action.

1.8 Personal Protective Equipment at Work Regulations

PPE is equipment that will protect the user against health or safety risks at work. It can include items such as safety helmets and hard hats, gloves, eye protection, high-visibility clothing, safety footwear and safety harnesses [HSE, 2013c].

PPE should be used as a last resort. Wherever there are risks to health and safety that cannot be adequately controlled in other ways, the Personal Protective Equipment at Work Regulations 1992 require PPE to be supplied. The Regulations also require that PPE is:

- Properly assessed before use to make sure it is fit for purpose
- Maintained and stored properly
- Provided with instructions on how to use it safely
- Used correctly by employees.

1.9 Control of Substances Hazardous to Health Regulations

The Control of Substances Hazardous to Health Regulations 2002 cover substances that are hazardous to health. Substances can take many forms and include:

- Chemicals
- Products containing chemicals
- Fumes
- Dusts
- Vapours

- Mists
- Gases and asphyxiating gases
- Biological agents (germs); if the packaging has any of the hazard symbols then it is classed as a hazardous substance.

Employers have a responsibility to manage and minimise the risks from work activities. They must develop suitable and sufficient control measures and ways of maintaining them by [HSE, 2013b]:

- Identifying hazards and potentially significant risks
- Taking action to prevent and control risks
- Keeping control measures under regular review.

To be effective in the long term, control measures must be practical, workable and sustainable.

Good practice in the control of substances hazardous to health can be encapsulated in the eight generic principles set out in the Control of Substances Hazardous to Health Regulations 2002:

- Design and operate processes and activities to minimise emission, release and spread of substances hazardous to health
- Take into account all relevant routes of exposure – inhalation, skin and ingestion – when developing control measures
- Control exposure by measures that are proportionate to the health risk
- Choose the most effective and reliable control options that minimise the escape and spread of substances hazardous to health
- Where adequate control of exposure cannot be achieved by other means, provide, in combination with other control measures, suitable PPE
- Check and review regularly all elements of control measures for their continuing effectiveness
- Inform and train all employees on the hazards and risks from substances with which they work, and the use of control measures developed to minimise the risks
- Ensure that the introduction of measures to control exposure does not increase the overall risk to health and safety.

2 Risk assessment

2.1 Learning objectives

By the end of this lesson you will be able to:

- Define the term 'risk'
- Describe the process of carrying out a risk assessment
- Explain the importance of carrying out a risk assessment
- Compare different uses of risk assessment in health and social care
- Explain why risk assessments need to be regularly reviewed and revised.

2.2 Introduction

All healthcare staff have a duty to protect patients, their colleagues and themselves as far as is 'reasonably practicable', by minimising the chance that they are harmed by something, whether that be a procedure, drug administration or dangerous environment.

It is helpful to understand what is meant by the terms 'hazard' and 'risk' [HSE, 2014a; NPSA, 2007]:

- A **hazard** is anything that might cause harm, such as chemicals, electricity, working from ladders, an open drawer etc.
- A **risk** is the chance, high or low, that somebody could be harmed by these and other hazards, together with an indication of how serious the harm could be
- A **clinical risk** or healthcare risk is the chance of an adverse outcome resulting from clinical investigation, treatment or patient care.

For an organisation like an ambulance service, there are other risks to consider:

- Injury and safety (patients, staff and the public)
- Legal and financial
- Service interruption
- Resource Escalatory Action Plan (REAP) level increases
- Regulatory requirements
- Reputation.

2.3 Risk assessment

Risk assessment does not have to be difficult. It can be distilled into five steps [NPSA, 2007]:

1. Identify the hazards (What can go wrong?)
2. Decide who might be harmed and how (What can go wrong? Who is exposed to the hazard?)
3. Evaluate the risk (How bad? How often?) and decide on the precautions (Is there a need for further action?)
4. Record your findings and your proposed action, and identify who will lead on what action. Record the date of implementation
5. Review your assessment and update, if required.

2.3.1 Identify the hazards

This step consists of working out what is likely to go wrong and why. Many hazards can be anticipated in advance, allowing time for a formal, written risk assessment to be completed, which is then kept on an organisation and/or departmental risk register. Items suitable for this include:

• Equipment
• Cleaning products
• Industrial action
• Resourcing Escalatory Action Plan (REAP) level increases [SECAmb, 2011]
• Adverse media coverage.

However, some risk assessments will have to be conducted quickly, and mentally, as there will be no time to conduct a formal written risk assessment. This dynamic risk assessment is the type you will perform as you arrive on scene at an incident and may well conduct a number of times during a patient episode, depending on the risk of harm and the volatility of the scene and/or patients and bystanders. You will learn more about this in the SCENE ASSESSMENT AND SAFETY lesson (chapter 7).

2.3.2 Decide who might be harmed and how

Consider who might be harmed by the hazard and the circumstances that might lead to harm occurring. This could be you, for example when assisting a senior clinician with an injection or cannulation attempt. Patients can be harmed in many ways, for example during manual handling or the administration of a drug. Your colleagues are also at risk during certain procedures, such as

when you are reversing the ambulance into the garage.

It is not usually necessary to identify the individual, just groups of people who may be at risk of harm from the hazard you are assessing. In addition to the examples listed above, consider other groups such as [HSE, 2014b]:

• Pregnant patients
• Children
• Non-English speakers
• People with a disability.

2.3.3 Evaluate the risk and decide on precautions

Evaluating risk is a skill that becomes easier with practice. To assist with the evaluation, it can be helpful to use a risk matrix (Table 2.1) to quantify the two aspects of risk evaluation [NPSA, 2008]:

• Consequence: How severe is the risk?
• Likelihood: How often is the risk likely to arise?

To calculate the risk rating, the consequence score is multiplied by the likelihood score. Consider the example of a staff injury at work. The consequence would be scored as follows:

1 = Minor injury requiring no medical intervention and no time off work
2 = Minor injury requiring some medical intervention and less than 3 days off work
3 = Moderate injury requiring hospital or other professional intervention and 4–14 days off work
4 = Major injury leaving the staff member with long-term incapacity and/or disability and more than 14 days off work
5 = Major injury resulting in death.

The likelihood scores are allocated as follows:

1 = Rare: Not expected to occur for years
2 = Unlikely: Expected to occur at least annually
3 = Possible: Expected to occur at least monthly
4 = Likely: Expected to occur at least weekly
5 = Almost certain: Expected to occur at least daily.

Precautions

Having identified risks and given them a risk rating, it is necessary to determine what precautions (controls) are most appropriate to try to reduce the likelihood of the risk occurring

Table 2.1: Risk matrix

Consequence	Likelihood				
	1	2	3	4	5
	Rare	Unlikely	Possible	Likely	Almost certain
5 Catastrophic	5	10	15	20	25
4 Major	4	8	12	16	20
3 Moderate	3	6	9	12	15
2 Minor	2	4	6	8	10
1 Negligible	1	2	3	4	5

[NPSA, 2008]. It is quite likely that there will already be policies and procedures in place, which as an employee you will be expected to be familiar with, although you may also need training to ensure you can comply with them. In addition, as an employee you are likely to have a responsibility to report any risks and not undertake any action which would knowingly cause harm to you or anyone else, including your employer [SWAST, 2014a].

When assessing the risks and deciding which precautions to take, consider the following [MOD, 2008]:

- Can the hazards be eliminated altogether?
- Can the risks be controlled to give the lowest risk rating?
- Is there a less risky alternative?
- Can access to the hazard be eliminated or reduced?
- Can work practices be changed to reduce the risk?
- Is personal protective equipment (PPE) required? This is generally considered a last resort and should not be preferred over other forms of risk elimination.

Finally, once you have decided on the most appropriate precautions to take, you should re-evaluate the risk on the basis that your precautions are undertaken.

2.3.4 **Record and implement findings**

Risk assessments and action plans need to be reviewed periodically (step 5), but this will not be straightforward unless the assessment has been well documented and is able to show that [NPSA, 2007]:

- A thorough check was made to identify all hazards and address the significant risks
- The precautions (controls) taken are reasonable and any residual risk is acceptable
- The solutions are realistic, sustainable and likely to be effective.

Dynamic risk assessments also need to be documented and this should take place as soon as possible after the incident. This will provide justification for actions taken in the event of any adverse outcomes as well as providing a starting point for future, formal risk assessments if the situation is likely to recur [MOD, 2008].

2.3.5 **Review and update**

Risk assessments need to be reviewed periodically as things change. New best practices emerge from research, equipment is updated or modified and new hazards may be identified. Examples of when risk assessments should be reviewed include [NPSA, 2007; MOD, 2008]:

- When you are planning a change
- When there has been a significant change
- Periodically, at least annually
- Following an accident or near-miss.

3 Infection prevention and control

3.1 Learning objectives

By the end of this lesson you will be able to:

- Explain what is meant by infection and how infections can occur and be transmitted
- Identify a number of microorganisms, the illnesses they cause and how they can enter the body
- Describe how to manage and dispose of sources of infection safely while avoiding causing harm to self or others
- Outline the current regulations, legislation and responsibilities relating to infection control
- Describe the different types of personal protective equipment (PPE) and how to use them appropriately
- Describe the key principles of good personal hygiene
- Describe the correct sequence for handwashing and when it should be carried out.

3.2 Introduction

An infection is the body's adverse response to the presence of a pathogen, or disease-causing microorganism [Betsy, 2012]. Damage to tissues caused by an infection can either be limited to the site of infection (localised) or spread throughout the body, typically via the blood (systemic). Sometimes, however, a pathogen in or on the body may not lead to an infection. This is known as colonisation [Weston, 2014].

A healthcare-associated infection (HCAI) is any infection acquired as a result of a healthcare-related intervention or an infection acquired during the course of healthcare that the patient may reasonably expect to be protected from. HCAI has replaced the term 'hospital-acquired infection', since many healthcare interactions take place outside of hospital (such as in your ambulance) [Dougherty, 2011]. The scale of the problem is staggering, with an estimated 300,000 patients each year in England acquiring an HCAI, with a significant number of deaths and a cost to the NHS of around £1 billion [NICE, 2012]. This is why infection prevention and control is so important.

Infection prevention and control is a collective term for those activities intended to protect people from infections [Dougherty, 2011].

3.3 Regulations and legislation

In the HEALTH AND SAFETY POLICIES AND LEGISLATION lesson, some of the relevant legislation relating to infection prevention and control was reviewed, in particular the Health and Safety at Work etc. Act 1974. This requires employers to provide training and appropriate personal protective equipment (PPE) to prevent harm, and employees to follow the training that they have received, use PPE provided, and report any situations where they believe that patients' and/or staff's health and safety are at serious risk.

However, the Health and Social Care Act 2008 specifically highlights infection prevention and control and also makes the Care Quality Commission responsible for ensuring that ambulance (and other care) services meet the requirements of the code of practice that accompanies the legislation. This code specified 10 key elements that ambulance services must demonstrate that they comply with [DoH, 2011]:

1. Systems to manage and monitor the prevention and control of infection. These systems use risk assessments and consider how susceptible service users are, as well as any risks that their environment and other users may pose to them

2. Provide and maintain a clean and appropriate environment in managed premises that facilitates the prevention and control of infections

3. Provide suitable accurate information on infections to service users and their visitors

4. Provide suitable accurate information on infections to any person concerned with providing further support or nursing/medical care, in a timely fashion

5. Ensure that people who have or develop an infection are identified promptly and receive the appropriate treatment and care to reduce the risk of passing on the infection to other people

6. Ensure that all staff and those employed to provide care in all settings are fully involved in the process of preventing and controlling infection

7. Provide or secure adequate isolation facilities

8. Secure adequate access to laboratory support as appropriate

9. Have and adhere to policies designed for the individual's care that will help to prevent and control infections

10. Ensure, so far as is reasonably practicable, that care workers are free of, and are protected from exposure to, infections that can be caught at work and that all staff are suitably educated in the prevention and control of infection associated with the provision of health and social care.

There is also additional legislation that does not apply exclusively to the healthcare setting, but is intent on reducing the risk of infection. This includes regulations relating to food hygiene (Food Safety Act 1990), water supply [DWI, 2012] and waste management (Hazardous Waste Regulations 2005 and the Control of Substances Hazardous to Health Regulations 2002).

3.4 Microorganisms

Microorganisms are very small organisms that live outside and inside larger organisms such as the human body. The four main types that enter the body and cause infection are:

- Bacteria
- Viruses
- Fungi
- Parasites.

Bacteria

These are probably the most important microorganisms in relation to infection control as they are responsible for many opportunistic infections in healthcare. There are around ten times as many bacteria as there are cells in the human body and many have functions that are essential, such as *Escherichia coli (E. coli)*, which aids digestion in the gut. However, it can cause a urinary tract infection (UTI) if it gains access to the urinary tract [Dougherty, 2011].

Bacteria are fairly simple, single-celled microorganisms and are often classified by their shape. For example, they may be termed bacillus (rodlike), coccus (spherical or ovoid) or spiral (corkscrew or curved). Examples of common bacteria include streptococcus A, which can cause throat and ear infections, and

staphylococcus, which can cause impetigo and pneumonia. You may have heard of a particularly troublesome strain of staphylococcus, which is resistant to many antibiotics and is called meticillin resistant *Staphylococcus aureus* (MRSA) [Betsy, 2012].

Viruses

Viruses are even smaller than bacteria and have no cellular structure. They typically just consist of a core containing genetic material such as deoxyribonucleic acid (DNA) or ribonucleic acid (RNA) and are sometimes surrounded by a membrane called an envelope. Viruses can reproduce only by using the cellular machinery of other organisms and so are rather like parasites [Tortora, 2013].

Common viruses include the rhinovirus which is responsible for the common cold, respiratory syncytial virus (RSV) which can cause serious respiratory tract infections in infants and children, and the Varicella-zoster virus (VZV) which causes chickenpox and shingles [Betsy, 2012].

Fungi

You are probably most familiar with fungi as mushrooms or as yeast used in breadmaking and brewing. Some fungi are responsible for opportunistic infections, such as dermatophytes, which can cause athlete's foot, and *Candida albicans*, a yeast which can cause vaginal thrush [Dougherty, 2011].

Parasites

Parasites are organisms that live at the expense of another organism or host. Pathogenic parasites include bacteria, viruses, protozoa (animal-like single-cell microorganisms) and animals such as roundworms, flatworms and arthropods. Examples of parasitic infections include malaria and toxoplasmosis [Betsy, 2012].

3.5 Infection

Chain of infection

Transmission of infection is a complex process, involving a number of factors, which must all be present and are collectively known as the chain of infection (Figure 3.1) [Ross, 2014; Dougherty, 2011].

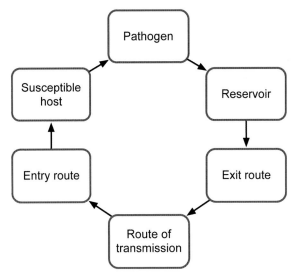

Figure 3.1 The chain of infection

Pathogen

An infectious agent is required, such as a bacterium, virus, fungus or parasite. This link can be broken by cleaning, sterilisation of equipment and the treatment of the patient, using antibiotics for bacterial infections, for example.

Reservoir

A reservoir is a place where the pathogen can live and replicate; it includes the human body, but also animals, water and the soil, for example. This link can be broken by cleaning equipment and the environment (such as the ambulance) and removing stagnant water by running low-use taps and showers, for example.

Exit route

The exit route is a method for the pathogen to leave its reservoir. In humans, this usually involves urine, faeces, vomit, sputum and in aerosolised form, such as after sneezing or coughing. Asking a patient with active tuberculosis to wear a mask would help break this chain.

Route of transmission

The transmission route can be direct, such as through touching, sexual intercourse and faecal-oral via ingestion, or indirectly via contaminated bedding, clothing, blood and bodily fluids and then the hands of healthcare workers. One of the most effective ways of breaking this chain is with good hand hygiene.

Entry route

Entry routes include the respiratory, gastrointestinal and genitourinary tracts, but also mucous membranes and via the skin. Direct access to the blood is also possible if the pathogen is inadvertently injected into a person. Ensuring that a paramedic who cannulates a patient uses an aseptic technique would be an example of breaking this chain.

Susceptible host

Some people are more vulnerable to infection than others, for example those with a weak immune system due to old age, medication or pre-existing disease. Others may have their natural defences compromised by wounds, surgery, intravenous cannulas and urinary catheters. This chain can be broken by ensuring that healthcare workers are vaccinated and that adequate nutrition and personal hygiene is provided to vulnerable groups.

3.6 **Personal hygiene**

Personal hygiene is defined as the physical act of cleansing the body to ensure that the hair, nails, ears, eyes, nose and skin are maintained in an optimum condition. It also includes mouth hygiene, which is the effective removal of plaque and debris to ensure that the structures and tissues of the mouth are kept in a healthy condition. In addition, personal hygiene includes ensuring the appropriate length of nails and hair [DoH, 2010a].

Good personal hygiene habits include [DoH, 2010b; Dougherty, 2011]:

- Having a shower or bath every day
- Brushing your teeth at least once (but preferably twice) a day
- Washing your hair with soap or shampoo at least once a week
- Washing your hands after going to the toilet
- Washing your hands with soap before preparing and/or eating food
- Wearing clean clothes.

3.7 **Hand hygiene**

Good hand hygiene is the primary measure to reduce HCAIs. It is a straightforward method and inexpensive, but poor compliance among healthcare workers is a worldwide problem [WHO, 2009].

You should clean your hands in the following circumstances [NICE, 2012]:

- Immediately before every episode of direct patient contact or care, including aseptic procedures
- Immediately after every episode of direct patient contact or care
- Immediately after any exposure to body fluids
- Immediately after any other activity or contact with a patient's surroundings that could potentially result in hands becoming contaminated
- Immediately after removal of gloves.

Use an alcohol-based handrub to decontaminate your hands, except when your hands are visibly soiled or potentially contaminated with body fluids, and when it is suspected that alcohol-resistant organisms (such as *Clostridium difficile* or other organisms that cause diarrhoeal illness) are involved.

In order to ensure that you can clean your hands while at work, you should [NICE, 2012]:

- Be 'bare below the elbows' when delivering direct patient care
- Not wear any wrist or hand jewellery
- Ensure that fingernails are short, clean and free of nail polish
- Cover cuts and abrasions with waterproof dressings.

3.7.1 **Alcohol handrub**

Procedure

This is the World Health Organization (WHO) recommended procedure for hand hygiene with handrub. This procedure should take 20–30 seconds [WHO, 2009].

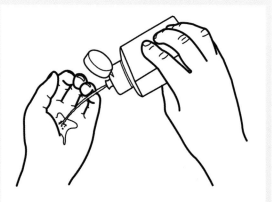

1. Apply a palmful of the alcohol rub in a cupped hand, covering all surfaces

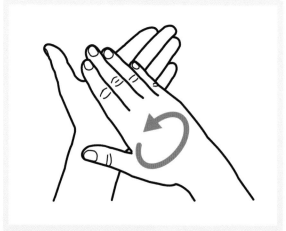

2. Rub hands palm to palm

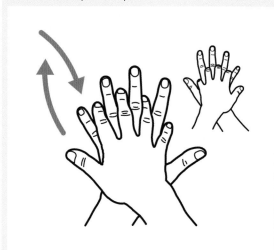

3. Right palm over left dorsum with interlaced fingers and vice versa

Procedure continued →

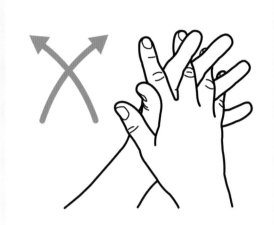

4. Palm to palm with fingers interlaced

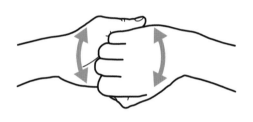

5. Backs of fingers to opposing palms with fingers interlocked

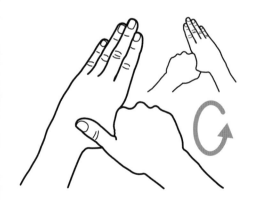

6. Rotational rubbing of left thumb clasped in right palm and vice versa

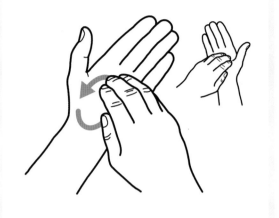

7. Rotational rubbing, backwards and forwards with clasped fingers of right hand in left palm and vice versa

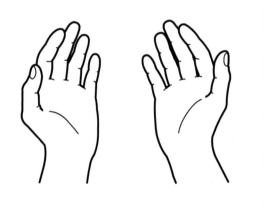

8. Once dry, your hands are safe
Based on the 'How to Handrub' poster. © World Health Organization 2009. All rights reserved.

3.7.2 Handwashing

Handwashing procedure

This is the WHO recommended procedure for hand washing. This procedure should take 40–60 seconds. [WHO, 2009]

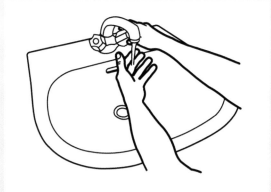

1. Wet hands with water

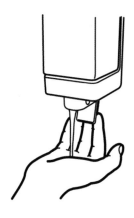

2. Apply enough soap to cover all hand surfaces

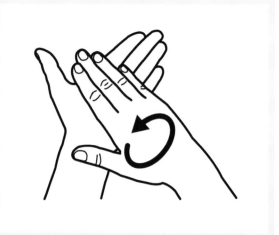

3. Rub hands palm to palm

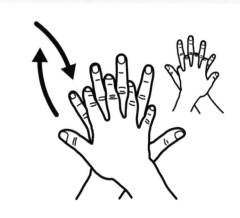

4. Right palm over left dorsum with interlaced fingers and vice versa

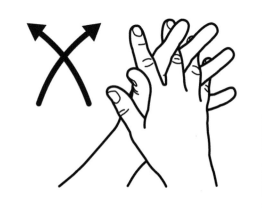

5. Palm to palm with fingers interlaced

Procedure continued →

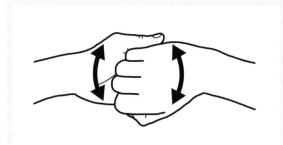

6. Backs of fingers to opposing palms with fingers interlocked

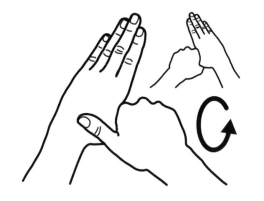

7. Rotational rubbing of left thumb clasped in right palm and vice versa

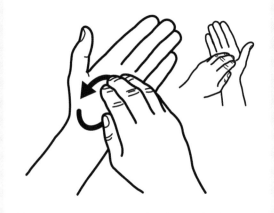

8. Rotational rubbing, backwards and forwards with clasped fingers of right hand in left palm and vice versa

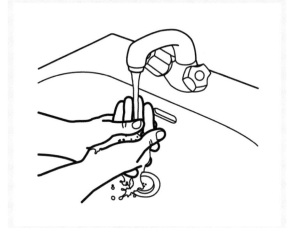

9. Rinse hands with water

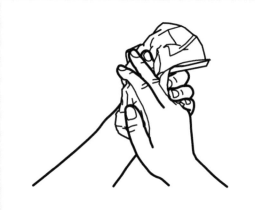

10. Dry hands thoroughly with a single use towel

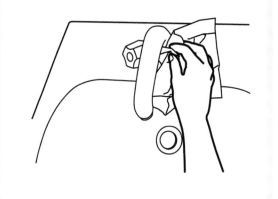

11. Use towel to turn off taps

Procedure continued →

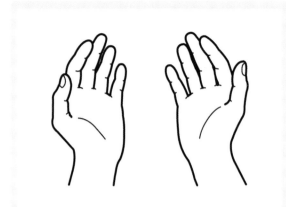

12. Your hands are now safe

3.8 Personal protective equipment

Personal protective equipment (PPE) is used to prevent the spread of infection to you, your colleagues, patients and other members of the public. Your choice of PPE (including not wearing any) should be based on an assessment of the risk of transmission of infection [DoH, 2010c].

Typical items of PPE to prevent infection include:

* Gloves
* Aprons
* Face masks
* Eye protection
* Sleeve protectors
* Protective suits (these are generally only for specially trained personnel, such as hazardous area response team (HART) members, and are not covered in this text).

3.8.1 Gloves

Gloves should only be worn (Figure 3.2):

* If there is a risk of contact with blood and/or bodily fluids
* When sharp and/or contaminated items are handled
* If there is likely to be contact with non-intact skin or mucous membranes during contact with a patient.

Gloves should not be worn longer than required and never when driving from scene. Don't forget that hand hygiene is required before and after wearing gloves. Put gloves on immediately prior

to patient contact and change them between each patient task, when caring for different patients and as soon as they are contaminated. Once you have removed your gloves, treat them as clinical waste and discard appropriately [DoH, 2010c].

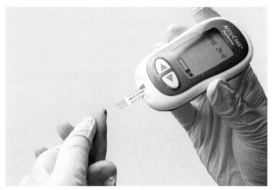

Figure 3.2 Non-latex disposable gloves should be worn when there is a risk of contact with blood, such as when checking a patient's blood sugar

3.8.2 Aprons

Aprons should be worn in the following situations:

* Your uniform is likely to be contaminated with blood and/or other bodily fluids
* Carrying out cleaning that may lead to contamination of your uniform
* Transporting infectious patients.

Aprons should be disposed of as clinical waste following a single use. Unfasten or break the ties and then pull the apron away from your neck and shoulders. Only touch the inside of the apron. Once away from your body, turn it inside out and then fold it into a bundle before discarding appropriately [DoH, 2010c].

3.8.3 Face masks

There are two types of face mask in common use by ambulance services (Figure 3.3):

* Surgical face mask
* Filtering face piece (FFP3) mask.

Surgical face masks are ineffective against airborne infection, but provide protection against splashes of blood and bodily fluids onto the face and into the mouth and nose. In addition, they are also useful for patients who are prone to bouts of coughing and sneezing.

FFP3 masks, when fitted correctly, provide protection against airborne infections such as severe acute respiratory syndrome (SARS) [NHS England, 2013].

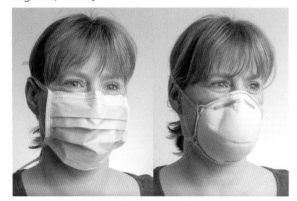

Figure 3.3 Surgical face mask (left) and FFP3 mask (right)

3.8.4 Eye protection

Eye protection, such as goggles, should be worn if a procedure being undertaken is likely to lead to splashing of bodily fluids, including blood, into the eyes, e.g. when assisting the paramedic with intubation. Ideally, the eye protection used should be single-patient use, but if this is not the case, wash the eye protection in hot soapy water, dry and store for subsequent use [NEAS, 2010].

3.8.5 Sleeve protectors

Most ambulance services have a 'bare below elbows' policy, making contamination of long-sleeved uniform less likely. However, cross-contamination can occur if you are manual handling multiple patients while wearing long-sleeved clothing such as your hi-visibility jacket or fleece. Sleeve protectors can help protect your uniform from wrist to elbow.

They are for single-patient use, can be worn over the top of gloves and should be disposed of as clinical waste [DoH, 2010c].

3.8.6 Wearing and removing PPE

The amount of PPE required will vary depending on the patient and not all items are always required. In the event that an apron, mask and eye protection are required, adopt the following procedures for putting on and removing PPE [DoH, 2009]:

Procedure

Take the following steps when putting on PPE:

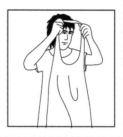

1. Put on apron as shown and fasten at back of waist

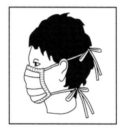 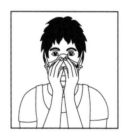

2. Apply face mask:
- Secure ties or elastic bands at middle of head and neck
- Fit flexible band to nose bridge
- Fit snug to face and below chin
- Fit check if using a respirator [NHS England, 2013]

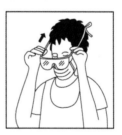 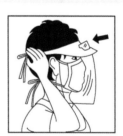

3. Put on eye protection. Place over face and eyes and adjust to fit

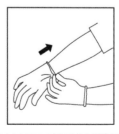

4. Put on disposable gloves. Extend to cover wrists

Procedure

Take the following steps to remove PPE:

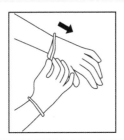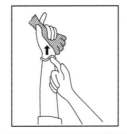

1. Remove gloves:

- Grasp the outside of the glove with the opposite gloved hand; peel off
- Hold the removed glove in the gloved hand
- Slide the fingers of the ungloved hand under the remaining glove at the wrist
- Peel the second glove off over the first glove and discard appropriately

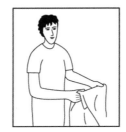

2. Remove apron:

- Unfasten ties
- Pull the apron away from the neck and shoulders, touching the inside of the apron only
- Turn the apron inside out, fold or roll into a bundle and discard

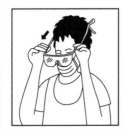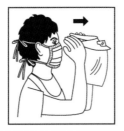

3. Remove eye protection. Handle by headband or earpieces and discard appropriately

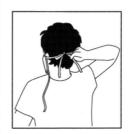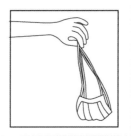

4. Remove face mask. Untie or break bottom ties, followed by top ties or elastic. Remove by handling ties only and discard appropriately.

3.9 **Managing healthcare waste**

Healthcare waste must be segregated immediately by the person generating the waste into appropriate colour-coded storage or waste disposal bags or containers and labelled, stored, transported and disposed of appropriately [NICE, 2012].

Table 3.1 provides examples of typical waste arising from ambulance service activity. Ambulance services should have the following items available for staff use [DoH, 2013a]:

- Yellow-lidded sharps receptacles
- Orange waste receptacles for infectious waste
- Black or clear waste receptacles for domestic waste
- Yellow/black waste receptacles for offensive waste (Figure 3.4).

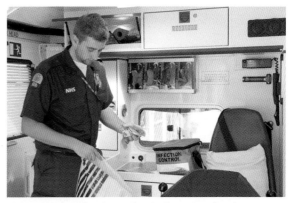

Figure 3.4 Offensive/unhygienic waste that is not infectious can be disposed of in a yellow and black striped ('tiger') bag

Table 3.1: Types of waste arising from ambulance service activity

Activity	Waste type	Receptacle/bag	Justification	Disposal route
Injections	Contaminated sharps or syringes with medicine residue	Yellow-lidded sharps receptacle	Potentially contaminated with medicinal products	Incineration
Treating patients	Medicines and medicated intravenous bags	Yellow-lidded receptacle, clearly labelled NOTE: Liquids may be placed only in containers which are leak-proof and designed for liquids	Medicinal products require segregation	Incineration
Items/equipment for treating patients	Contaminated packing, gloves, aprons, other PPE, dressings, airways, suction liners, laryngoscope blades	Infectious waste in orange waste receptacles	Due to lack of patient records/ screening, unlikely to be able to classify as non-infectious	Alternative treatment or incineration
Items/equipment for treating patients	Uncontaminated aprons, other PPE, non-medicated intravenous bags, non-infectious urine, faeces, vomit and their containers	Offensive/ unhygienic waste disposed of in yellow and black striped ('tiger') bags (Figure 3.4)	Risk assessment to determine no possible contamination and non-infectious	Non-hazardous municipal incineration/energy from waste or landfill NOTE: Liquids (including body fluids) are banned from landfill
Waste packaging as a result of treating patients	Contaminated packaging: plastic and cardboard	Infectious after use, disposed of in orange bag	Due to lack of patient records/ screening, unlikely to be able to classify as non-infectious	Alternative treatment or incineration
Refuse/rubbish	Uncontaminated packaging and refuse/rubbish	Non-infectious, black or clear bag	Used packaging, while patient treatment is being carried out in the vehicle, will usually not be infectious/ clinical waste	Non-hazardous municipal incineration/energy from waste, materials recycling facilities or landfill

4 Fire safety

4.1 Learning objectives

By the end of this lesson, you will be able to:

- Describe practices that prevent fires from:
  - Starting
  - Spreading
- Explain emergency procedures to be followed in the event of a fire in the work setting.

4.2 Introduction

Fire is a chemical reaction that requires three elements:

- Heat
- Oxygen
- Fuel.

Together, they make up the fire triangle (or triangle of combustion, Figure 4.1). For combustion or burning to occur, oxygen must combine with a fuel. Fuels can be in solid, liquid or gas form to start with, but for flaming combustion to occur, a solid or liquid fuel must be converted into a vapour, which then reacts with oxygen. An oxygen concentration of about 16% is required for combustion to occur and air contains 21%, which is plenty [HMFSIPS, 1998].

4.3 Fire prevention

Prevention is better than cure and there are a number of things you can do to prevent fires from starting [HMG, 2006]:

- Do not smoke in the workplace. The NHS has prohibited smoking in all areas other than those dedicated as smoking zones. Take care with cigarettes and matches, always discard in a suitable place and ensure they are fully extinguished
- Do not allow the build-up of rubbish or other combustible materials in your work area, corridors or stair enclosures as this is fuel and may create an obstruction to escape routes
- Do not have fabric, paper or other readily combustible material near electric fires or portable gas heaters
- Do not leave hotplates or containers, e.g. frying pans, unattended when in use
- Flammable gases and liquids should be stored in the designated location, e.g. the medical gases store

- Defective electrical wiring or equipment must be turned off immediately, marked as defective and reported to the Estates Department. If possible, also remove from general access
- Switch off all electrical and gas appliances when they are not in use
- Check your working area before you leave for the day
- Ensure that manual fire-fighting equipment is accessible, undamaged and maintained.

4.4 What to do in case of fire

If you discover a fire [DoH, 2013]:

- Stay safe: Never compromise your own safety
- Raise the alarm: Press your thumb against the glass of the nearest and safest fire call point (fire break glass). Alternatively, repeatedly shout 'FIRE' to warn others
- Phone 999 (or 9 999 from some phones) and request the fire service: Activation of a building fire alarm does not mean the fire and rescue service is automatically alerted, you should make the emergency call every time
- Get out and close the door: Go to the designated fire assembly point immediately.

If you hear the fire alarm you should [DoH, 2013]:

- Leave your place of work: Close windows and doors behind you if this can be done quickly
- Calmly exit: Make your way to the nearest and

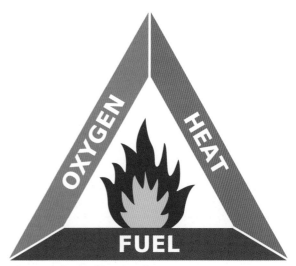

Figure 4.1 The fire triangle
"Fire triangle". Licensed under CC BY-SA 3.0 via Wikimedia Commons.

safest fire exit. Do not run or stop to collect personal belongings

- Encourage others to exit: Attempt to offer assistance to anyone who appears to be confused or having difficulties, especially people with disabilities. If your usual exit route is blocked by smoke or flames, stop, change direction and find an alternative escape route. You should still meet at the normal assembly point for your workplace

- Do not use lifts: Their movement assists fire travel and they may stop suddenly if there is a power failure. They may also take you to the scene of the fire. Use the stairs at all times

- Move to your designated assembly point: Make yourself known to the fire marshal or person who is coordinating the evacuation. Note that fire marshals are typically only appointed in larger premises (i.e. not ambulance stations) and are identified by a yellow tabard

- Form an orderly group: Remain together until a head count is established and until further instructions are given.

Vehicle fires

If a fire breaks out in a vehicle, take the following actions [SCAS, 2013]:

1. Stop
2. Switch off the ignition and press the battery isolator button (if the vehicle has one)
3. Release the bonnet, DO NOT open
4. Get everyone out of the vehicle
5. Remove medical gas cylinders if possible
6. Move any patients, crew and yourself to a place of safety in case the burning vehicle explodes. This may be as much as 200 metres away
7. Warn oncoming traffic
8. Summon help by dialling 999 and requesting the fire and rescue service. Inform the emergency operations centre
9. If and only if you believe it is safe to do so, attempt to put out the fire with the dry powder extinguisher provided. If the fire is in the engine compartment, do not open the bonnet: use the extinguisher through the grill or under the edge of the bonnet. Use with caution, and if in doubt do not attempt to tackle the fire.

5 Stress

5.1 Learning objectives

By the end of this lesson, you will be able to:

- Describe common signs and indicators of stress
- Compare strategies for managing stress.

5.2 Introduction

Stress is the adverse reaction people have to excessive pressures or other types of demand placed on them. There is a clear distinction between pressure, which can create a 'buzz' and be a motivating factor, and stress, which can occur when this pressure becomes excessive [HSE, 2007]

Six broad areas have been highlighted as being the primary sources of stress at work [HSE, 2007]:

- Demands: This includes issues such as workload, work patterns and the work environment

- Control: How much say the person has in the way they do their work

- Support: This includes the encouragement, sponsorship and resources provided by the organisation, line management and colleagues

- Relationships: This includes promoting positive working to avoid conflict and dealing with unacceptable behaviour

- Role: Whether people understand their role within the organisation and whether the organisation ensures they do not have conflicting roles

- Change: How organisational change (large or small) is managed and communicated in the organisation.

5.3 Signs of stress

Stress can cause changes in those experiencing it, making it important for everyone to look out for changes in a person's or a group's behaviour, particularly in NHS ambulance services, where half of employees experience work-related stress [PIE, 2014]. However, in many cases, only you will notice the changes that occur as a result of the stress you experience [HSE, 2008].

Stress can show itself in many different ways and people will exhibit different signs and symptoms.

Some of the well-known signs and symptoms of stress include [HSE, 2014]:

- Changes to behaviour such as:
  - Difficulty sleeping
  - Altered eating habits
  - Smoking and/or drinking more
  - Avoiding friends and family
  - Sexual problems
- Physical symptoms:
  - Tiredness
  - Indigestion and nausea
  - Headaches
  - Aching muscles
  - Palpitations
- Mental:
  - Increased indecision
  - Difficulty in concentrating
  - Poor memory
  - Feeling inadequate
  - Low self-esteem
- Emotional:
  - Mood swings, becoming irritable or angry
  - Increased anxiety
  - Feeling numb
  - Hypersensitivity
  - Feeling drained and listless.

5.4 **Managing stress**

Although stress is not an illness, it can cause serious illness if not identified and managed. The success of coping strategies to help reduce the effects of stress will vary from person to person. Consider some of the strategies that have been recommended [NHS Choices, 2014]:

- If you're not sure about the trigger for your stress, keep a diary of stressful episodes for 2–4 weeks
- Take action to help relieve stress:
  - Exercise: Physical activity can help remove some of the emotional intensity of stress
  - Eat and drink healthily: Eat a balanced diet and avoid excessive amounts of caffeine and alcohol
  - Take control: This can be easier said than done in the ambulance service, but identify problems and think about possible solutions. Having a suggestion adopted by an organisation to help in your daily work, particularly when it is benefiting patients, is very satisfying [Pilbery, 2013]
  - Talk to someone: Sharing work troubles can help ease the stress as well as provide an opportunity for others to understand how you are feeling and help you see things a different way
  - Avoid unhealthy habits: Don't rely on alcohol, smoking and caffeine as a method of coping. The temporary relief they provide can lead to long-term health problems
  - Accept the things you can't change: There are inevitably going to be aspects of the job that you cannot change. Accept those and focus on areas where you can have an impact and take control.

Chapter 6: **Manual Handling**

1 **Musculoskeletal anatomy and physiology**

1.1 **Learning objectives**

By the end of this lesson you will be able to:

- Identify and describe the anatomy and physiology of the musculoskeletal system and its relation to safe moving and handling.

1.2 **Introduction**

Although often considered together, the skeleton is usually considered to be a system, whereas skeletal muscle (as opposed to smooth muscle found in blood vessels, for example) is a tissue and not a system. However, both are closely related as can be seen by their respective functions.

The skeletal system serves six basic functions [Tortora, 2008]:

- Support: It is the structural framework for the body, supporting soft tissues and providing points of attachment for tendons and the majority of the skeletal muscles
- Protection: Many of the most important internal organs are protected by the skeleton, for example the brain, heart, lungs and spinal cord
- Movement: Since the majority of skeletal muscles attach to bones, when they contract, bones are made to move
- Mineral storage: Bones store a number of minerals, mostly calcium and phosphorus, which can be released as required
- Blood cell production: Some bones contain red bone marrow, which produces red and white blood cells, and platelets
- Energy storage: Bone containing yellow bone marrow, which is mostly made up of fat, provides an energy reserve.

Skeletal muscle performs a range of functions, either through sustained contraction, or by alternating contraction and relaxation [Marieb, 2013]:

- Body movement: This is not just a function of

muscles on their own, but an integrated process of bones, muscles and joints
- Stability of body position: Skeletal muscle contractions stabilise joints and maintain body posture, such as sitting upright, or keeping the head upright
- Storage and movement of internal substances: Ringlike bands of muscles, known as sphincters, help keep contents of hollow organs contained within. This includes keeping urine in the bladder and food in the stomach
- Generating heat: Contracting muscular tissue generates heat, known as thermogenesis. Involuntary skeletal muscle contraction to generate heat is better known as shivering.

1.3 **Anatomical terms**

In order to be able to accurately describe the location of an organ or a wound, or the movement that resulted in an injury, it is necessary to be able to use terms that describe position and direction. These always relate to the standard anatomical position (Figure 1.1). When referring to left and right, it is always the patient's right and left, not yours.

Terms of position and direction

Common terms used to describe position and direction include [Kapit, 2001; Tortora, 2008]:

1. Superior: Also referred to as cranial or rostral. Towards the head or upper part of a structure or the body; above. For example, the head is superior to the abdomen
2. Inferior: Away from the head or towards the lower part of a structure or the body; below. For example, the abdomen is inferior to the head
3. Anterior: Towards or at the front of the body. For example, the sternum is anterior to the spine
4. Posterior: Sometimes also called dorsal. Towards or at the back of the body; behind. For example, the heart is posterior to the sternum
5. Medial: Towards or at the midline of the body. For example, the heart is medial to the lungs

6. Lateral: Away from the midline of the body. For example, the arms are lateral to the chest

7. Proximal: Closer to the point of attachment of a limb to the body torso. For example, the elbow is proximal to the hand

8. Distal: Further from the point of attachment of a limb. For example, the knee is distal to the hip

9. Superficial: Towards or at the body surface. For example, the skin is superficial to the skeletal muscles

10. Deep: Away from the body surface. For example, the lungs are deep to the skin

Terms of motion

Common terms used to refer to motion of the body and/or limbs include [Kapit, 2001]:

- Extension: Normally, straightening of a joint. Extreme (abnormal) extension is called hyperextension. At the ankle and wrist, extension is called dorsiflexion

- Flexion: Bending a joint, or reducing the angle between the bones of a joint. Flexion of the ankle joint is called plantar flexion

- Abduction: Movement of a joint that results in a bone moving away from the midline

- Adduction: Movement of a joint that results in a bone moving towards the midline

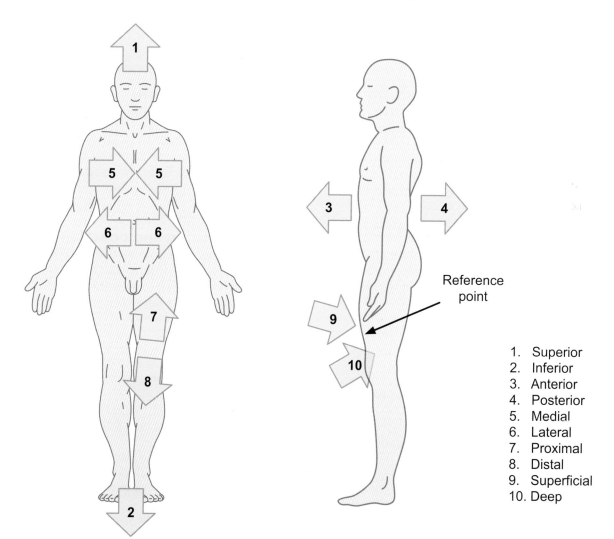

Reference point

1. Superior
2. Inferior
3. Anterior
4. Posterior
5. Medial
6. Lateral
7. Proximal
8. Distal
9. Superficial
10. Deep

Figure 1.1 Anatomical terms of position and direction

- Circumduction: A circular motion, which consists of flexion, abduction, extension and adduction undertaken in sequence. This can be achieved with ball and socket, ellipsoid and saddle joints
- Rotation: Movement of a joint that causes the moving bone to turn on its axis. If this is towards the body it is called internal rotation and if away, external rotation
- Supination: External rotation of the radiohumeral joint
- Pronation: Internal rotation of the radiohumeral joint
- Inversion: Turning the sole of the foot inward so that the medial border of the foot is elevated
- Eversion: Turning the sole of the foot outward so that the lateral border of the foot is elevated.

1.4 Joints

Since bones do not bend without getting damaged, connective tissues form joints that keep the bones together, while allowing some degree of movement (usually). There are three basic types [Tortora, 2008; Kapit, 2001]:

- Fibrous: These joints have limited or no movement, such as the sutures that hold the bones of the skull together
- Cartilaginous: As with fibrous joints, these permit little or no movement. An example of this type of joint is the intervertebral disc
- Synovial: These are freely moveable joints which contain a cavity between the articulating bones. The ends of the bones within the joint are covered in a smooth, slippery articular cartilage, which reduces friction and helps to absorb shocks.

Synovial joints

There are different types of synovial joint; Table 1.1 describes four of these and gives examples of where they can be found in the body [Kapit, 2001].

1.5 The skeletal system

There are 206 bones in the adult human skeleton and they are generally split into two groups: the axial and appendicular skeleton (Figure 1.2). The axial skeleton consists of 80 bones, including the skull, vertebrae, hyoid, sternum and ribs. The appendicular skeleton consists of the remaining 126 bones, including the pectoral (shoulder) and pelvic girdles and bones of the arms, wrists, hands, thighs, legs and feet [Kapit, 2001].

Breaks in bones (fractures) are more common in the appendicular skeleton, but tend to be more serious if they occur in the axial skeleton [Tortora, 2008].

1.5.1 Types of bones

Virtually all of the bones in the human body can be classified by their shape (Table 1.2) [Tortora, 2008].

1.5.2 Skull

The skull is made up of 22 bones, with 8 forming the cranial cavity, and the remainder, the facial bones, forming the face (Figure 1.3). Regions of the brain, which are located within the cranial bones, are generally named after the cranial bone which is located superficially, for example the front and temporal lobes.

1.5.3 Vertebral column

The vertebral column (spine) is made up of 33 irregular bones known as vertebrae (Figure 1.4) [Kapit, 2001]:

Table 1.1: Types of synovial joint

Joint name	Movement	Example location
Ball and socket	All directions	Hip and shoulder
Hinge	One direction; flexion; extension	Elbow
Pivot	Rotation	1st and 2nd cervical vertebrae
Gliding	Gliding movements over two flat articulating surfaces	Acromioclavicular joint

- 7 cervical
- 12 thoracic
- 5 lumbar
- 5 sacral – although these usually fuse into a single bone, the sacrum
- 4 coccygeal – again, these normally fuse to form the coccyx.

It functions as a strong, flexible rod that allows for a range of movements, while supporting the head, protecting the spinal cord and providing points of attachment for the ribs, pelvis and back muscles.

In between the vertebrae are intervertebral discs, which consist of an outer fibrous ring (annulus fibrosus) and a soft, pulpy core (nucleus pulposus). These form strong joints, allowing for a range of movements while absorbing vertical forces. When compressed, the discs flatten, but in some cases they can bulge or protrude, leading to compression of spinal nerve roots. In this case, they are said to be a prolapsed (or slipped) disc [Tortora, 2008].

1.5.4 **Thoracic cage**

The thoracic cage is the bony part of the thorax, which is usually used to refer to the whole chest.

It encloses the organs and vessels within the thoracic cavity and is made up of the sternum (consisting of the manubrium, body and xiphoid process), costal cartilages, ribs and thoracic vertebrae (Figure 1.5) [Tortora, 2008].

There are 12 pairs of ribs, with the first 7 known as true ribs as they physically connect with the sternum thanks to a strip of costal cartilage. The remaining pairs of ribs are called false ribs as they do not directly connect with the sternum, or (as in the case of the 11th and 12th pairs of ribs) do not connect with the sternum at all [Marieb, 2013].

1.5.5 **Shoulder girdle**

The shoulder (pectoral) girdle consists of two scapulae (shoulder blades) and two clavicles (collarbones, Figure 1.6). The clavicles articulates with the manubrium of the sternum, forming the sternoclavicular joint. The scapula articulates with the clavicle at the acromioclavicular joint, and with the humerus at the glenohumeral (shoulder) joint. The shoulder girdle does not articulate with the vertebral column, but instead is positioned by means of muscle attachments [Tortora, 2008].

Table 1.2: Types of bones

Bone type	Description	Example
Long	As their name suggests, these bones are longer than they are wide. They are made up of a shaft (diaphysis) and a variable number of ends (epiphyses) and are slightly curved to increase their strength	Humerus (upper arm)
Short	These are more cube-like bones of almost equal length and width, and make up many of the bones in the wrist and ankle	Trapezoid (wrist)
Flat	These bones provide protection for underlying organs and a point of attachment for muscles. Examples include the skull and sternum	Sternum
Sesamoid	These develop in tendons that are subject to high levels of friction, tension and stress, such as the palms of the hand and soles of the feet. They do not develop in everyone, with the exception of the patella (knee cap), which virtually everyone possesses	Patella (knee cap)
Irregular	Bones are considered irregular if they have a complex shape that does not fit in any of the other categories. Examples include the vertebrae and hip bones	Vertebra

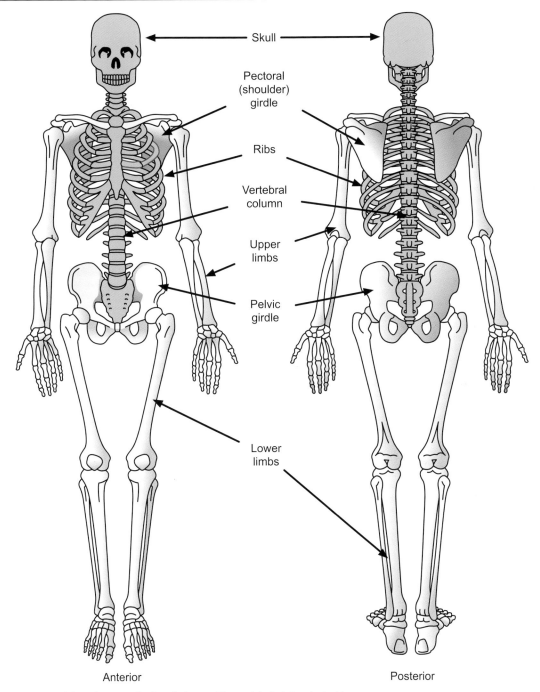

Skull

Pectoral
(shoulder)
girdle

Ribs

Vertebral
column

Upper
limbs

Pelvic
girdle

Lower
limbs

Anterior

Posterior

Figure 1.2 Axial and appendicular skeleton. The axial skeleton is in blue

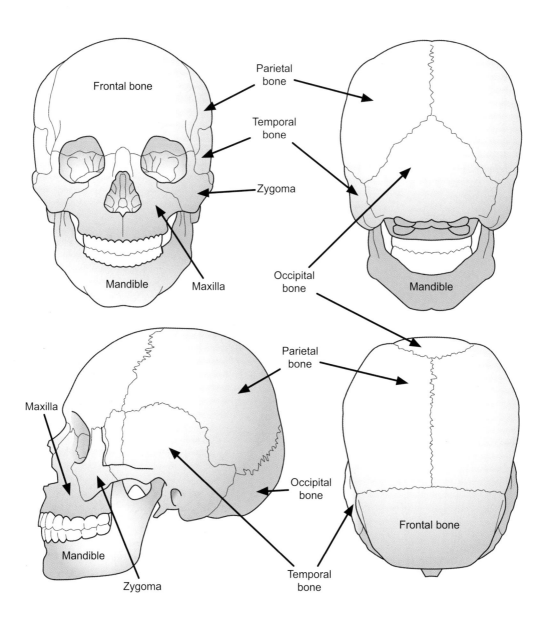

Figure **1.3** Views of the skull. Anterior (top left), posterior (top right), lateral (bottom left) and superior (bottom right)

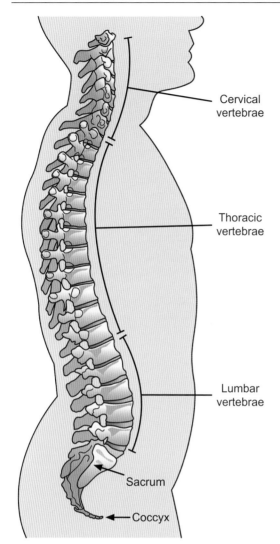

Figure 1.4 The vertebral column

Cervical vertebrae

Thoracic vertebrae

Lumbar vertebrae

Sacrum

Coccyx

1.5.6 Upper limbs

The upper limb consists of 30 bones (Figures 1.7 and 1.8) [Kapit, 2001]:

- 1 in the upper arm (humerus)
- 2 in the lower arm (radius and ulna)
- 8 in the wrist (carpal bones)
- 5 in the palm (metacarpals)
- 14 in the fingers (phalanges).

1.5.7 Pelvic girdle

The pelvic girdle comprises of two hip bones (sometimes called coxal bones), which themselves are composed of three bones, which fuse by the time adulthood is reached (Figure 1.9): ilium,

ischium and pubis. Anteriorly, the hip bones meet at the pubic symphysis joint, and posteriorly, with the sacrum at the sacroiliac joints. Together, these bones form a bowl-like structure known as the bony pelvis [Tortora, 2008].

1.5.8 Lower limbs

Each of the lower limbs consists of 30 bones (Figure 1.10) [Tortora, 2008]:

- 1 femur (thigh)
- 1 patella (kneecap)
- 1 tibia and 1 fibula (lower leg)
- 7 tarsals (ankle)
- 5 metatarsals and 14 phalanges (foot).

1.6 Skeletal muscle

It's not necessary to remember all of the skeletal muscles of the body, but knowing the location and name of some of them, particularly those which you can feel, is helpful. Figures 1.11 and 1.12 highlight a number of these muscles.

Skeletal muscles produce movement by exerting a force on tendons, which pull on bones or other structures. They do this by contracting, and since the two articulating bones do not generally move equally, the point of attachment of the muscle tendon to the bone that initiates the movement is called the origin. The point of attachment to the other bone is called the insertion [Tortora, 2008].

1.6.1 Mechanics of movement

To produce movement, bones act as levers and joints as the fulcrum, the fixed point which the lever (bone) can move around. A lever is affected by two forces: the effort, which causes movement (the muscles), and the load, or resistance, which acts in opposition to the effort [Tortora, 2008].

A lever allows a given effort to move a heavier load, or move it further or faster, than it could without the lever [Marieb, 2013]. If the load is close to the fulcrum and the effort applied is far away, a small effort over the large distance will move a heavier object over a small distance. This lever is said to operate at a mechanical advantage, or is a power lever. Conversely, if the load is far from the fulcrum and the effort applied is near, the effort required must be

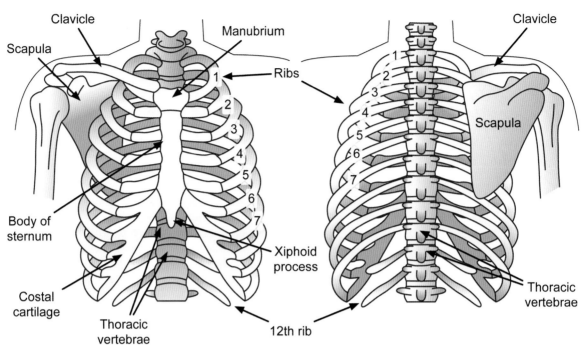

Figure 1.5 The anterior (left) and posterior (right) thorax

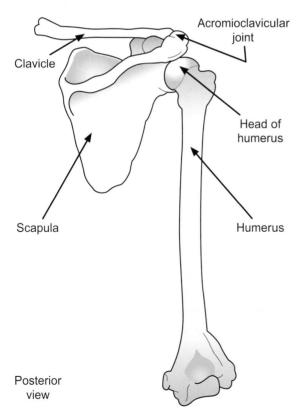

Posterior view

Figure 1.6 The shoulder girdle

greater than the load for movement to occur. This lever is said to operate at a mechanical disadvantage and is called a speed lever. This is because this lever can move a small load rapidly over a large distance [Tortora, 2008]. There are three types of levers, determined by the position of the fulcrum (F), effort (E) and load (L), as shown in Table 1.3.

2 Principles of manual handling

2.1 Learning objectives

By the end of this lesson you will be able to:
- Explain principles for safe moving and handling
- Describe what action should be taken if the individual's wishes conflict with their plan of care in relation to health and safety and their risk assessment.

2.2 Introduction

Manual handling of patients places staff and the patient at risk of injury. Proportionally, injuries to ambulance staff are much more frequent compared with other professions. In 2012/13, there were 659 handling injuries sustained by

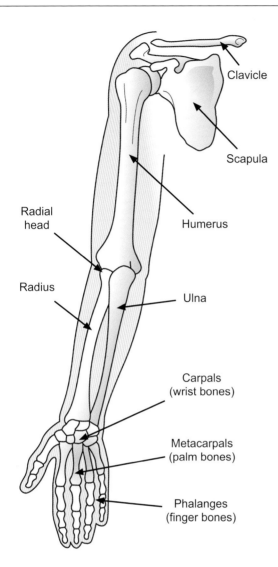

Figure 1.7 The upper limb – anterior view

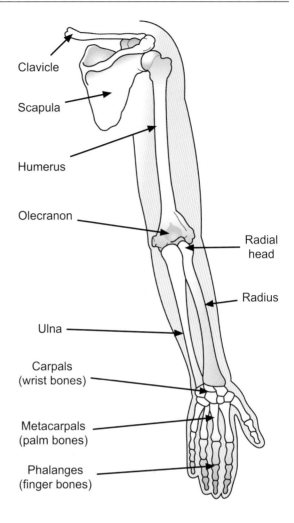

Figure 1.8 The upper limb – posterior view

ambulance staff that were either classed as major (led to a fracture, amputation or dislocation, for example) and/or led to an absence from work of more than 7 days [HSE, 2013]. There are around 17 Reporting of Injuries, Diseases and Dangerous Occurrences Regulations (RIDDOR) reportable handling injuries per 1,000 ambulance staff [HSE, 2013], but this could be as high as 178 per 1,000, with 90% of these injuries occurring in accident and emergency crews as opposed to the patient transport service [Ferreira, 2005].

2.3 **Risk assessment**

In the HEALTH AND SAFETY chapter you learned about RISK ASSESSMENT, and manual handling is a perfect example of a set of actions that need a risk assessment to be undertaken **before** taking action. The difficulty in emergency situations is that the time available to make this risk assessment may be short.

There are 5 steps to take [HSE, 2006]:

1. Identify the hazards
2. Decide who might be harmed and how
3. Evaluate the risk and decide on precautions
4. Record your findings and implement them
5. Review your assessment and update if necessary.

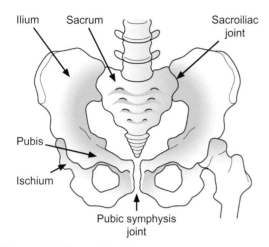

Figure 1.9 The pelvic girdle

This is not very user-friendly or specific to manual handling, and so these steps can be encapsulated in the TILEE acronym [HSE, 2011; Gregory, 2010b]:

- **T**ask: Consider whether the lift involves:
  - Holding the load away from the body
  - Involves long distances
  - Requires strenuous effort or twisting
- **I**ndividual: Consider whether the lift:
  - Requires specialist training
  - Presents a hazard
  - If you and your colleagues are capable of performing the lift
- **L**oad: Is the load:
  - Heavy
  - Difficult to get hold of
  - Unstable
  - Unpredictable
  - Harmful
  - Likely to grab out when alarmed at being carried down the stairs
- **E**nvironment: Determine the presence of:
  - Constraints on posture, e.g. low ceiling, confined spaces
  - Poor, uneven flooring
  - Hot/cold/wet weather
  - Poor lighting
  - Noise

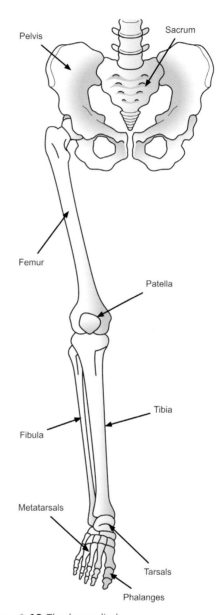

Figure 1.10 The lower limb

- **E**quipment: Consider what equipment:
  - Is available
  - Will reduce risk to you and the patient
  - Is safe to use
  - You are trained and competent in the use of.

2.3.1 **Reducing risk**

Once you have identified a risk relating to manual handling, you will need to determine

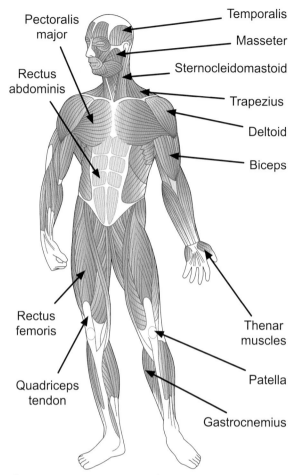

Pectoralis major

Rectus abdominis

Rectus femoris

Quadriceps tendon

Temporalis

Masseter

Sternocleidomastoid

Trapezius

Deltoid

Biceps

Thenar muscles

Patella

Gastrocnemius

Figure 1.11 Anterior view of the superficial muscles

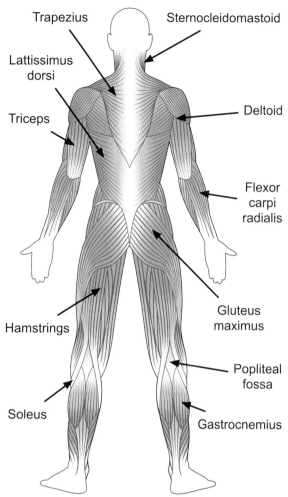

Trapezius

Lattissimus dorsi

Triceps

Hamstrings

Soleus

Sternocleidomastoid

Deltoid

Flexor carpi radialis

Gluteus maximus

Popliteal fossa

Gastrocnemius

Figure 1.12 Posterior view of the superficial muscles

how best to manage this. Strategies for managing risk are best considered in advance, for example during your training or by consulting manuals or guidance provided by your service and the Health and Safety Executive. When you are at the patient's side, however, these approaches are not suitable. You will seldom, if ever, work alone, so ask colleagues for advice and don't be afraid to ask for additional help if your risk assessment suggests this would be beneficial.

You should not use equipment you are not familiar with, but some equipment does come with a manual or simple diagrams printed on its surface, which you can use to remind yourself about the correct way round it should be used, or the sequence of actions required, for example. Don't forget that other manual handling equipment may be available in your location,

such as hoists, which can help reduce the risk to you and the patient. However, this will usually rely on a trained member of staff being available to help you.

Patients who refuse manual handling aids

It is unlikely during the course of your work that you will encounter patients who refuse to be transferred or lifted using manual handling aids. However, some policies are unlawful in relation to a patient's human rights, such as blanket no-lifting policies, no lifting unless life or limb are at risk, and no lifting if equipment could physically effect the transfer [A & Ors v East Sussex CC].

This does not mean, however, that patients have a right to be manually handled without aids, just that consideration needs to be given to

Table 1.3: Classes of lever

Class of lever	Mechanism	Examples
First	Effort and load opposite each other with the fulcrum in the middle	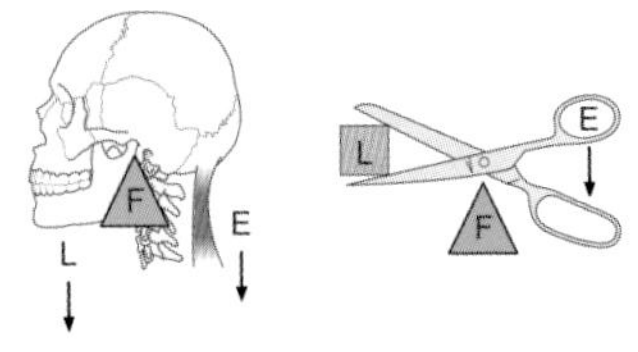
Second	Effort applied at one end, with fulcrum at the other end and load in the middle. Uncommon in the human body	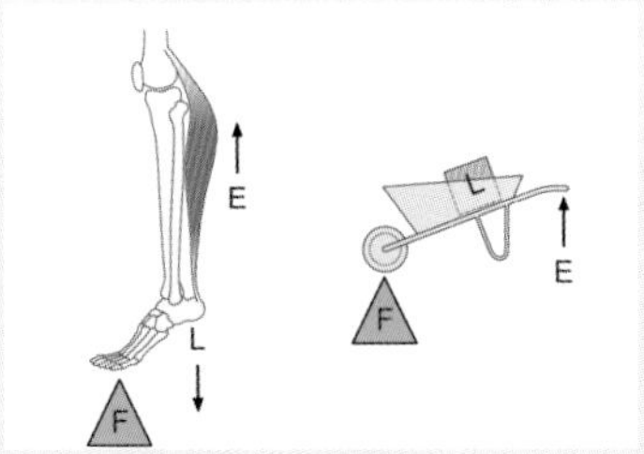
Third	Effort between load and fulcrum. Allows for rapid and extensive movements, such as throwing	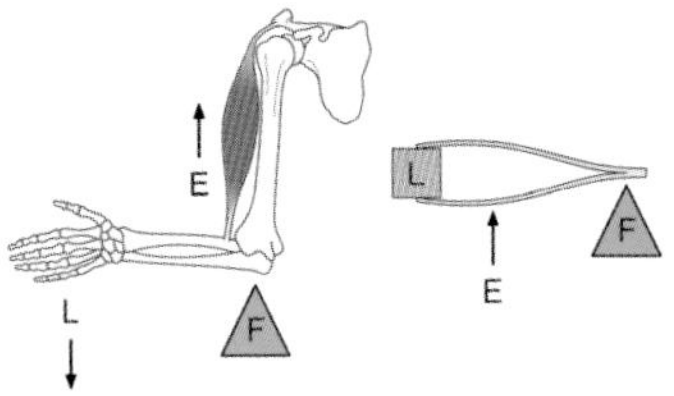

alternatives on a case by case basis. For example, a patient who refuses to be hoisted up off the floor does not have a right to be lifted by the ambulance crew, but an alternative, such as a lifting cushion, could be utilised instead [HSE, 2004]. In the event that a compromise cannot be reached, contact your line manager while on scene to assist with decision-making.

2.4 Biomechanics

Biomechanics is the application of the physical laws of mechanics to the human body. In order to reduce the risk of injury and facilitate manual handling, it is important to be aware of the following mechanical principles [Smith, 2011b]:

- Force
- Gravity and equilibrium
- Friction
- Stress and strain
- Pressure
- Levers
- Moment of force or turning force
- Stability and equilibrium.

2.5 General principles

You are going to learn about specific MOVING AND HANDLING EQUIPMENT AND TECHNIQUES in the next lesson, but it is helpful to know the basic principles to adopt when approaching a manual handling task [HSE, 2003].

Procedure

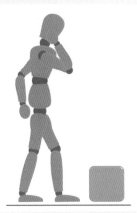

1. Think before lifting/handling. Plan the lift. Can handling aids be used? Where is the load going to be placed? Will help be needed with the load? Remove obstructions such as discarded wrapping materials. For a long lift, consider resting the load midway on a table or bench to change grip.

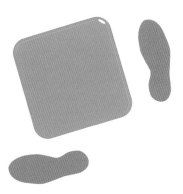

2. Adopt a stable position. The feet should be apart with one leg slightly forward to maintain balance (alongside the load, if it is on the ground). The worker should be prepared to move their feet during the lift to maintain their stability. Avoid tight clothing or unsuitable footwear, which may make this difficult.

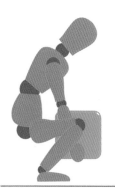

3. Start in a good posture. At the start of the lift, slight bending of the back, hips and knees is preferable to fully flexing the back (stooping) or fully flexing the hips and knees (squatting).

Don't flex the back any further while lifting. This can happen if the legs begin to straighten before starting to raise the load.

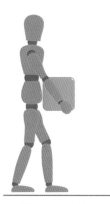

4. Keep the load close to the waist. Keep the load close to the body for as long as possible while lifting. Keep the heaviest side of the load next to the body. If a close approach to the load is not possible, try to slide it towards the body before attempting to lift it.

Procedure continued →

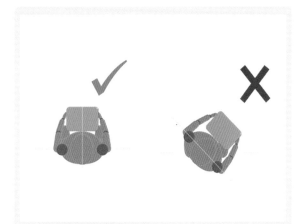

5. Avoid twisting the back or leaning sideways, especially while the back is bent. Shoulders should be kept level and facing in the same direction as the hips. Turning by moving the feet is better than twisting and lifting at the same time.

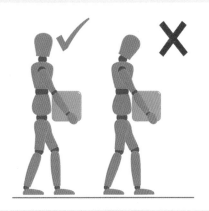

6. Keep the head up when handling. Look ahead, not down at the load, once it is held securely.

Move smoothly. The load should not be jerked or snatched as this can make it harder to keep control and can increase the risk of injury.

Don't lift or handle more than can be easily managed. There is a difference between what people can lift and what they can safely lift. If in doubt, seek advice or get help.

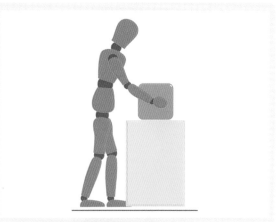

7. Put down, then adjust. If precise positioning of the load is necessary, put it down first, then slide it into the desired position.

There is no such thing as a completely 'safe' lift, but try to keep the weights for lifting and lowering in the zones shown in Figure 2.1. If you are twisting, reduce weights by 10% if you are required to twist beyond 45° and by 20% if you must twist beyond 90° [HSE, 2012].

2.6 **Lifting aids**

As you found out in the HEALTH AND SAFETY POLICIES AND LEGISLATION lesson, The Manual Handling Operations Regulations 1992 (as amended), The Lifting Operations and Lifting Equipment Regulations 1998 and The Provision and Use of Work Equipment Regulations 1998 all require that your employer provides aids to assist in manual handling.

In the ambulance service, this may include:

• Patient handling slings
• Handling belts
• Slide sheets
• Transfer (banana) boards
• Turntables
• Lifting cushions
• A carry chair
• Powered ambulance stretcher
• Tail-lift on the back of the ambulance.

Although not typically available on your ambulance, hoists are regularly used in hospitals and nursing homes and you may be able to utilise these if a suitably qualified member of staff is available.

Women

Men

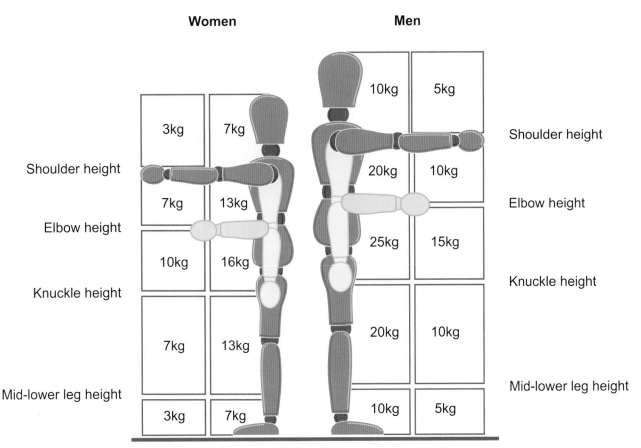

Figure 2.1 Guideline weights for lifting and lowering
All illustrations are public sector information published by the Health and Safety Executive and licensed under the Open Government Licence

3 Moving and handling equipment and techniques

3.1 Learning objectives

By the end of this lesson you will be able to:

- Describe the aids and equipment that may be used for moving and positioning
- Describe the impact of specific conditions on the correct movement and positioning of an individual.

3.2 Introduction

This lesson provides guidance on different techniques that can be utilised for moving and handling patients. The choice of technique will depend on the urgency of the move, the number of staff and equipment availability as well as the wishes and capabilities of the patient.

3.3 Patients on the floor

The usual advice from a call handler in RESPONSE TO A 999 CALL (chapter 2) is to advise the caller not to move the patient. However, once an assessment has been completed by a crew on scene, the patient may no longer be required to stay immobile and certainly shouldn't remain on the floor.

If they need to remain flat, then an orthopaedic stretcher is helpful, if there is room. In confined spaces, a slide sheet can help to manoeuvre them to another location with more space, but a carry sheet should be used if you are intending to lift the patient.

If your patient cannot get themselves up off the floor, but is able to sit up, either with or without your support, a lifting cushion such as the Mangar ELK is ideal. However, you may find that your patient can get themselves off the floor, with guidance and assistance from you.

3.3.1 Instructing a patient to get off the floor – one-chair method

In order to undertake this procedure, the patient needs to be able to roll onto their side and be able to kneel, so it may not be suitable for patients with knee and hip problems.

Procedure

Take the following steps to instruct a patient to get off the floor using a single chair [Smith, 2011b]:

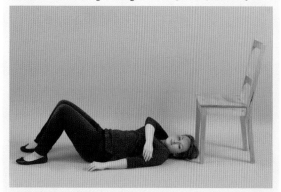

1. Position a chair at the head end of the fallen patient. Instruct them to bend their knees up and to bring one arm across their chest

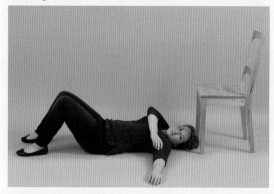

2. Instruct the patient to move their other arm away from the body

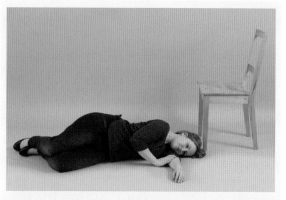

3. Instruct the patient to roll onto their side, and to bring their arm over their body so that it is flat on the floor

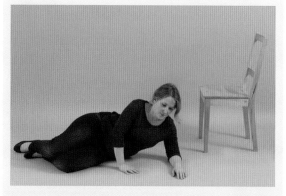

4. Instruct the patient to push up on their hand and at the same time push up on their forearm that is resting on the floor, until they are half-sitting

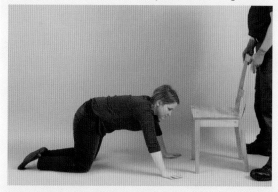

5. Continue to verbally support the patient as they continue to push upwards, until they end up on all fours facing the chair

Procedure continued →

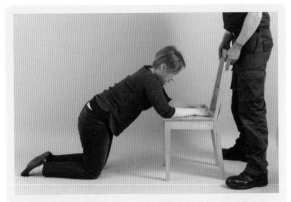

6. While holding the chair steady, instruct the patient to lower their arms onto the chair and ask them to lean onto the seat of the chair

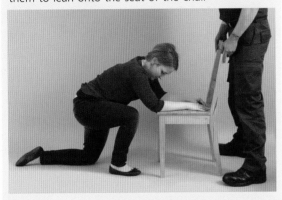

7. Instruct the patient to raise their stronger leg and place the foot of that leg on the floor

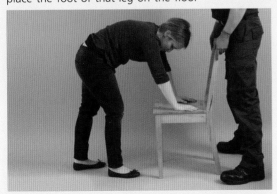

8. Instruct the patient to push up and straighten their legs

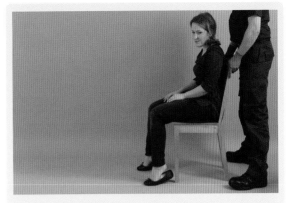

9. Instruct the patient to sit on the chair

3.3.2 Instructing a patient to get off the floor – two-chair method

This procedure is preferred when the patient cannot kneel and requires no physical intervention by the ambulance crew member.

Procedure

Take the following steps to instruct a patient to get off the floor using two chairs [Smith, 2011b]:

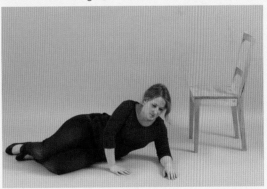

1. Position a chair at the head end of the fallen patient. Instruct them to bend their knees up and roll into side lying. They should then bring one arm over the chest until their hand is flat on the floor. Instruct them to push up with one hand and lower arm into a side sitting position as in the one-chair method

Procedure continued →

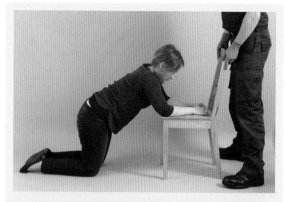

2. Instruct the patient to face the chair and place their forearms on the chair

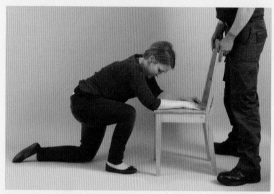

3. Instruct the patient to bend one knee and place the foot of that leg onto the floor, while at the same time pushing up on their forearms and hands

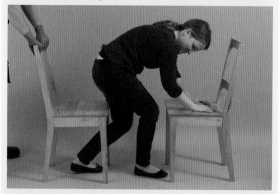

4. Place a second chair behind the patient, ensuring it is under their hips

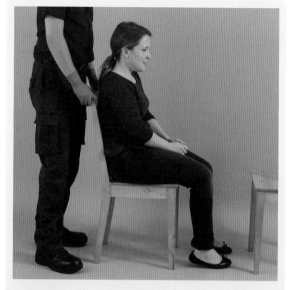

5. Instruct the patient to sit backwards onto the chair

3.3.3 Lifting cushion

If a patient cannot get themselves off the floor using the one- or two-chair method, a lifting cushion (Figure 3.1) may be helpful. The patient does need to be able to partly assist with a transfer, for example, by shuffling/rolling onto the cushion. They also need to have sitting balance if using a cushion with no back [Smith, 2011b].

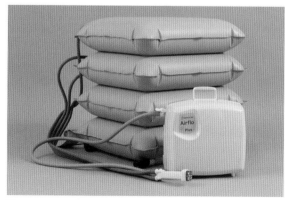

Figure 3.1 The Mangar ELK lifting cushion

Mangar ELK Procedure

Take the following steps to assist a patient from the floor using the Mangar ELK [Mangar International, 2012; Smith, 2011b]:

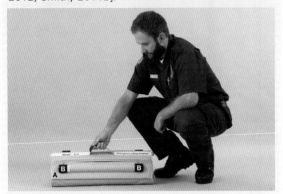

1. Unroll the ELK by unclipping the flap (A) from the ends of the stability bar (B)

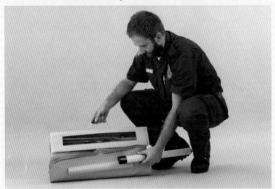

2. Remove the end cap and then the stability bar from its pocket (B) in order to provide a more comfortable transfer for the patient

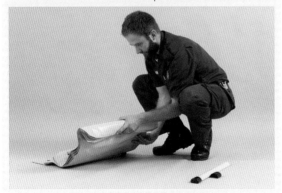

3. Fold the edge of the ELK underneath itself, by folding along the line of the stability bar pocket

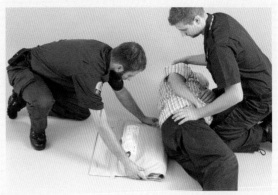

4. One crew member should roll the patient onto their side. A second crew member should position the ELK so that its 'upper' edge is approximately level with and tight up against the patient's waistband. If the patient cannot sit up on their own, consider inserting a handling sling level with their shoulder blades, so you can assist them to sit up. **Note**: Place a blanket, groundsheet, towel or similar under the ELK if using it on a rough surface

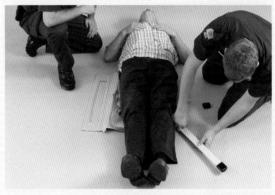

5. Roll the patient over onto the ELK until they are lying fully and squarely on the cushion. Unfurl the edge of the ELK, replace the stability bar and fit the end cap

Procedure continued →

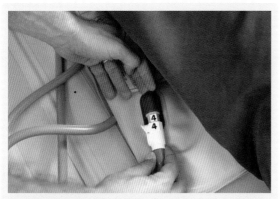

6. Connect the four distribution hoses from the 4-Way Hand Control to the four connectors on the ELK. The ends of the hoses are colour coded and numbered to match the corresponding ELK connectors (No. 4 is the top compartment; No.1 the bottom). **Note:** If the fallen person is very large, it is recommended to connect the compressor and the hand control before the person is rolled onto the ELK

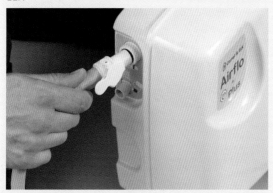

7. Position the Airflo compressor at the side of the ELK ensuring that it will not be in the way while lifting and supporting the patient.Connect the hose from the 4-Way Hand Control to the air outlet socket on the Airflo compressor and select the AUTO function on the Airflo compressor by pressing the power button until the LED light comes on

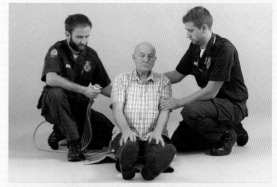

8. Kneeling beside the patient, place them in a seated position on the ELK. If necessary, place a transfer belt (with looped handles) around the patient's chest and adjust to fit. You may find a slide sheet useful. Explain to the patient what to expect when the ELK elevates

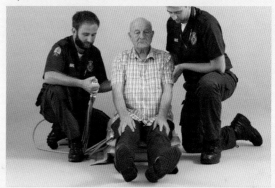

9. Press the number 1 button on the 4-Way Hand Control. Steady the patient as the ELK lifts. Stop inflation when the first (bottom) compartment becomes hard. The compressor will automatically stop as each compartment becomes fully inflated

Procedure continued →

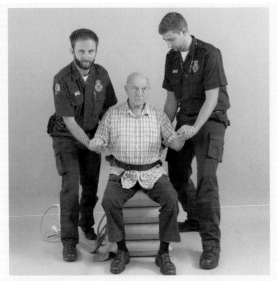

10. Continue to operate buttons 2, 3 and 4, in sequence, in exactly the same manner. Support the patient at all times. Always inflate the ELK sections from the bottom up. When all four compartments are inflated, the patient may be helped to stand or to transfer

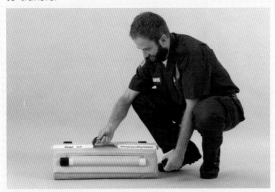

11. To deflate, disconnect each of the air hoses from the ELK. After use, roll the ELK up with the 4-Way Hand Control and re-secure the flap around the ends of the stability bar

The following video from the manufacturer demonstrates safe use of the Mangar ELK:

ELK Emergency Services

3.3.4 Fall in confined space

If the patient has fallen in a confined space, such as a bathroom or small bedroom, manual handling is more hazardous. The most practical way to manage these situations is to move the patient to an alternative location while they are still on the floor.

Procedure

Take the following steps to move a patient in a confined space [NEAS, 2014; Smith, 2011b]:

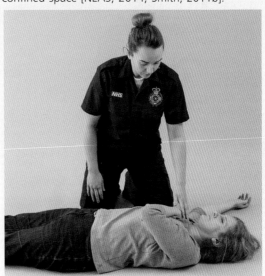

1. Assist the patient to position the arm further away from you across their chest and bring the nearer arm away from the patient's body so that it does not get trapped during rolling

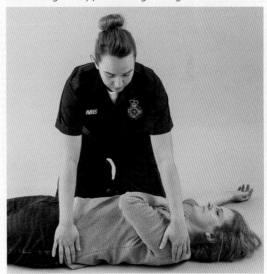

2. Start in a high-kneeling position and support the patient's hip and shoulder

Procedure continued →

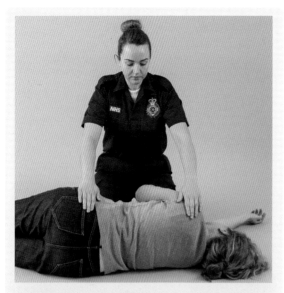

3. Roll the patient onto their side, sitting back into a low-kneeling position as you do so

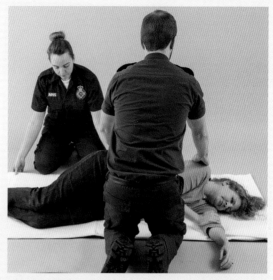

5. Lower the patient and roll them again onto their other side and smooth out the sliding sheets

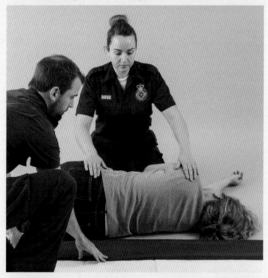

4. Now that the patient is on their side, a second crew member should roll two full-length slide sheets, or a slide sheet and carry sheet, with the carry sheet next to the patient, or a tubular slide sheet, and place them lengthways and half under the patient

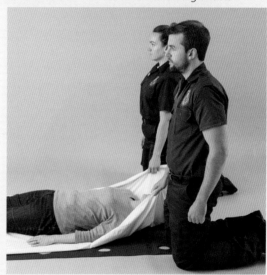

6. Lay the patient supine and position yourself and another crew member, if required, in a high-kneeling position at one end of the patient, whichever is closer to the nearest open space

Procedure continued →

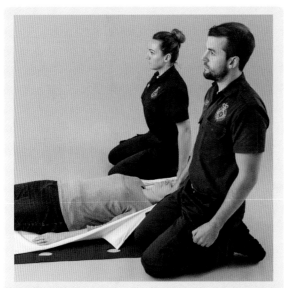

7. Decide which crew member is to issue instructions for the move. Hold the top slide sheet, or the carry sheet, or the top layer of a tubular sheet and transfer your weight so that you end in a low-kneeling position. Repeat until an open space is reached

3.4 Seated patients

Many patients will be seated, on the toilet, a chair or their bed, when you need to either assist them to stand or transfer them onto a carry chair or ambulance trolley. As before, you should see what the patient is capable of as they may be able to stand with no or minimal assistance.

3.4.1 Sitting to sitting transfer

A transfer board (also called a banana board, on account of the curved shape and yellow colour of some boards!) can enable the patient to transfer from a chair or bed onto the carry chair or vice versa. In order to use this technique, the patient must be able to [Smith, 2011b]:

- Flex forward and transfer their weight laterally
- Place their feet on the floor
- Use their body strength to assist and understand what is required of them
- Place their arm towards the end of the board and assist with movement across it.

A crew member can assist by bringing the patient's feet around (although a turntable can assist with this) and helping to transfer the patient's weight laterally. However, if the patient requires help with their feet and support to sit, then a second crew member should be used, preferably with a handling belt applied.

Procedure

Take the following steps to assist a patient to use a transfer board [Smith, 2011b; EEAST, 2014]:

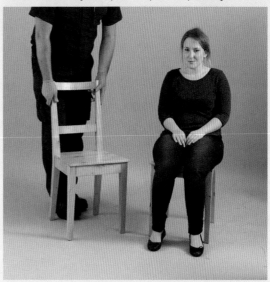

1. Explain the procedure to the patient and ensure they have suitable footwear. Place the destination chair at the correct angle (this will vary depending on the board used)

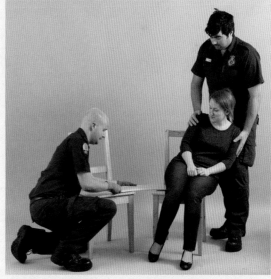

2. Ask the patient to lean away from the transfer side and insert about a third of the board under the patient's buttock. Ensure that a third of the board rests on the destination chair. Ensure the board is level

Procedure continued →

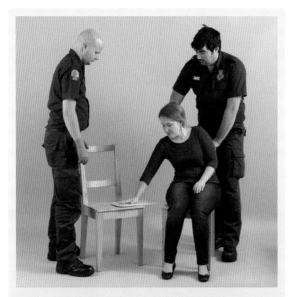

3. Instruct the patient to place their hand towards the far end of the board and lean towards it. Ensure the patient's fingers are not under the board

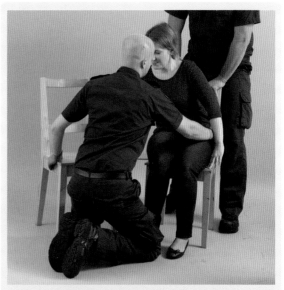

5. Once the patient has transferred onto the destination chair, they should be instructed to lean away from the board to allow its removal. Remove the turntable if used

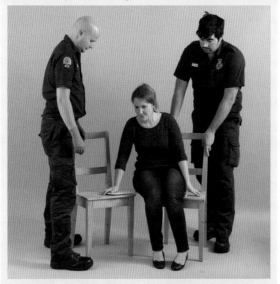

4. The patient should now shuffle across the board, using their other hand and feet to push. If they have reduced ability to push through their legs, use a turntable

3.4.2 **Sitting to standing transfer**

Standing up out of a chair can be a challenge for some patients, even though they may be able to walk once they are upright.

Procedure

Take the following steps to assist a patient to transfer from a sitting position to standing [Smith, 2011b; EEAST, 2014]:

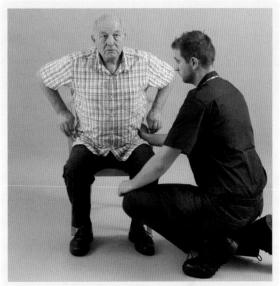

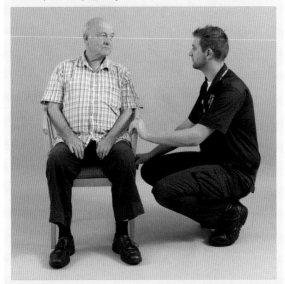

1. Explain the procedure to the patient and ensure they have suitable footwear. Instruct the patient to lean forward so that their back is off the back of the chair. Then instruct them to shuffle their bottom towards the front of the chair/edge of the bed and ensure that both of their feet are firmly on the floor

2. Instruct the patient to place their hands on the arms of the chair, or the mattress if on a bed, or crew member's hands. Instruct the patient to lean forward so that their chin is over their knees and encourage them to look up and not at the floor. Instruct them that you will give the command "Ready, steady, stand" and on "Stand", the patient should push up on the arms of the chair/mattress. The patient should keep their strongest leg close to their body, with the other foot slightly in front

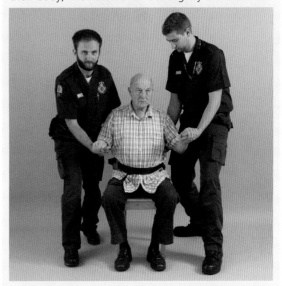

3. Alternatively, if there are no arms on the chair or the patient requires additional assistance, place a handling belt around the patient. Position yourself and another crew member either side of the patient, with your inside hand taking hold of the handling belt and your outer hand in a palm-to-palm hold (Figure 3.2). Instruct the patient as in step 2

Procedure continued →

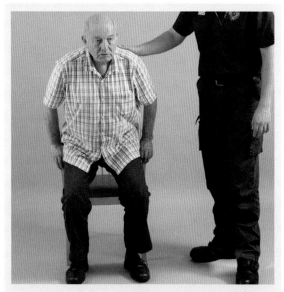

4. Give the command "Ready, steady, stand". If you are assisting the patient, a gentle rocking motion can help, and then on "stand", move forward and then upwards with the patient as they stand

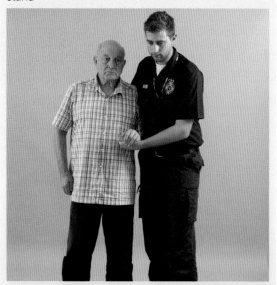

5a. If the patient normally walks with a frame, provide this to them. It may help the patient's confidence if you walk slightly behind and to one side, with your hands just above the patient's hips

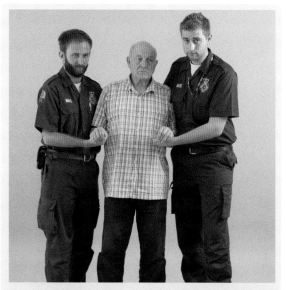

5b. Alternatively, two crew members can walk with the patient, taking care not to impede the patient's natural step and allowing them to move their feet in their own time

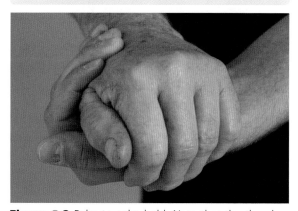

Figure 3.2 Palm-to-palm hold. Note that the thumbs are unlinked

3.5 Patients in bed

You will frequently encounter patients in bed or on a hospital trolley who require transferring from either bed to ambulance trolley or bed to chair.

3.5.1 Patient transfer board

A patient transfer board is often available in hospitals and nursing homes to enable the transfer from bed to ambulance trolley and vice versa. An alternative is to use a hoist, if available and patient condition allows.

Procedure

Take the following steps to transfer a patient from bed to trolley using a patient transfer board [NEAS, 2014]:

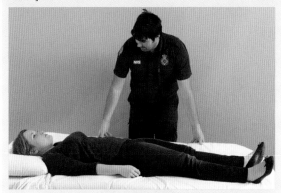

1. Explain the procedure to the patient and gain consent where possible. Place the ambulance trolley next to the bed

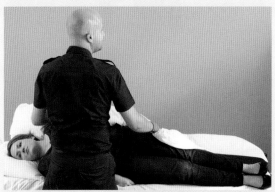

2. Using the sheet on the bed/trolley, one crew member should grip the sheet at the level of the patient's shoulders and roll the patient towards themselves

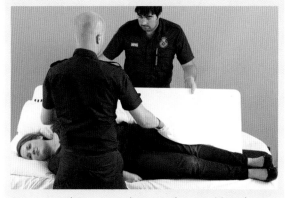

3. A second crew member can then position the board between the patient and the trolley

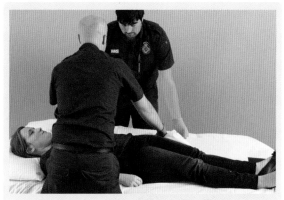

4. The first crew member lowers the patient onto their back while the second maintains the position of the board. The patient's feet should be on the lower end of the sheet

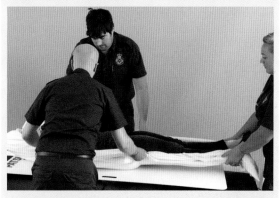

5. With both crew members gripping the sheet at the patient's shoulder and hip, slide the patient across the board and onto the trolley. Additional crew members are helpful to ensure that the patient's legs and feet transfer smoothly

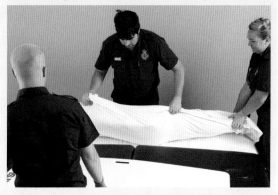

6. After ensuring the patient is centrally positioned, roll them to one side and remove the board

Procedure continued →

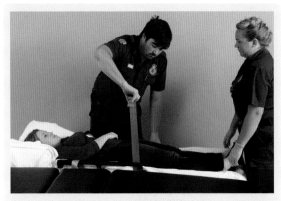

7. Roll the patient onto their back and secure them to the trolley. Don't forget to clean the board

3.6 Carry chair

The carry chair is an important manual handling aid, used by ambulance services as the primary method for transporting patients up and down stairs and into the ambulance. However, it is associated with a high risk of low back injury when used to lift patients [Ferreira, 2005]. In addition, the carry chair is not a wheelchair, so plan movements to keep the distance to be travelled to a minimum.

The procedure below relates to the Ferno Compact 2 carrying chair, commonly found on ambulances. However, there are many models, including those with tracks to assist with descending stairs, so ensure you are appropriately trained, particularly in the lifting techniques required for these chairs, as they are not covered here.

Ferno Compact 2 procedure

Take the following steps to prepare and transport a patient on the Ferno Compact 2 carry chair [EEAST, 2014]:

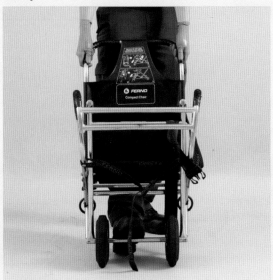

1. Unroll the carry chair by placing it on the ground. With your foot on the chair's foot bar, lift the back up and rearward

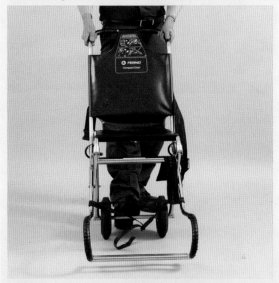

2. Completely unfold by firmly pushing up the back until an audible click is heard

Procedure continued →

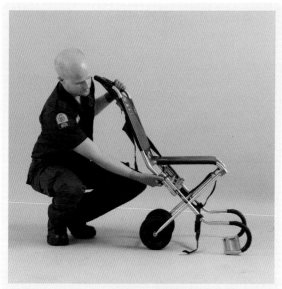

3. Once the chair is locked, move both of the safety rings down over the hinge bracket

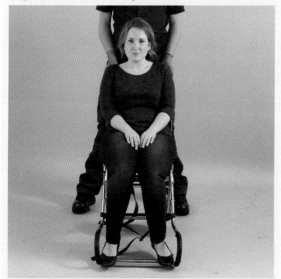

4. When a patient is on the carry chair, ensure that one crew member has a firm grip on the back of the chair at ALL times

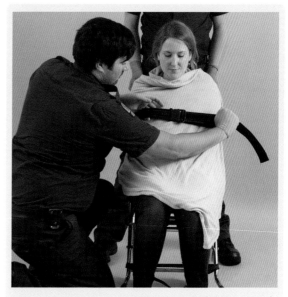

5. Secure the patient onto the chair by using the chest restraint. A leg restraint is also provided, which can be used if deemed necessary. Blankets can be used with the chair and are helpful for improving patient comfort, but ensure that they are clear of moving parts

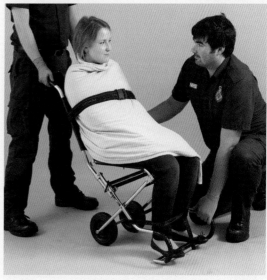

6. Once the patient is secured on the chair, crew members need to position themselves at the back and front of the chair. Instruct the patient not to grab out with their arms during the manoeuvre

Procedure continued →

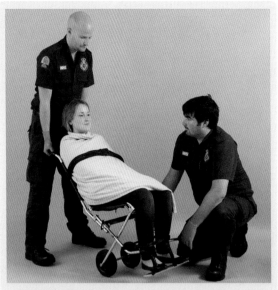

7. Explain to the patient that you are about to tip them backwards, but reassure them that they will not fall. The crew member at the back of the chair then tilts the chair backwards, until the weight of the chair and patient are balanced on the wheels. The chair can be rolled without lifting, but uneven terrain is likely to require the assistance of one or more additional crew members to ensure the chair does not tip over

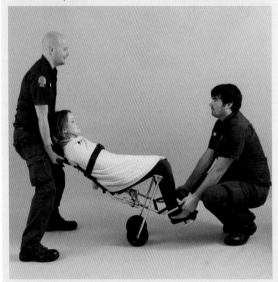

8. To carry the chair, it should be tilted backwards as before, and then crew members should grasp the front and back carrying handles and lift simultaneously

3.7 Ambulance trolley

There are a wide range of ambulance trolleys available, so ensure you are familiar with the one on your ambulance. Basic pre-shift checks common to most trolleys include [EEAST, 2014]:

- Check that the mattress and restraining system is properly installed. Damaged mattresses present an infection control risk and should be replaced
- Check that the ambulance trolley sides raise, lower and lock in position
- Check that the ambulance trolley can raise and lower satisfactorily
- Check that the wheels and brakes of the trolley are effective
- Ensure that the trolley locks properly into the ambulance locking device
- If the trolley has push/pull handles, check their operation and stow them away
- If the trolley has a headrest, check that it locks in position when attached to the trolley.

Trolley positioning

Ambulance trolleys can be placed in a range of positions to improve patient comfort and clinical condition. The positions may need to be adopted and changed quickly as the patient's condition changes, so ensure you are familiar with how to place the trolley into and out of these positions.

Trolley positions

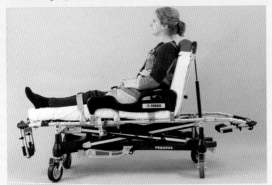

Upright position. This is preferred for patients with breathing problems

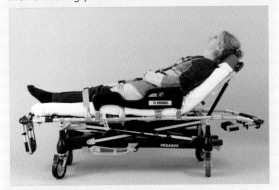

Semi-recumbent position. This consists of placing the patient's head and torso at an angle of 45°

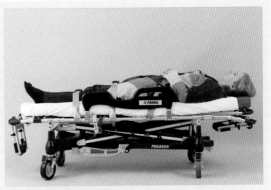

Recumbent position. This is the preferred position for patients with suspected spinal injuries and/or shock

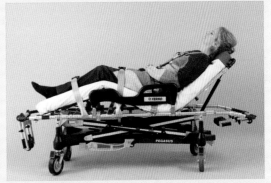

Fowler position. This position can help relieve tension on abdominal muscles, which may make abdominal illness and injuries less painful

Procedure continued →

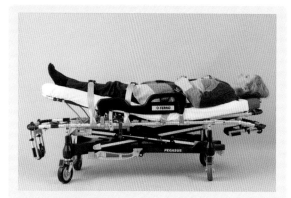

Lower limbs raised. This is helpful for controlling bleeding in lower leg injuries, and will increase cardiac output for several minutes in hypovolaemia [Geerts, 2012]

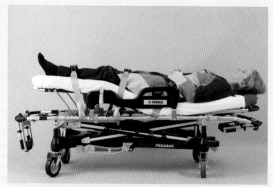

Trendelenburg. This position is frequently taught but has been found to have a temporary effect on blood pressure and no effect on cardiac output. In addition, this position may aggravate an already impaired ventilatory function due to the weight of the abdominal contents resting on the diaphragm. It may also increase intracranial pressure in patients with a traumatic brain injury [NAEMT, 2014; Peña, 2012; Johnson, 2004]

Chapter 7: **Scene Assessment**

1 **Scene assessment and safety**

1.1 **Learning objectives**
By the end of this lesson you will be able to:
- Outline and explain the parts of an initial scene assessment
- Explain the importance of ensuring scene safety prior to approaching any incident for:
  - Patients
  - Yourself
  - Your colleagues
  - Bystanders.

1.2 **Introduction**
Despite the name, scene assessment begins before you physically arrive at the patient's location. You will be passed details of the incident, although initially this may only include the address, with further details provided as you respond. The address may be recognised as belonging to a frequent and/or violent caller, having access issues and/or a location prone to high-speed road traffic collisions, for example [Bledsoe, 2014].

To help you cover the essential aspects of a scene assessment, consider using the SCENE mnemonic [AACE, 2013]:
- **S**: Safety
- **C**: Cause including the nature of illness (NOI) or mechanism of injury (MOI)
- **E**: Environment
- **N**: Number of patients
- **E**: Extra resources needed.

1.3 **Safety**
Maximising the safety of everyone on scene requires RISK ASSESSMENT (chapter 2). The ambulance service has many formal, written risk assessments, but these cannot legislate for all eventualities. In order to reduce the risk to you, your colleagues, patients and bystanders, it is necessary to undertake a more fluid and mental (i.e. in your head as opposed to a written down) risk assessment. This is known as a dynamic risk assessment (DRA) and relates to the fact that the environment or situation is dynamic, rather than the risk itself. DRA underpins subsequent decision making and is focused on thinking **before** you act, and not the other way around [Ashbury, 2014].

One simple tool to help you structure DRA is the US Navy's Time Critical Risk Management (TCRM) ABCD tool [US Navy, 2009]:
- A: Assess the situation
- B: Balance resources and options
- C: Communicate intentions
- D: Do and debrief.

Assess the situation
Situation awareness is a fancy term for knowing what is going on around you. It consists of gathering relevant information, interpreting it and anticipating what might happen in the future [Ashbury, 2014]. This is important, because scene safety is not just something you should assess on arrival and then fail to re-evaluate. Instead, you should be constantly reviewing the environment/situation to identify signs that the risk to your safety and that of those around you is increasing.

Balance resources and options
In an ideal situation, you would have unlimited staff, equipment and expertise available on scene. However, that is unlikely to happen, so it is important that you review your options based on what you have available now and/or what can be made available and the timeframe involved. For example, an obese patient stuck in the bath may prove difficult to extricate with just two members of the ambulance crew. In this situation, you would be likely to contact the emergency operations centre (EOC) and request another crew to assist, and consider use of a lifting cushion. A wait of 30 minutes (or more) might be acceptable if the patient was kept warm. However, if the house were to catch fire then this clearly would be too long and alternative options would have to be considered.

Communicate intentions

Once you have made a plan, it is important to communicate that to the patient and your colleagues as well as others, for example the EOC, other emergency services etc. It also presents an opportunity for other team members to identify potential problems with your plan. Although you may not be the primary decision-maker, you may well spot something that someone else has missed, particularly if they are under a lot of pressure, for example because the patient is very sick and requiring ongoing treatment.

Do and debrief

In time-critical situations, you will have to get on and 'do the job' to the best of your abilities and with the minimum amount of risk given the circumstances. However, once the incident is over, it is important to review how things went, whether the actions taken did reduce the risk, how well the team communicated and what aspects you would change next time. This should involve everyone and be documented, should you subsequently be required to justify the actions you took.

Given the nature of emergency work, it is unlikely that risk can be completely eliminated, but by taking a few moments to think before taking action, you can minimise the chance of harm coming to your patient, your colleagues and/or anyone else on scene.

1.4 Cause

Although you are likely to have been passed some details about the incident or call you are attending, you should not be completely led by this. Establishing the presenting complaint from the patient's perspective will come later on in the assessment process, but you may be able to determine what has happened from the scene, particularly in trauma cases, such as when viewing the wreckage of two cars that have collided. However, it is important to keep an open mind even at this stage. For example, although you are attending a road traffic collision, your patient may have suffered from a medical problem, such as a cardiac arrest, which led to their losing control of the car. Conversely, a medical-sounding call, such as a patient with low blood sugar, may also have a traumatic

component if, for example, they fell and injured themselves as a result [Pilbery, 2013].

In trauma cases, find out about the mechanism of injury (MOI), which you will cover in the TRAUMA chapter. Knowledge of the MOI can assist in determining what injuries may have been sustained. Equally, for medical patients, establishing the nature of illness (NOI) can assist with the diagnosis, particularly in cases where bystander and/or patient information is limited (for example if the patient was discovered unresponsive). Clues from the scene, for example medical equipment such as home oxygen or hoists, medication and/or care notes may provide clues as to the underlying problem [Bledsoe, 2014].

1.5 Environment

Consider whether there are any environmental factors that need to be taken into account. These may complicate your extrication by affecting access to and from the scene and/or increase the risk of harm to the patient due to the development of hypothermia, for example. Incidents involving water can be hazardous for patient and crew alike. In these cases you remember to 'call, reach, throw, wade and row' (covered in the DROWNING lesson). The terrain may be an issue, particularly if the patient is located well away from roads that are suitable for an ambulance. In these cases, helicopters and/or mountain rescue teams can prove useful.

Other risky environments include confined spaces, where there may be risk of low levels of oxygen and/or the presence of toxic/explosive substances or, in the case of buildings or other structures, further collapse. These require specialist equipment and rescue knowledge that is typically provided by hazardous area response teams (HART) or the fire and rescue service [Bledsoe, 2014].

1.6 Number of patients

Determine the number of patients early on in your assessment to help you decide whether you can manage the scene on your own. It may also help to identify patients who have either wandered off from scene or who have been ejected from a vehicle, for example, and are currently hidden from view.

In addition, since most acts of terrorism are covert (i.e. there is often no prior knowledge of the time, location or nature of the attack), it is possible that you could be responded first to the aftermath of a terrorist attack. In these cases, the number of patients involved may provide the most important indication that a chemical, biological, radiological or nuclear (CBRN) event has occurred [Pilbery, 2013]. In these cases, you should use the STEP 1-2-3 Plus method [JESIP, 2013]:

- Step 1: One casualty and no obvious reason. Approach using normal procedures
- Step 2: Two casualties and no obvious reason. Approach with caution, consider all options. Provide a report on arrival to the emergency operations centre (EOC)
- Step 3: Three or more casualties in close proximity and no obvious reason. Use caution and follow Plus, the Joint Emergency Services Interoperability Programme (JESIP) first responder flowchart.

1.7 Extra resources

Depending on the number of patients, the severity of their injuries and the nature of the incident, you may need additional help and/or equipment from other emergency services. For example, you may require the police to keep a scene safe, or additional ambulances, including the air ambulance, for patient transport, or the fire and rescue service to stabilise a car that has rolled. Don't forget others, such as the coastguard, mountain rescue, utility and public transport companies. Request help early as it may take time for messages to be passed on and the relevant staff to arrive on scene.

2 Major incidents

2.1 Learning objectives

By the end of this lesson you will be able to:
- Define a major incident
- State the ambulance service responsibilities with regard to a major incident
- State who can declare a major incident
- State the role of the attendant (paramedic) of the first crew on scene
- List the responsibilities of the driver of the first crew on scene
- List the responsibilities of subsequent ambulance crews on scene
- Describe the potential roles for ambulance officers on scene
- Identify, and propose solutions to, risks which threaten the coherence of the response being provided to the major incident/situation
- Describe how to contribute to the safety of yourself and others
- State the role of strategic, tactical and operational commanders.

2.2 Introduction

Emergency

According to the Civil Contingencies Act 2004 an emergency is defined as:

- An event or situation which threatens serious damage to human welfare in a place in the UK
- An event or situation which threatens serious damage to the environment of a place in the UK
- War, or terrorism, which threatens serious damage to the security of the UK.

To distinguish this definition of emergency from the regular emergency work of the ambulance service, the term used most often is **major incident**.

Major incident

A major incident is commonly defined in the NHS as any occurrence that presents a serious threat to the health of the community, disruption to the service, or causes (or is likely to cause) such numbers or types of casualties as to require special arrangements to be implemented by hospitals, ambulance trusts or primary care organisations [DoH, 2005].

Details of the exact number of major incidents declared nationally by ambulance services are hard to determine in the absence of a national database. Estimates from work done in the 1990s suggest 4–6 major incidents per year [Carley, 1998], although a more contemporary audit places the average around 15 major incidents per year [NAO, 2002].

2.3 Classification of incidents

Major, mass and catastrophic incidents

NHS organisations are required to develop emergency preparedness arrangements for three levels of incident [DoH, 2007]:

- Major: Involving tens of patients and handled by individual trusts. An example is the Suffolk train crash on August 17th, 2010
- Mass: Involving hundreds of patients and requiring mutual aid response from neighbouring trusts. An example would be the July 7th, 2005 London bombings
- Catastrophic: Involving thousands of patients and severely disrupting health and social care and other support functions. An example would be the Great East Japan Earthquake on 11th March, 2011.

Types of incident

Major incidents are often divided into a number of types [SWAST, 2014; EEAST, 2013]:

- Big bang: A serious transport accident, explosion, or series of smaller incidents
- Rising tide: A developing infectious disease epidemic, or a capacity/staffing crisis
- Cloud on the horizon: A serious threat such as a major chemical or nuclear release developing elsewhere and needing preparatory action
- Headline news: Public or media alarm about a personal threat
- Internal incidents: Fire, breakdown of utilities, major equipment failure, hospital acquired infections, violent crime and internal security issues
- Deliberate: Release of chemical, biological, radiological and nuclear (CBRN) materials
- Mass casualties
- Pre-planned major events that require planning: Demonstrations, sports fixtures, air shows.

2.4 Role of the ambulance service

National Health Service (NHS) Ambulance Trusts have the responsibility for alerting, mobilising and co-ordinating the NHS response to short notice or sudden impact emergencies. This includes [NARU, 2012]:

- Initiating and maintaining a Command and Control System to provide appropriate support and guidance to all NHS responders and other agencies
- Co-ordinating all NHS communications on scene
- Managing the health, safety and welfare of all NHS responders
- Providing casualty triage, treatment and transport, including the selection of appropriate receiving hospitals
- Provision of specialist incident response capabilities, including hazardous area working, decontamination of casualties and active shooter incident.

During a major incident, the response of the ambulance service revolves around seven key principles [Mackway-Jones, 2012]:

- Command and control: Each emergency service on scene has an incident commander, but the police usually take overall command
- Safety: Personal safety is paramount and the appropriate personal protective equipment (PPE) must be worn. This does not always happen when crews are faced with a major incident. Of particular concern are hazardous materials or CBRN incidents
- Communication: This is the most common failing at major incidents [Mackway-Jones, 2012; JCO, 2010a]. The terrestrial trunk radio (TETRA) network should in theory alleviate some of the problems that have occurred in the past, but the use of runners should be considered if required
- Assessment: A rapid initial assessment of the scene can provide an estimate of the number of those injured and the severity of their injuries. This can be refined as the incident unfolds
- Triage: The dynamic process by which casualties are sorted into priorities for treatment. It needs to be repeated frequently
- Treatment: 'Do the most for the most' is the standard mantra. This depends on skills of the providers, severity of injuries and time on scene. The nature of the environment and casualty load may restrict the ability of the providers to give 'gold standard' care

- Transport: Most patients will probably be transported to hospital by ambulance, but alternative methods of transport can be used. The aim is to get the right patient to the right place at the right time.

2.5 Incident command and control

The ambulance service employs a 3-tier command system comprising a strategic commander, tactical commander and an operational commander. This is a hierarchical system whereby individuals are empowered through their role within the structure, providing them with specific authority over others for the duration of the event [NARU, 2012].

Strategic

The strategic commander is in overall charge of each service, responsible for formulating the strategy for the incident. Each strategic commander has overall command of the resources of their own organisation, but delegates tactical decisions to their respective tactical commander(s) [LESLP, 2012].

During major incidents, the strategic commander's responsibilities include [SWAST, 2014]:

- Establish a framework for the overall management of the incident
- Assess and assure the effectiveness of the response
- Determine strategic objectives and priorities
- Rapidly formulate and implement an integrated media and communications plan
- Ensure clear lines of communication with the tactical commander and external agencies
- Instigate further contingency and recovery planning as required
- Ensure the long-term resourcing and expertise for command resilience
- Decide on what resources or expertise can be made available (mutual aid)
- Undertake liaison with strategic commanders in other agencies
- Plan beyond the immediate response phase from recovering from the emergency to returning to or towards a new state of normality.

Tactical

The tactical commander works at the tactical level and is also known as the ambulance incident commander (AIC). Their responsibilities include [NARU, 2012]:

- Obtain sufficient information to determine the current status of the response. This should include ensuring that a detailed and formal handover is received from the acting ambulance incident commander (AIC) and that the whole command chain is aware that such a handover has taken place and appropriate log entries are made
- Formulate a tactical plan which takes account of all available information, including any pre-determined emergency plans, and anticipated risks
- Implement tactics in a timely manner, confirming roles, responsibilities, tasks, and communication channels
- Conduct on-going risk assessment and management in response to the dynamic nature of emergencies
- Review tactics with relevant others including key personnel involved in command, control and co-ordination
- Ensure actions to implement tactics are carried out, taking into account the impact on individuals, communities and the environment
- Determine priorities for allocating available resources
- Anticipate likely future resource needs, taking account of the possible escalation of emergencies
- Work in cooperation and communicate effectively with other responders
- Liaise with relevant organisations to address the longer-term priorities of restoring essential services and helping to facilitate the recovery of affected communities
- Obtain and provide technical and professional advice from suitable sources to inform decision making where required
- Provide accurate and timely information to inform and protect communities, working with the media where relevant
- Monitor and maintain the health, safety and welfare of individuals during the response
- Review actions taken at operational level

- Identify where circumstances warrant a strategic level of management and engage with the strategic level as required
- Ensure that any individuals under their area of authority are fully briefed and debriefed
- Evaluate the effectiveness of tactics and use this information to inform future practice
- Fully record decisions, actions, options and rationale in accordance with current information, policy and legislation
- Ensure engagement with multi-agency responders, providing a joined up and proportionate response
- Request Airwave interoperability where appropriate
- Ensure appropriate control measures are employed to manage all identified risks, reviewing and updating logs and risk assessments as appropriate
- Follow any action cards specific to the tactical commander role as issued by the host ambulance trust.

Operational

The operational commander has responsibility for the activities undertaken at the scene. They are usually located at the incident scene, ideally alongside the operational commanders of the other responding agencies at the forward command post [SWAST, 2014].

Responsibilities of the operational commander include [NARU, 2012]:

- Make an initial assessment of the situation and report this to other responders in accordance with established procedures
- Ensure a METHANE message is communicated to the relevant Emergency Control Centre
- Prepare and implement an initial plan of action
- Ensure actions are carried out, taking into account the impact on individuals, communities and the environment
- Conduct on-going risk assessment and management in response to the dynamic nature of emergencies
- Work in co-operation and communicate effectively with other responders
- Confirm the availability and location of relevant services and facilities

- Identify any resources required and deploy them to meet the demands of the response
- Ensure the establishment of the functional roles required to manage the incident and that appropriately trained individuals undertake each role
- Communicate any resource constraints to the relevant person, or find suitable alternatives
- Monitor and protect the health, safety and welfare of individuals during the response
- Deal with individuals in a manner which is supportive and sensitive to their needs
- Liaise with relevant organisations as required for an effective response
- Identify where circumstances warrant a tactical level of management and engage with the tactical level as required
- Implement the tactical plan where applicable, within a geographical area or functional area of responsibility
- Ensure that any individuals under their area of authority are fully briefed and debriefed
- Fully record decisions, actions, options and rationale in accordance with current information, policy and legislation
- Follow any action cards specific to the operational role as issued by the host ambulance trust.

2.5.1 Roles

A key principle of any command system is limiting how much responsibility a single person has to contend with. In order to achieve this at a major incident, commanders will often delegate responsibilities for tasks to others. There are a number of roles and responsibilities that can be delegated by operational commanders; these are shown in Figure 2.1 and explained in further detail below.

Additional support roles are not always required and/or may be undertaken by a single officer, depending on workload. They include [NARU, 2012]:

- Safety officer: Responsible for the health and safety of all NHS responders entering and working within the cordons of the incident
- Parking officer: Responsible for creating and maintaining a clear and functional parking area. They will ensure vehicles and crews are

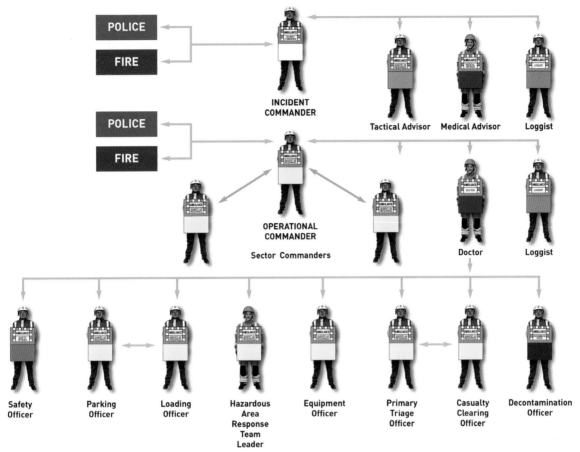

Figure 2.1 An incident command structure showing examples of the additional support roles that may be required. Reproduced by the kind permission of the National Ambulance Resilience Unit (NARU)

logged into the area and direct resources to the casualty clearing station (CCS) when casualties need removing from the incident

- Loading officer: Responsible for keeping a log of the number and destinations of casualties transported from the CCS
- Primary triage officer: Responsible for co-ordinating the triage of all casualties at the incident
- Casualty clearing officer (CCO): Responsible for the management of the CCS. Works closely with the triage, parking and loading officers to ensure an efficient triage and treatment of all casualties and the appropriate use of available transport resources
- Equipment officer: Responsible for ensuring the supply and re-supply of equipment to all responding NHS resources
- Hazardous area response team leader (HART):

Provides direct line management for all HART resources.

2.6 First crew on scene

As Peter Taylor found out on July 7th, 2005, you could be first on scene at a major incident [JCO, 2010b]. Your role as first on scene is laid out in your organisation's major incident plan and you should familiarise yourself with it **before** you are called to a major incident.

The first vehicle on scene needs to park up close to police control, if present, and as close to the incident as possible upwind and uphill. As part of a double manned ambulance (DMA), the driver will assume the role of communications officer until relieved. They will remain with their vehicle, securing the doors to prevent the ambulance from being inadvertently loaded with casualties.

Gathering appropriate resources to cope with a major incident takes time, so it's important to request help early. You **do not** have to wait until an officer arrives on scene to declare a major incident. It is likely that your senior colleague will make the decision, but as the communications officer, you will relay the message.

2.6.1 Attendant's role

The attendant will be the ambulance incident commander until relieved. If there is one on the ambulance, they should put on a green and white chequered tabard and wear appropriate personal protective equipment (PPE). They must NOT get involved in the treatment of any casualties.

Actions they will take include:

- Making a detailed reconnaissance of the incident, using the mnemonic METHANE to collate the information necessary for the driver to report back to the emergency operations centre (EOC)
- Working with other services, establish [LESLP, 2012; Pilbery, 2013]:
  - Access to and egress from the incident
  - An initial rendezvous point
  - An ambulance parking point
  - A casualty clearing station
- Co-ordinating the commencement of primary triage, treatment and removal of casualties
- Briefing the senior officer on arrival and complying with their requests.

2.6.2 Driver's role

Your actions as driver are as follows:

- Stay with the vehicle
- Do not attempt to treat casualties
- Leave the rooftop blue lights illuminated and instruct subsequent crews to turn off their blue lights
- Don your personal protective equipment (PPE)
- Secure the doors of your vehicle to ensure patients are not inadvertently loaded
- Maintain contact with the emergency operations centre (EOC)
- Relay a METHANE report to the EOC once the attendant has provided you with the necessary details.

METHANE

The mnemonic METHANE is designed to provide the initial communication surrounding details of the major incident. It consists of [NARU, 2012]:

- **M**ajor incident declared or standby. The person making the report should be explicit whether this is a major incident declaration or a standby in anticipation of the occurrence of a major incident
- **E**xact location of the incident. Where possible the grid reference or GPS co-ordinates should be included, along with any landmarks or iconic sites
- **T**ype of incident. What is the exact nature of the incident? For example rail, chemical, road or terrorist
- **H**azards. What hazards are known to be present or could potentially manifest themselves?
- **A**ccess and egress. What are the agreed or best routes to and from the scene?
- **N**umber of casualties. How many casualties are there and, if possible to determine, what are the level and severity of injuries?
- **E**mergency services. Which emergency services are present and which are required? Include specialist resource request if known.

2.7 Subsequent crews on scene

Additional crews should report their presence to the communications officer once on scene. In addition, they will be required to do the following [LESLP, 2012]:

- Turn off the ambulance blue lights
- The driver should stay with the vehicle unless advised otherwise
- Both crew members should wear appropriate personal protective equipment (PPE)
- Radio communications should be kept to a minimum and all radio messages passed to the incident communications centre on the designated radio channel
- If required to move casualties, place on the appropriate equipment

• If on scene, the casualty clearing station officer or medical incident commander will nominate the hospital to which the casualties will be taken but it is likely that, in the initial stages, all casualties will be transported to the nearest primary receiving hospital

• Once the patient is handed over, recover any essential equipment or replacement before leaving the hospital

• When clear, contact the emergency operations centre for further instructions.

2.8 Triage

The aim of triage is to do the most for the most and it should be used any time that the number of casualties exceeds the number of skilled rescuers. It is a dynamic process and therefore needs to be repeated many times during the care of each casualty.

Triage sieve and sort

There are two phases to triage. The first, the triage sieve (Figure 2.2), takes place where the casualty is found [NASMeD, 2013]. This is a fast, physiological assessment of the casualty. The second, more in-depth assessment, is called the triage sort and generally takes place at the casualty clearing station. The triage sort usually adopts the Triage Revised Trauma System [Champion, 1989], which utilises respiratory rate, systolic blood pressure and Glasgow Coma Scale (GCS), with scores attached to ranges of values. The total score identifies the patient category.

The triage sieve and sort are not the only primary and secondary tools that have been developed. Although none is evidence-based, this has not stopped their widespread use in civilian and military major incident management [Jenkins, 2008].

Over- and under-triaging

A key aspect of triaging is not under- or over-triaging, i.e. making sure that the right priority is identified for any casualty. An example of over-triage would be a patient who is not breathing, even with airway opened, but has a pulse. This patient should be triaged as dead, but this can be difficult to reconcile with ambulance crews, who ordinarily would attempt to resuscitate this patient [JCO, 2010b; Kilner, 2002].

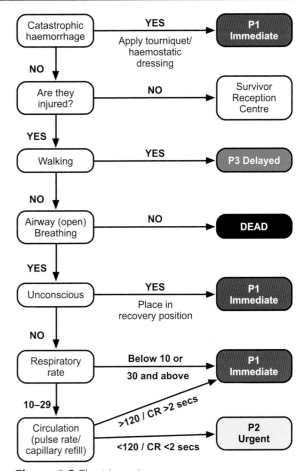

Figure 2.2 The triage sieve.
Copyright National Ambulance Resilience Unit, 2014

Another cause of over-triaging is to use the adult triage sieve on children. This can be avoided by use of a specific children's triage sieve. The most common in the UK is probably the paediatric triage tape (PTT), but there are other systems in use worldwide [Wallis, 2006]. However, if this is not available, children should be triaged using the adult triage sieve, as this will avoid under-triage [SWAST, 2014].

Over-triage is dangerous as it puts pressure on already scarce resources and has been adversely linked to critical mortality (the number of deaths in critically injured survivors) [Frykberg, 1988].

Under-triage can occur when triaging casualties with normal physiological observations (i.e. respiratory rate of 10–29 breaths per minute and heart rate less than 120 beats per minute or capillary refill time less than two seconds) but who are unable to walk. The triage sieve makes no allowance for patients who cannot normally walk, for example casualties who require a wheelchair to mobilise or babies who have not yet learned how to walk.

Under-triage can also occur when the casualty has a normal respiratory rate and is triaged without consideration given to their pulse rate or capillary refill time, which are abnormal. This results in the casualty being triaged as Urgent instead of the correct category, Immediate [Kilner, 2002].

Treating and triaging

Purists would argue that no treatment should be carried out during the triage sieve. In reality, simple interventions such as the insertion of basic airway adjuncts or turning an unconscious patient into the recovery position can be justified. Catastrophic haemorrhage should also be controlled [SCAS, 2010; SWAST, 2014].

Recording your findings

There are various triage tagging systems in use. The simplest are 'slapper bands', which are in use by several ambulance services in the UK. More commonly, you will find triage labels, with space to allow the recording of findings and provide a means to identify the patient (Figure 2.3). It doesn't matter which system your service uses as long as you know where the tags are and how to use them!

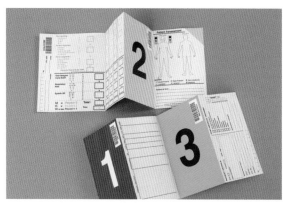

Figure 2.3 A triage label

2.8.1 Vulnerable populations

The Civil Contingencies Act 2004 identified vulnerable persons as a priority in emergencies. Therefore major incident plans need to take account of specific groups such as children, non-English speakers and people with learning difficulties and mental illness [DoH, 2005].

Children

The injured casualties in a major incident may be children only, a mixture of adults and children, or adults only with children who need caring for. As far as is practically possible, families should be kept together, but this may not be possible depending on resources and the severity of injuries.

The Children Act 2004 Section 11 requires ambulance services to safeguard the well-being of children. When children are unaccompanied but uninjured, the local authority is responsible for the child. Since social workers may not be immediately available, children may need to be cared for by the ambulance service or police. Children should not be entrusted to adults with no connection with the child, however well-meaning.

Check with your service to find out exactly what procedures are in place for children at a major incident.

3 Hazardous materials

3.1 Learning objectives

By the end of this lesson you will be able to:

- Describe the systems for labelling hazardous substances
- Describe how to find out information about a hazardous substance
- Describe the risks when attending a hazardous substance incident
- Describe actions which need to be undertaken when attending a hazardous substance or CBRN incident.

3.2 Introduction

There's a good chance if you have a look in the cupboard under your kitchen sink or shed/garage that you will find a hazardous/dangerous substance. Since the key component of scene assessment is safety for yourself, your colleagues, patients and bystanders, it is important that you appreciate how readily available hazardous substances are. Patients who are contaminated with a hazardous substance can easily contaminate others. On a grander scale are incidents involving transport vehicles, most commonly on the road, but also by rail, sea and air. You are unlikely to become heavily involved with these types of incidents as you will not have the training or equipment to be able to safely do so. These are incidents for the fire and rescue service and hazardous area response team (HART) to deal with. However, if you can identify the hazardous substance early, this can assist commanders in determining what resources are required.

Information about the hazardous material can be obtained from a number of sources [HSE, 2014d]:

- The packaging and associated warning labels
- Emergency telephone advice from services such as Chemsafe or TOXBASE (typically accessed through the emergency operations centre)
- The driver and the documentation being carried in the case of vehicular incidents.

3.3 Labelling hazardous substances

In June 2015, the Classification, Labelling and Packaging (CLP) Regulations came into force, which define what information must be provided on the label of a hazardous substance or mixture (Figure 3.1). This includes [ECA, 2011]:

- Name, address and telephone number of the supplier(s)
- The nominal quantity of the substance or mixture in the package where this is being made available to the general public, unless this quantity is specified elsewhere on the package
- Product identifiers
- Hazard pictograms, where applicable
- The relevant signal word, where applicable
- Hazard statements, where applicable
- Appropriate precautionary statements, where applicable
- A section for supplemental information, where applicable.

This replaced the former regulations, the Dangerous Substances Directive (DSD) and Dangerous Preparations Directive (DPD). However, it is likely that you will encounter packaging with both, so it is important that you are familiar with them.

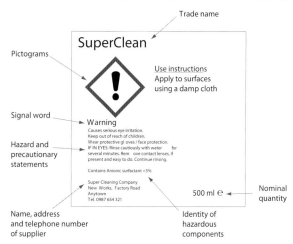

Figure 3.1 An example label for a hazardous mixture [EC, 2013]

3.3.1 CLP pictograms

The CLP has introduced nine pictograms, which have replaced the older orange square warning symbols (Table 3.1). In addition, there are two signal words that accompany the pictograms [EC, 2013]:

- **Danger**: Substances and mixtures with the most severe hazards
- **Warning**: Substances and mixtures with less serious hazards.

3.4 Transporting hazardous substances

Road and rail vehicles registered in Great Britain on domestic journeys are required to display a hazard warning panel with an emergency action ('Hazchem') code, United Nations (UN) number, danger label, contact number and (optionally) company name or logo (Figures 3.2 and 3.3) [NCEC, 2013].

Table 3.1 CLP pictograms and sample hazard statements

CLP pictogram	Example hazard statement	Old DSD/DPD symbol
	Explosive; mass explosion hazard	
	Extremely flammable gas/aerosol	
	May cause or intensify fire; oxidiser	

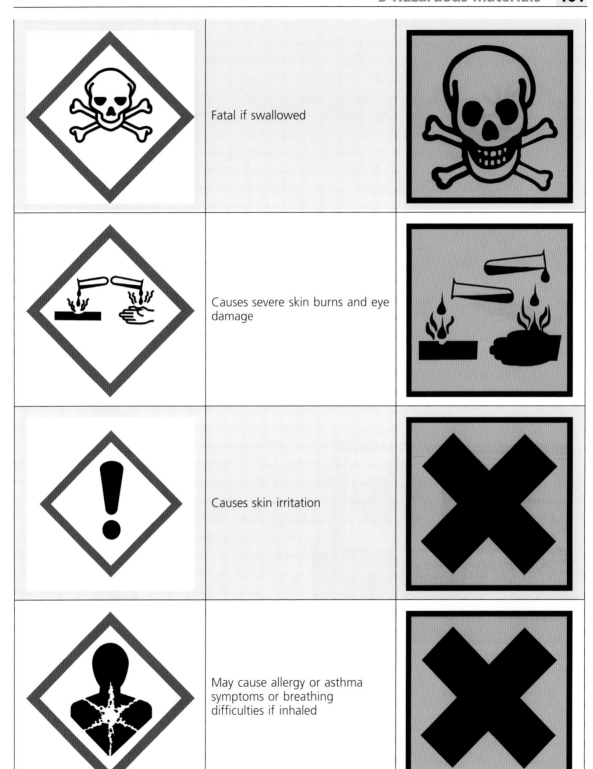

	Fatal if swallowed	
	Causes severe skin burns and eye damage	
	Causes skin irritation	
	May cause allergy or asthma symptoms or breathing difficulties if inhaled	

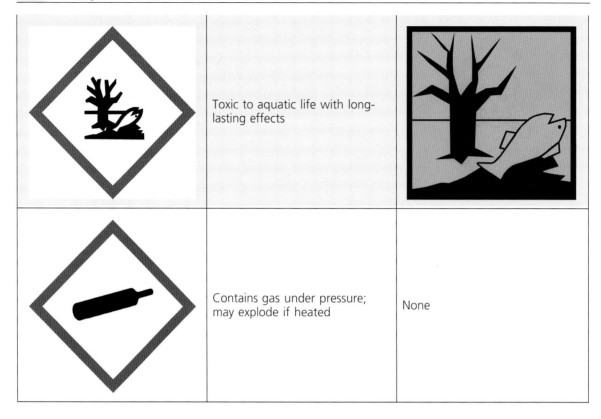

	Toxic to aquatic life with long-lasting effects	
	Contains gas under pressure; may explode if heated	None

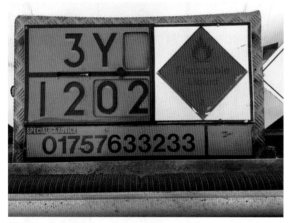

Figure 3.2 A hazard warning panel from a diesel tanker

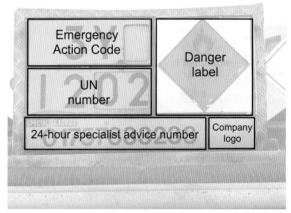

Figure 3.3 Annotated hazard warning panel

International journeys

Vehicles on international journeys must display the Hazard Identification Number (HIN) on an orange coloured plate. This also contains information about the hazardous properties of the substance, as well as its UN number (Figure 3.4).

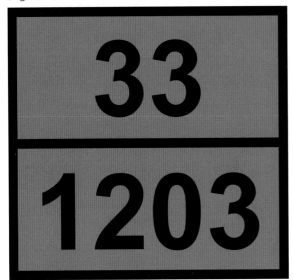

Figure 3.4 Orange plate with HIN (top) and UN number (bottom)

3.5 Danger labels

Danger labels are displayed on vehicles and packaging/containers of dangerous goods that are to be transported (Figure 3.5).

3.6 Ambulance crew actions at scene

In the event that an 'ordinary' emergency call turns out to involve hazardous substances, or you come across an incident that appears to involve hazardous substances, previous guidance for unprotected ambulance staff was to withdraw and await specialist teams, such as the hazardous area response team (HART) [HPA, 2009].

However, following research conducted as part of the Optimisation through Research of Chemical Incident Decontamination Systems project, it has become apparent that additional lives can be saved by the rapid (within 15 minutes of exposure) implementation of a number of measures, including the removal of patient's outer clothing [HPA, 2009a]. This has led to a change in the guidance for all emergency service personnel who are the first response to a CBRN incident.

3.6.1 Arrival

It is possible that the emergency operations centre (EOC) will have made you aware that you are attending a CBRN incident, but in the early stages, this may be hard to determine.

Signs of a CBRN release include [JESIP, 2013]:

• Dead or distressed people, birds and animals
• Multiple individuals showing unexplained signs of:
    • Skin, eye or airway irritation
    • Vomiting
    • Sweating
    • Pin-point pupils
    • Runny nose
    • Disorientation
    • Breathing difficulties
    • Seizures
• Presence of hazardous or unusual materials/equipment
• Unexplained vapour/mist clouds and/or oily droplets or film on surfaces of water
• Withered plant life or vegetation.

Provide a situation report to EOC using the METHANE mnemonic.

3.6.2 Hazard assessment

If there are three or more patients in close proximity with no obvious cause, you should conduct a hazard assessment, preferably with other emergency services if they are on scene. This hazard assessment should include:

• CBRN release indicators
• Patient numbers (walking and non-walking)
• Signs and symptoms of casualties
• Weather conditions
• Hazards present or suspected
• Location: Is it a likely target for terrorists or a hazardous material incident?
• Built environment: Is it city centre, open space, underground?
• Presence of perpetrators.

This will enable a decision on the hazard area and on the safe working area, and enable a joint operational plan.

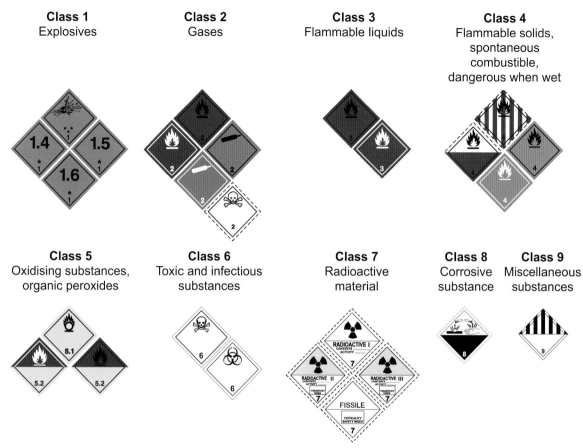

Figure 3.5 Danger labels

3.6.3 **Evacuate, disrobe and decontaminate**

Encourage patients to move away from the main area of contamination (hot zone) into an area which, ideally, should be uphill and upwind (warm zone). However, you should avoid physical contact where possible. Once in the warm zone, patients need to undress to their underwear. Skin, hair, clothing and items like jewellery are all likely to be contaminated and need to be removed. Advise patients that they should not remove clothing over their heads, but cut them if necessary. Absorbent materials such as paper towels, towels and medical dressings can be used to remove contaminants from exposed skin. If you have disrobing packs, distribute them to patients, but alternative clothing or blankets can be used to protect patients from hypothermia and maintain dignity. However, patients must leave all items removed during the disrobing procedure where they are removed.

Patients and ambulance crew must not eat, drink or smoke and must avoid touching their faces to reduce the risk of ingesting or transferring hazardous materials.

Communication

Asking patients to remove their clothes, particularly in public, requires trust. One method to achieve this is to communicate clearly with patients. You should ensure that you tell patients [JESIP, 2013]:

- Why and how patients need to be undressed and decontaminated

- To assist others if they can

- That additional help and resources are on the way

- That they should not eat, drink or smoke and avoid touching their face.

Chapter 8: **Patient Assessment**

1 **Patient assessment process**

1.1 **Learning objectives**

By the end of this lesson you will be able to:

- State the components of the patient assessment process
- Describe the ABCDE approach to initial patient assessment including:
  - Airway
  - Breathing
  - Circulation
  - Disability
  - Exposure/Environment
- State the components of the tool AVPU to assess level of consciousness
- Outline how to obtain a patient history using the acronyms SAMPLE, OPQRST and SOCRATES
- Describe the steps in a 'head-to-toe' assessment.

1.2 **Introduction**

Once you have completed your scene assessment, the next step is to conduct a patient assessment. This chapter will break down the patient assessment process into its separate parts so you can explore them further. Figure 1.1 shows the patient assessment process from start to finish. This chapter and some of the subsequent chapters are going to cover this in some detail, so just concentrate on the order of the assessment process, rather than on what it is you are expected to do during each stage [Pilbery, 2013; AACE, 2013].

1.3 **Primary survey**

The primary survey (Figure 1.2) is a swift patient assessment and management process, which can be completed within 60–90 seconds. It is designed to be a step-wise approach, meaning that any abnormalities identified in one step should be addressed before moving on to the next. Patients who have suffered traumatic injuries should have a check for life-threatening (or catastrophic) haemorrhage, before you check

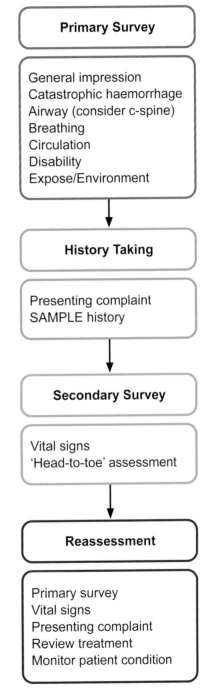

Figure 1.1 The patient assessment process

Primary Survey

General impression
Catastrophic haemorrhage
Airway (consider c-spine)
Breathing
Circulation
Disability
Expose/Environment

Figure 1.2 The primary survey

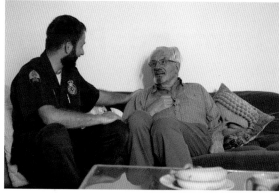

Figure 1.3a General impression. Compare this patient to the one in Figure 1.3b

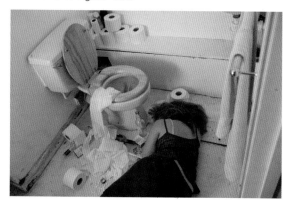

Figure 1.3b General impression

the patient's airway. In addition, in this group of patients you should give consideration to the patient's cervical spine and avoid unnecessary movement of the head and neck. This is covered in more detail in the ASSESSMENT AND MANAGEMENT OF THE TRAUMA PATIENT lesson (chapter 15).

1.3.1 General impression

The general impression is your first and immediate assessment of the patient and their current location, which will give you an early indication as to how sick and/or injured your patient is. Some of this information you will have already gathered from your scene assessment. However, now your focus is on the patient. Note the patient's approximate age, gender and ethnicity as your management and expectations of what the patient can do will vary. For example a 1-year-old child will not present in the same way as an adult. In addition, patient positioning can give you early clues. Is the patient sitting up and smiling (Figure 1.3a) or are they lying apparently lifeless on the floor (Figure 1.3b)? This step relies heavily on experience and intuition and you may find this challenging as a new SW [NAEMT, 2011].

This is also your chance to assess how responsive the patient is. If the patient is awake, introduce yourself with "Hello, my name is ..." and identify yourself as being from the ambulance service. Ask how they would prefer to be addressed.

If the patient appears not to be awake or is unconscious, check for responsiveness by asking

them if they are alright, or try giving them a command like "Open your eyes". If they do not respond, gently shake the patient's shoulders. Patients who fail to respond are critically ill until proven otherwise [Nolan, 2012].

1.3.2 Airway

Assessment of the airway involves three steps:
• **Look** for signs of airway obstruction
• **Listen** for noisy or absent breathing
• **Feel** for air movement as the patient breathes.
Remember, the primary assessment proceeds in a step-wise manner. Any signs of obstruction such as snoring or gurgling sounds need to be addressed now, before moving on to breathing. You will learn how to deal with airway problems in the MANAGING THE AIRWAY lesson (chapter 9).

1.3.3 **Breathing**

Once you have a patent (open) airway, you are ready to move on to breathing. As with the airway, you will adopt a look, listen, feel approach.

The first question you should ask is whether the patient is breathing. If they aren't, then you will have to provide breaths for the patient, i.e. ventilate them. If they are breathing, you will need to decide whether it is adequate. You can start with the respiratory rate and depth of breathing (indicated by chest movement), but the ASSESSMENT OF BREATHING lesson (chapter 10) will also explain about other methods of assessing breathing, including pulse oximetry, accessory muscle use and auscultation.

1.3.4 **Circulation**

In medical patients, circulation is the next step following airway and breathing. You can obtain a good idea of the patient's circulation by looking at the colour of their limbs (usually the hands as they are most accessible and normally visible). Feeling for a pulse is a skill which you will cover in the ASSESSMENT OF CIRCULATION lesson (chapter 11); it can tell you the heart rate and adequacy of the cardiac output, particularly if distal pulses such as the wrist are absent when a central pulse (such as found in the neck) is palpable. Clearly, a patient who does not have a pulse needs CPR immediately! This is covered in the ADULT BASIC LIFE SUPPORT and PAEDIATRIC BASIC LIFE SUPPORT lessons later on in the course (chapter 21).

1.3.5 **Disability**

Disability in the primary assessment refers to the patient's level of consciousness, or how awake they are. There are many causes of unconsciousness and these are covered in the ASSESSMENT OF DISABILITY later on in the course (chapter 12). During the primary assessment, you will need to check three things to assess the patient's disability [AACE, 2013; Pilbery, 2013]:

- Level of consciousness
- Pupils
- Blood sugar.

Level of consciousness

A rapid assessment of the patient's level of consciousness (LOC) can be undertaken using the acronym AVPU:

- **A**: Alert
- **V**: Responds to verbal stimulus
- **P**: Responds to pain
- **U**: Unresponsive.

Pupils

When looking at a patient's pupils, you are interested in whether they are of equal size and react to light. There are a number of reasons why this may not be the case and you'll find out about these in the DISABILITY chapter later on.

Blood sugar

Hypoglycaemia, or low blood sugar, is a cause of reduced level of consciousness, which can usually be corrected by the administration of glucose, either orally (by mouth) or intravenously. In addition, there are drugs which can mobilise the body's own glucose stores and you'll be learning about these in the DIABETES lesson (chapter 14).

1.3.6 **Expose/Environment**

You will undertake a full 'head-to-toe' assessment later on in the patient assessment process, but a quick look early on will provide you with clues to obvious illness/injury that needs to be managed quickly. For example, some types of rashes (e.g. non-blanching) signal serious illness such as sepsis or anaphylaxis. It also provides a chance to identify sites of hidden bleeding that you did not pick up on earlier on in your assessment.

Working out of hospital, however, you do need to be mindful about maintenance of patient privacy by not unnecessarily exposing them in public as well as ensuring that they do not lose body heat. This is particularly important in trauma as patients are three times more likely to die if they are hypothermic (their body temperature is below 35°C) [Ireland, 2011].

1.4 History taking

Presenting complaint

The presenting complaint is usually the reason you have been called to the patient (Figure 1.4). The majority of presenting complaints fall into the categories of pain, discomfort and/or abnormal body function. Sometimes this is explicit ("I have terrible chest pain") but can be vague, particularly in the elderly ("I just don't feel right today") [Gregory, 2010b; Pilbery, 2013]. Avoid using words like problem or complaint when finding out the reason for the emergency call.

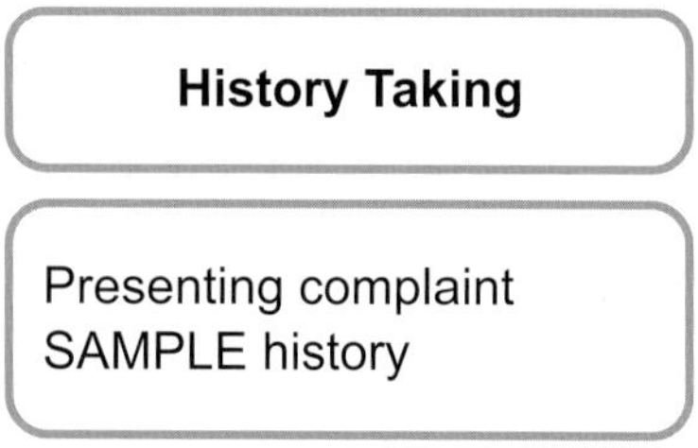

History Taking

Presenting complaint
SAMPLE history

Figure 1.4 History taking

S A M P L E history

Once you know the presenting complaint, you will need to ask further questions. At the bare minimum, this should include the parts of the SAMPLE acronym [Pilbery, 2013]:

- **S**: Signs and symptoms of the presenting complaint
- **A**: Allergies (particularly to medication, food allergies might be relevant)
- **M**: Medications
- **P**: Past medical history
- **L**: Last oral intake
- **E**: Events that led to the current illness or injury.

Note that when you are working with a clinician, such as a paramedic, you may find that they use and document a different method, made up of the following components [Douglas, 2005]:

- History of presenting complaint
- Past medical history
- Drug history including allergies
- Family history
- Social history
- Systematic enquiry.

Signs and symptoms of the presenting complaint

To help you organise the signs and symptoms of the presenting complaint, there are two acronyms that you can use: OPQRST [Wardrope, 2008] and SOCRATES. These were originally designed with assessment of pain in mind, but can be helpful for other presenting complaints. OPQRST:

- **O**: Onset. When did it (the presenting complaint) start?
- **P**: Provocation/palliation. What makes it worse/better? Include self-treatment such as taking analgesia
- **Q**: Quality. How does the patient describe their symptom, particularly pain? Is it sharp or dull, for example?
- **R**: Region/radiation/referral. Where is the symptom located? In the case of pain, does it stay in one place (can the patient point to it with one finger) or does it go elsewhere?
- **S**: Severity. On a scale of 0 to 10, where 0 is no pain and 10 is the worst pain imaginable, what score does the patient give it now?
- **T**: Time. How long has the patient had it and if it has been relieved, what time was this? In the case of pain, also consider whether the pain is intermittent (comes and goes).

SOCRATES is very similar:

- **S**: Site
- **O**: Onset
- **C**: Character. Same as Quality above
- **R**: Radiation
- **A**: Association. Are there any other signs and symptoms associated with the presenting complaint?
- **T**: Timing
- **E**: Exacerbating/relieving factors. Same as Provocation/palliation above
- **S**: Severity.

1.4.1 Allergies and medication

Allergies

The range of drugs that you can administer as an SW is limited and these are typically safe. However, you should always ask the patient about any allergic reactions to medication they have received in the past. It is also a good idea to ask about other allergies, such as those caused by food, animals, pollen or metal [Douglas, 2005].

Medication

Write down all of the patient's medication including the dose and frequency of administration. Just writing 'drugs with patient' or similar is not acceptable.

It is also a good idea to ask about any over-the-counter medicines (i.e. those not prescribed by a doctor, but obtained from a pharmacist or supermarket), as well as herbal and homeopathic remedies [Pilbery, 2013].

Strictly speaking there are no drugs called 'over-the-counter'. They are either General Sales List medications, which can be sold without the supervision of a pharmacist, or Pharmacy medicines, which, as the name suggests, require a pharmacist to oversee the purchase, usually because it is necessary to check that they are appropriate for the patient.

1.4.2 Past medical history

You will probably cover some of the patient's medical history while obtaining the history of the presenting complaint, but the following questions will help you uncover other medical illnesses or surgery that may prove helpful [Douglas, 2005; Gregory, 2010b]:

- Have you had any illnesses that you saw your GP about?
- Have you had to take any time off work because of ill health?
- Have you had any operations?
- Have you been admitted to hospital, and if so, why?
- Have you suffered any injuries?

1.4.3 Last oral intake and events leading to illness/injury

Last oral intake

Find out when the patient last had anything to eat or drink. This information is useful for patients who are unconscious or deteriorate on the way to hospital, or who may require surgery, as patients with a full stomach are at risk of aspiration. Also, you may be able to identify the onset of food poisoning and/or food allergies [Gregory, 2010b].

Events leading to the illness or injury

This is also known as the history of the presenting complaint and if you have used either of the OPQRST or the SOCRATES acronyms, you will have already obtained most of the information required.

Additional information that is useful to obtain includes [Gregory, 2010b]:

- Associated symptoms: For example, does the patient have shortness of breath and nausea with their chest pain?
- Previous episodes: Find out what happened last time, including any diagnoses made or hospital admissions
- Effect on daily living: Does the presenting complaint interfere with getting to the toilet or making a cup of tea, for example?

1.5 Secondary survey

The secondary survey is often tailored to your findings from the primary survey and history (Figure 1.5). For example, if the presenting complaint is shortness of breath, then you are going to ensure that you obtain a respiratory rate and oxygen saturations, and auscultate the lungs.

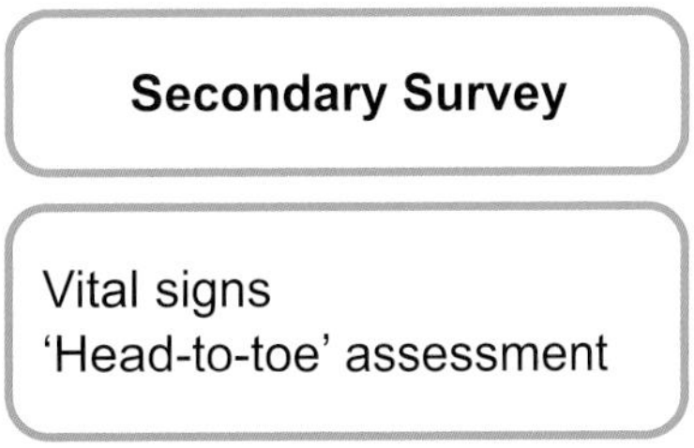

Secondary Survey

Vital signs
'Head-to-toe' assessment

Figure 1.5 Secondary survey

Vital signs

If you have not already been instructed to do so, now is the time to obtain some physiological observations from the patient, or obtain vital signs. Your ambulance service may have a specified minimum set of observations to obtain, but this will generally include:

- Respiratory rate
- Oxygen saturations
- Pulse rate
- Blood pressure
- Glasgow Coma Scale score (often just referred to as GCS)
- Blood sugar
- Temperature.

Depending on the patient's presenting complaint and the management plan, you may also obtain an electrocardiogram (ECG).

Being able to record vital signs accurately is a fundamental skill of the SW and these will be explored in depth in the relevant chapters as you progress through the course.

'Head-to-toe' assessment

It is not always appropriate to perform a 'head-to-toe' or full-body examination for every patient, but in cases of multiple injury, or in cases when the patient is found collapsed and the history is limited or non-existent, it can be helpful to identify signs of injury, or illness. The assessment outlined here is a rapid full-body assessment which should take around 60–90 seconds to complete. Clinicians that you work with are likely to perform more thorough assessments on specific areas of the body depending on the presenting complaint.

Procedure

Take the following steps to perform a 'head-to-toe' assessment [Pilbery, 2013]:

1. Look at the face for obvious injuries such as lacerations, bruising, fluid and deformities
2. Inspect the area around the eyes and eyelids
3. Check the eyes for redness and the presence of contact lenses
4. Assess the pupils with a pen torch, to ensure that they react to light
5. Look behind the ears for bruising and in the ear for signs of fluid or blood leaking out
6. Look for bruising, lacerations and deformity around the head and then gently feel for tenderness and depressions of the skull
7. Feel the cheekbones for tenderness, symmetry and instability
8. Feel the maxilla (the bone just below the nose)
9. Check the nose for blood and fluid leaking out
10. Feel the jaw
11. Assess the mouth and nose for cyanosis (blue-tinged skin), foreign bodies (including loose teeth and/or dentures), bleeding, lacerations and deformities
12. Smell the patient's breath for specific odours (such as pear-drops, which can be present in some diabetic patients)
13. Look at the neck and note any obvious lacerations, bruises and/or deformity. Look for

bulging veins in the neck and feel the trachea to ensure it is centrally located

14. Feel the back of the neck for tenderness and deformity
15. Look at the chest for any obvious injury and watch the chest rise and fall as the patient breathes
16. Gently feel the ribs to ensure they are intact and to identify if they are tender. Don't press over any obvious bruising or fractures
17. Listen for breath sounds
18. If safe to do so, log roll the patient and listen to the back of the chest. Also, look for injuries and feel for deformities and tenderness.
19. Check the abdomen and pelvis for obvious injury and gently feel the abdomen, which should be soft and non-tender
20. Look at the pelvis for signs of injury, then gently feel the iliac crests for signs of instability, tenderness or crepitus. Do not compress the pelvis (sometimes called 'springing')
21. Check the extremities (arms and legs) for lacerations, bruises, swelling, deformities and the presence of medical bracelets. Feel for distal pulses and check motor and sensory function. Compare the right and left sides.

1.6 Reassessment

The first thing you'll probably notice about the Reassessment section is that it contains many of the things you have already undertaken as part of the patient assessment process (Figure 1.6). As with scene safety, a patient's clinical condition is dynamic and frequently changes, either due to the illness and/or injury they have acquired, or as a result of an intervention you have performed, such as defibrillation, or drug administration. Frequent reassessment will mean that you will not miss these changes.

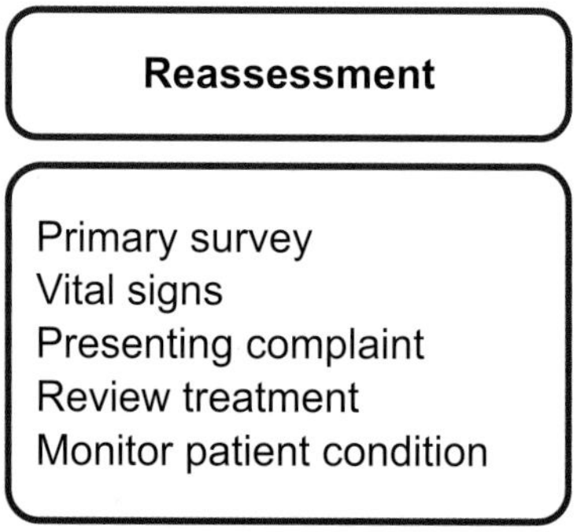

Reassessment

Primary survey
Vital signs
Presenting complaint
Review treatment
Monitor patient condition

Figure 1.6 Reassessment

Chapter 9: **Airway**

1 **Airway anatomy**

1.1 **Learning objectives**
By the end of this lesson you will be able to:
* Identify and describe the structures of the upper and lower airway.

1.2 **Introduction**
The respiratory system is made up of a number of structures (Figure 1.1):
* Nose
* Pharynx (throat)
* Larynx (voicebox)
* Trachea (windpipe)
* Bronchi
* Lungs.

Structurally, the respiratory system is split into two halves: the upper and lower respiratory systems. The upper consists of everything above the larynx, and the lower, everything below the pharynx.

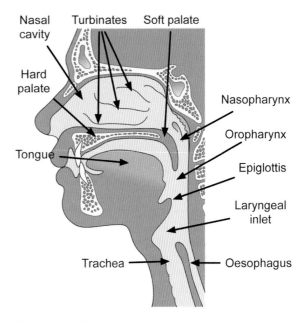

Figure 1.2 The upper airway

1.3 **Upper airway**
Nose
This is mostly constructed from cartilage, and is external to the skull. Its orifices (nostrils, or nares) open into the nasal cavity of the skull, which is divided by the nasal septum. The nasal cavity contains the superior, middle and inferior turbinates (Figure 1.2), which increase the internal surface area of the nasal cavity, which in turn increases the temperature and humidity of air that passes through during breathing [Drake, 2005].

Nasopharynx
This is the area at the back of the nasal cavities, above the level of the soft palate. It is bordered by the sloping base of the skull above, and mostly skeletal muscle on either side, forming a domed vault at the top of the pharyngeal cavity.

Elevation of the soft palate during swallowing helps to ensure that food does not rise up into the nasal cavity. The tissues that cover the top of the nasopharynx contain the pharyngeal tonsil.

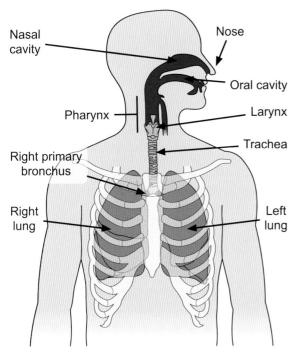

Figure 1.1 The structures of the respiratory system

Enlargement of this is known as adenoids and can, in severe cases, block the nasopharynx.

Mouth

The mouth (or oral cavity) starts at the lips and is continuous with the oropharynx posteriorly. The roof of the mouth is made up of the hard and soft palates, with the floor made up of mostly soft tissue, including the tongue. The tongue is a muscular, non-compressible tissue that attaches to the mandible bone, stylohyoid process and hyoid bone. The tongue, in the past, has been accused of being the most common cause of obstruction. However, research conducted on adult anaesthetised patients has demonstrated that it is usually the soft palate and epiglottis that cause obstruction of the airway, not the tongue [Nolan, 2012].

Oropharynx

This is the area posterior to the oral cavity, below the level of the soft palate but continuous with the nasopharynx, and above the margin of the epiglottis (which marks the start of the laryngopharynx). Anteriorly, the palatoglossal folds mark the boundary between the oral cavity and oropharynx.

Laryngopharynx

This is continuous with the oropharynx, running from the superior margins of the epiglottis to the top of the oesophagus around the level of the sixth cervical vertebra (spinal bone) in adults. Just anterior to the laryngopharynx are a pair of mucosal pouches called valleculae (where the tip of a curved laryngoscope blade goes).

1.4 Lower airway

Larynx

The larynx is a hollow structure made up of muscles and ligaments, and heralds the start of the lower respiratory tract. In adults, it is cylindrical in shape, with the narrowest part of the airway at the level of the vocal cords. It is continuous with the trachea below and opens into the laryngopharynx posteriorly.

The larynx is suspended from the hyoid bone above, and trachea below, by a series of membranes and ligaments, which makes it very mobile within the neck (Figure 1.3). During swallowing, it moves upwards and forwards causing the epiglottis to swing downwards,

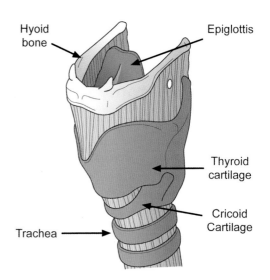

Figure 1.3 The larynx

effectively closing the laryngeal inlet while at the same time opening the oesophagus.

As well as acting as a valve to close off the respiratory tract during swallowing, the larynx also produces sound for speech, singing etc. It is the most heavily innervated sensory structure, and stimulation (by a laryngoscope, for example) can result in a doubling of heart rate and blood pressure. However, in children, stimulation can sometimes cause bradycardia, which, if severe, results in asystole [Walls, 2012].

Bronchi

The trachea divides into the left main bronchus and right main bronchus (together, the bronchi) at the carina (Figure 1.4). These bronchi split into secondary bronchi, tertiary bronchi, the brochioles, and finally the terminal bronchioles. The right main bronchus is more vertical, wider and shorter than the left, which explains why objects that are inhaled (foreign bodies) tend to end up here. In a similar design to the trachea, the main bronchi are incomplete rings of cartilage.

Lungs

The lungs are a pair of spongy, cone-shaped organs located in the thoracic (chest) cavity. They are separated by the mediastinum, a region in the thoracic cavity that contains the heart, major vessels, oesophagus and trachea, among others. This means that in the event that one lung

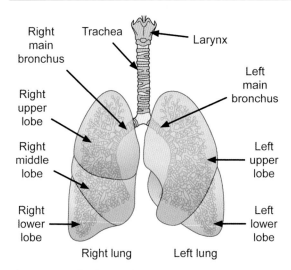

Figure 1.4 The lower airway

collapses, due to air entering the thoracic cavity after a traumatic injury, for example, the other lung may remain inflated.

The lungs are covered by the pleura, which consists of two layers: the parietal pleura, which covers the wall of the thoracic cavity, and the visceral pleura, which covers the lungs. In between is the pleural cavity, a small space filled with a fluid to prevent friction and allow the lungs to slide over each other during breathing. It also helps the membranes stick together due to the surface tension of the water, in a similar way that a glass with a wet bottom lifts the coaster it was sitting on.

The lungs extend from the diaphragm to just above the clavicles. The left lung is smaller than the right due to the space taken up by the heart. It also has only two lobes, the upper and lower, whereas the right lung has three, the upper, lower and middle lobes [Tortora, 2008].

2 Managing the airway

2.1 Learning objectives

By the end of this lesson you will be able to:

- Explain factors that affect airway patency and the step-wise approach to airway management
- Explain how to perform a range of manual airway manoeuvres
- Describe the equipment required for suction and its safe use.

2.2 Introduction

More often than not, your patient will be conscious and able to talk, scream or cry, indicating that they have a patent airway. For some, however, you will need to assist them in opening and maintaining their airway. Basic manoeuvres with nothing more than your hands are often enough to open and keep open a patient's airway, but things can change and it is important that you frequently reassess airway patency.

In this section, you are going to explore the following airway manoeuvres, which may be familiar if you have undertaken a first aid course:

- Head tilt–chin lift
- Jaw thrust
- Jaw thrust with head tilt
- Recovery position.

Once these have been covered, we will move on to more invasive procedures:

- Suction
- Oropharyngeal airways.

Endotracheal intubation and supraglottic airway device insertion are covered in the ASSISTING THE PARAMEDIC: AIRWAY lesson (chapter 16). Children and infants have a chapter all to themselves (chapter 18), since the management of the child's airway requires modification based on their age.

2.3 Manual airway manoeuvres

Manual airway manoeuvres can be achieved with just your (or a colleague's) hands. They are great for the initial management of the airway, and in some cases may be all that is required.

2.3.1 Head tilt–chin lift

When to do it (indications)

- An unresponsive patient who has an airway obstruction caused by loss of pharyngeal muscle tone.

When not to do it (contra-indications)

- If the patient has a suspected spinal injury.

Advantages

- No equipment is required
- Technique is simple and non-invasive.

Disadvantages

- Does not protect the airway from aspiration
- Not suitable for patients with cervical spinal injury.

Procedure

Take the following steps to perform a head tilt–chin lift [Pilbery, 2013; Nolan, 2012]:

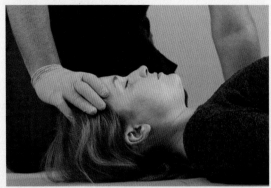

1. With your patient lying on their back (supine), position yourself at the patient's side. Place the hand closer to the patient's head on their forehead and gently tilt the head backwards

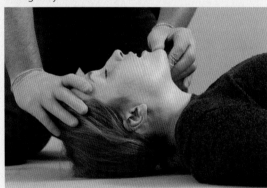

2. Place two fingers on the bony part of the chin and gently lift upwards

2.3.2 Jaw thrust

When to do it (indications)

- An unresponsive patient who has an airway obstruction caused by loss of pharyngeal muscle tone.

When not to do it (contra-indications)

- A responsive patient unless they have a fractured jaw.

Advantages

- No equipment is required
- Technique is simple and non-invasive
- Maintains neutral alignment of the head when cervical spinal injury suspected.

Disadvantages

- Does not protect the airway from aspiration
- Difficult to maintain for prolonged periods
- Requires second person to provide ventilations, if required.

Procedure

Take the following steps to perform a jaw thrust [Pilbery, 2013; Nolan, 2012]:

- With your patient lying on their back (supine), position yourself at the patient's head
- Identify the angle of the mandible
- Place your fingers behind the mandible and lift in an upwards and forwards direction (Figure 2.1)
- Using your thumbs, open the patient's mouth.

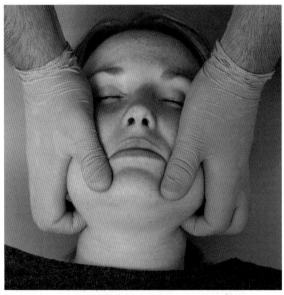

Figure 2.1 Lifting the mandible

2.3.3 Jaw thrust with head tilt

When to do it (indications)

- An unresponsive patient who has an airway obstruction caused by loss of pharyngeal muscle tone and jaw thrust alone is not sufficient to open the airway.

When not to do it (contra-indications)

• A responsive patient.

Advantages

• No equipment is required
• Technique is simple and non-invasive.

Disadvantages

• Does not protect the airway from aspiration
• Difficult to maintain for prolonged periods
• Requires second person to provide ventilations, if required.

Procedure

Take the following steps to perform a jaw thrust with head tilt [Pilbery, 2013]:

1. With your patient lying on their back (supine), position yourself at the patient's head
2. Identify the angle of the mandible
3. Place your fingers behind the mandible and lift in an upwards and forwards direction
4. Using your thumbs, open the patient's mouth
5. Tilt the head backwards.

2.3.4 Recovery position

There are a number of variations of the recovery position. This is the method that the European Resuscitation Council recommend [Koster, 2010]:

Procedure

Take the following steps to place a patient in the recovery position:

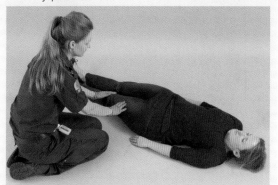

1. Kneel beside the patient and straighten both of their legs

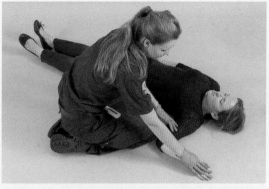

2. Place the arm nearer to you at right angles to their body, with the arm bent at the elbow and palm of the hand facing upwards

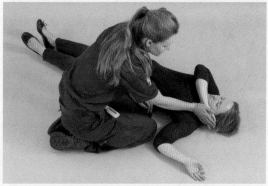

3. Bring the other arm across the chest and hold the back of their hand against the cheek that is nearer to you. Don't let go

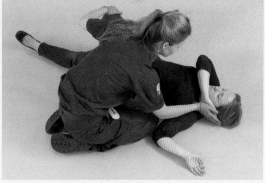

4. With your other hand, grasp the leg further away from you just above the knee and lift upwards so the leg flexes. Keep the foot on the ground

Procedure continued →

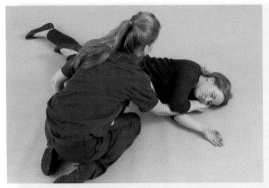

5. While supporting the head, pull the leg towards you, so that the patient rolls to face you

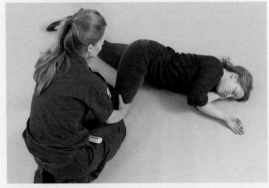

6. Adjust the uppermost leg so that the patient's hip and knee are bent at right angles

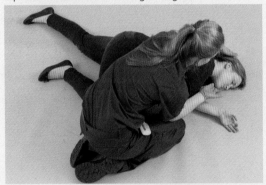

7.Tilt the head back to ensure the airway remains open

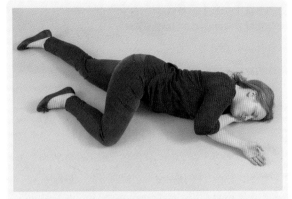

8. Adjust the patient's hand that is under their cheek, if required, to maintain head tilt and keep the patient facing slightly downwards, to allow free drainage of secretions from the mouth. Reassess frequently.
The Resuscitation Council UK published updated guidelines in October 2015. For access to the latest guidance visit: www.resus.org.uk/resuscitation-guidelines

2.4 Suction

If you can hear gurgling in the airway, then you should think suction. Suctioning an airway involves removing vomit, blood and secretions with suctioning equipment. On your ambulance, you will usually have a mains operated/battery powered suction unit (Figure 2.2) and a hand-operated device (Figure 2.3). Make sure you are familiar with the operating instructions for the devices you carry.

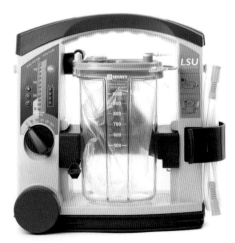

Figure 2.2 Mechanical suction device
Image reproduced by the kind permission of Laerdal Medical

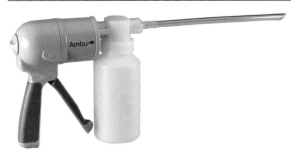

Figure 2.3 Hand-operated suction device
Image reproduced by the kind permission of Ambu A/S

Suction catheters

You are likely to have two types of suction catheters on the ambulance: a rigid, wide-bore catheter (sometimes called a Yankeur) and a smaller, flexible catheter which can fit down an oropharyngeal or nasopharyngeal airway, but is limited by its small size and is unsuitable for blood and vomit (Figure 2.4).

When to do it (indications)

• In patients who cannot maintain and clear their own airway and in whom vomit, blood or secretions are at risk of entering the lower respiratory tract.

When not to do it (contra-indications)

• In patients who can maintain and clear their own airway.

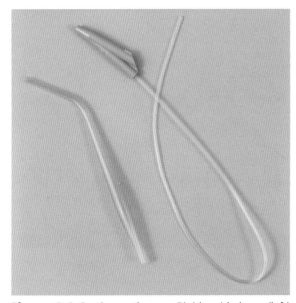

Figure 2.4 Suction catheters. Rigid, wide-bore (left) and flexible (right)

Advantages

• Prevents aspiration of vomit, blood and secretions.

Disadvantages

• Suctioning removes air as well as secretions. Keep suction times short.

Procedure

Take the following steps to perform suction using a mechanical suction device [Randle, 2009; Roberts, 2014]:

1. Prepare your equipment. You will need:
   • Suction unit
   • Yankeur and soft-tip catheters and suction tubing
   • Gloves
   • Protective eyewear
   • Oxygen
2. Explain the procedure to the patient and obtain consent if conscious
3. Pre-oxygenate if possible
4. Put on gloves and eyewear
5. Attach suction tubing and catheter and switch on suction unit if using a mechanical device
6. Open the patient's mouth and insert the catheter into their mouth without suctioning. Make sure you can visualise the end of the suction catheter at all times
7. Apply suction by occluding the control vent on the catheter (mechanical device) or squeezing the handle (hand-operated device) and gently withdraw the catheter. Suction for no more than 15 seconds
8. Re-oxygenate the patient and reassess the airway. Further suction attempts may be required.

Notes:

There is no clear guidance on suction pressures for the emergency management of patients. If you only need to clear small amounts of saliva, then a suction pressure of 150–200 mmHg is sufficient [Randle, 2009]. However, in cases where there is a large amount of blood or vomit, turn the suction up to maximum initially and adjust downwards, as required [NAEMT, 2014].

In cases of severe bleeding or active vomiting, positioning the patient to allow for postural drainage is more important: for example, turning a patient onto their side when they are immobilised on an orthopaedic stretcher.

Although prolonged suctioning will cause hypoxia (which is why suctioning for no more than 15 seconds is suggested), an airway obstructed by blood or vomit will not allow any air exchange and is likely to result in aspiration. In this case, patient positioning and aggressive suction will be required until the airway is at least partially clear. Re-oxygenation can then be performed and suction repeated as required. Follow the guidance of the senior clinician on scene [NAEMT, 2014].

2.5 Airway adjuncts

Airway adjuncts are devices that assist in airway management. Probably the most commonly used airway adjunct is the oropharyngeal airway (Figure 2.5), but there are others such as the nasopharyngeal airway and bougie, which you may see clinicians using.

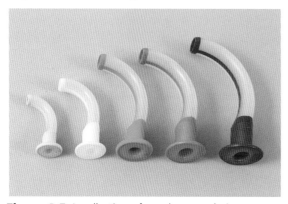

Figure 2.5 A collection of oropharyngeal airways

2.5.1 Oropharyngeal airway (OPA)

When to do it (indications)

- An unresponsive patient with an absent gag reflex.

When not to do it (contra-indications)

- Any patient who has a gag reflex.

Advantages

- Easy to place
- Technique is simple and non-invasive.

Disadvantages

- Tongue can be pushed back during insertion, making obstruction worse
- Does not protect against vomiting.

Procedure

Take the following steps to insert an oropharyngeal airway [Nolan, 2012]:

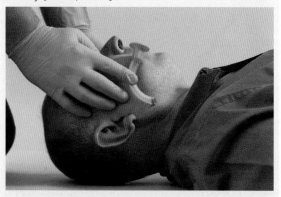

1. Select the correct size OPA by measuring the vertical distance between the patient's incisors and the angle of the jaw

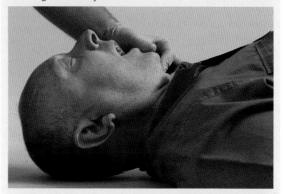

2. Open the patient's mouth and check it is clear of foreign bodies, vomit, blood or secretions. Suction if required

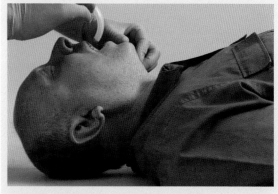

3. Insert the airway 'upside down' along the roof of the mouth until it reaches the soft palate

Procedure continued →

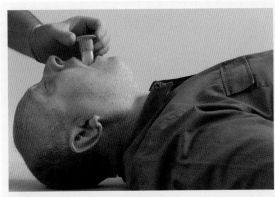

4. Rotate the OPA through 180°

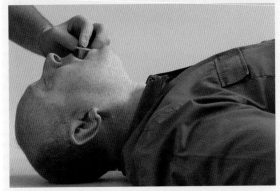

5. Advance the OPA until it rests in the pharynx. Remove immediately if the patient gags. Continue to provide manual manoeuvres such as head tilt–chin lift or jaw thrust as appropriate

3 Tracheostomies

3.1 Learning objectives
By the end of this lesson you will be able to:
- Explain the difference between laryngectomy and tracheostomy
- Describe how to manage the airway of a patient with a laryngectomy or a tracheostomy.

3.2 Introduction
A tracheostomy is an artificial opening made into the trachea through the neck (Figure 3.1). Patients have them inserted for a number of reasons including [Feber, 2006; Bowers, 2007]:
- Following trauma or surgery to the head and neck which leads to an airway obstruction
- Bypassing a tumour which obstructs the upper airway
- For prolonged ventilation

- For some types of chronic disease where minimising the anatomical dead space is beneficial
- To provide access to chest secretions in the event of respiratory insufficiency
- To protect from aspiration in the event of impaired swallow reflex (for example, neuromuscular disorders).

As the name suggests, a laryngectomy is the removal of the larynx. This is typically due to involvement of the larynx in oral, pharyngeal and laryngeal cancers. If the patient requires a total laryngectomy, the larynx is removed and the trachea cut and stitched to the front of the neck [NTSP, 2014]. This is important for subsequent management, because these patients cannot be ventilated from the mouth and/or nose (Figure 3.1).

3.3 Tracheostomy tubes
There are a wide variety of tracheostomy tubes, which can seem rather overwhelming. However, tubes are broadly classified into the following categories [NTSP, 2014]:
- Cuffed/uncuffed
- With/without inner cannula
- Fenestrated/unfenestrated.

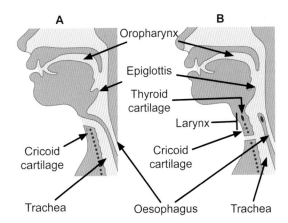

Figure 3.1 The anatomical differences between A) laryngectomy and B) tracheostomy

Cuffed/uncuffed tubes

As with adult endotracheal tubes, a cuffed tracheostomy tube has a soft balloon around the distal end, which is inflated by injecting air into the pilot balloon via the injection port (Figure 3.2). These are used when patients require positive pressure ventilation (PPV) and/or when the patient cannot protect their own airway from secretions. Note that if the cuffed tube is inflated and the lumen becomes blocked or occluded, the patient will not be able to breathe!

Uncuffed tubes tend to be used in longer-term patients, but since they lack the cuff, it is important that these patients have an effective cough and gag reflex to minimise the chance of aspiration. These tubes are not suitable for positive pressure ventilation.

Inner cannulas

Tracheostomy tubes with an inner cannula (sometimes called double-cannula or double-lumen tubes) consist of an outer tube or cannula which maintains airway patency, and an inner cannula, which can be removed for cleaning and/or disposed of and replaced (Figure 3.3). Uncuffed, double-cannula tracheostomy tubes are

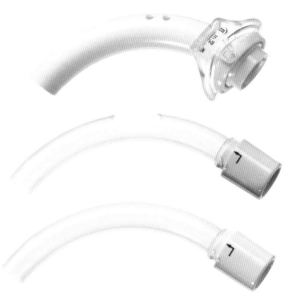

Figure 3.3 An uncuffed, fenestrated tracheostomy tube (top). Inner cannula with opening for fenestrations (middle). Inner cannula with no fenestrations (bottom)

the safest type to use in the community [NTSP, 2014].

Fenestrated tubes

These tracheostomy tubes have an opening on the outer cannula which allows air to pass through the patient's oropharynx and nasopharynx. This is helpful because it allows the patient to talk and produce an effective cough. However, fenestrations increase the risk of aspiration and prevent positive pressure ventilation unless a non-fenestrated inner cannula is used. Non-fenestrated inner cannulas should also be used if the patient requires suction (Figure 3.3).

3.4 Management of the tracheostomy patient

Patients with tracheostomies have a potentially patent upper airway, since the upper airway and trachea are anatomically connected. However, it is quite possible that the reason the patient had a tracheostomy in the first place is that their upper airway is difficult or impossible to manage [McGrath, 2012].

Help and equipment

The clinician will not be able to manage on their own and your assistance is vital. If a relative or

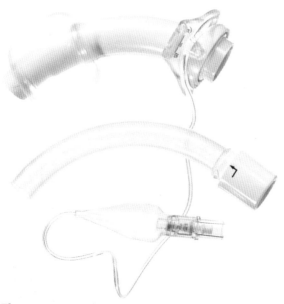

Figure 3.2 A cuffed, unfenestrated tracheostomy tube (top). Inner cannula with no fenestrations (middle). Pilot balloon and inflation valve for tracheostomy cuff (bottom)

carer is present, it is quite possible that they know more about tracheostomy management than you do, so listen to their advice and encourage them to help.

Patients may well have equipment to hand, such as replacement tubes, but you can manage with the equipment from your vehicle:

- Airway adjuncts such as oropharyngeal and nasopharyngeal airways
- Bag-valve-mask
- Supraglottic airway devices
- Laryngoscope and endotracheal tubes
- Gum-elastic bougie
- Monitor capable of waveform capnography.

Airway and breathing

Check and open the upper airway as normal. Look, listen and feel for breathing at the face and tracheostomy site for no more than 10 seconds. Apply waveform capnography to the tracheostomy tube as soon as possible [Whitaker, 2011].

If the patient is breathing, apply high-flow oxygen to both face and tracheostomy. This may require two cylinders, or the addition of a flowmeter into the Schrader valve of the oxygen cylinder. If the patient is not breathing, making agonal gasps or there are no signs of life, start chest compressions and follow the basic/advanced life support (BLS/ALS) algorithms while continuing to troubleshoot the tracheostomy, since this may be the cause of the cardiac arrest [Koster, 2010; Deakin, 2010].

Tracheostomy patency

Start by checking for and removing the following:

- Decannulation caps (used when removing tracheostomies) block the end of the tracheostomy
- Obturators (inserted inside the tracheostomy when first inserting a tube into the patient, Figure 3.4)
- Speaking valves, which should not be used with an inflated cuffed tube (Figure 3.5)
- Blocked humidification devices such as Swedish noses.

If the tracheostomy tube is a double-cannula design, remove the inner cannula, but remember that with some types of tubes the connector

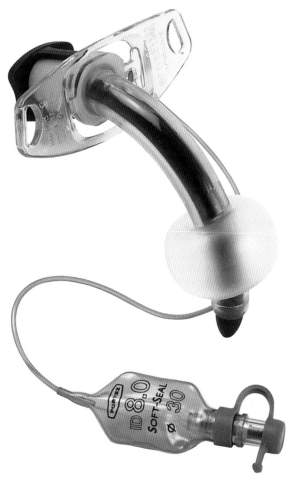

Figure 3.4 A tracheostomy tube with an obturator inside

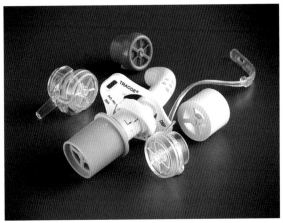

Figure 3.5 A selection of speaking valves. These should never be fitted to cuffed tubes

required for bag-mask ventilation is mounted on the inner cannula. Pass a suction catheter through the tube and into the trachea to check patency. It should pass easily through the tube. Don't use a gum-elastic bougie at this stage as it is more rigid than a suction catheter and might create a false passage in cases where the tube is misplaced. If the suction catheter passes through the tube, suction the tube and attempt to ventilate the patient. If this fails and the tube has a cuff, deflate it and reassess the patient using the same look, listen and feel technique as before at both the face and the stoma site.

Next steps

If everything attempted thus far has failed to improve the patient's condition, remove the tube. Reassess the patient again and hopefully they will be breathing. If the patient is in cardiac arrest continue with BLS/ALS. Attempt to oxygenate the patient via the oral route, but don't forget to cover the stoma site with swabs or a gloved hand. Use standard airway adjuncts to achieve effective ventilation. Alternatively, a paediatric face-mask or supraglottic airway device (SAD) can be placed over the stoma and the patient ventilated. If there is a large air leak from the mouth and/or nose, occlude them both during PPV.

If it is not possible to effectively ventilate the patient then a suitable clinician will need to attempt endotracheal intubation. This may be possible via the oral route, although they should expect it to be difficult. Use an uncut tube as it will need to be inserted further than normal in order to bypass the stoma.

In patients with an established tracheostomy or who have a known upper airway problem that is going to make intubation difficult, it can actually be more straightforward to simply insert another, smaller diameter tracheostomy or endotracheal tube into the stoma. Always use capnography as well as bilateral chest rise to confirm correct placement [Whitaker, 2011; Kodali, 2013].

3.5 Management of the laryngectomy patient

Unlike patients with a tracheostomy, laryngectomy patients do not have any connection between the upper airway and their lungs. Do not attempt to ventilate via the mouth/ nose. Laryngectomy patients do not normally have tracheostomy tubes either, but may have a tracheo-oesophageal puncture (TEP) valve fitted to allow for speech. This may be visible inside the stoma, but should not be removed. They are usually fitted with a one-way valve to prevent aspiration [NTSP, 2014].

Since these patients have, in effect, no upper airway, it cannot be obstructed by an inappropriate head position, and due to the reduction in anatomical dead space, chest compressions typically generate sufficient tidal volume to negate the need for PPV if this proves difficult to administer. Instead, just provide a supply of high-flow oxygen to the stoma site.

Tracheostomies are ten times more commonly performed than laryngectomies, so in the event that there is any uncertainty about whether the stoma is a laryngectomy or tracheostomy site, it is better to apply oxygen to both face and stoma.

Help and equipment

As with tracheostomy patients, these are not patients that the clinician can manage alone, and your assistance is vital. If a relative or carer is present, it is quite possible that they know more about laryngectomy management than you do, so listen to their advice and encourage them to help.

Patients may well have equipment to hand such as replacement tubes, but you can manage with the equipment from your vehicle:

- Airway adjuncts such as oropharyngeal and nasopharyngeal airways
- Bag-valve-mask
- Supraglottic airway devices
- Laryngoscope and endotracheal tubes
- Gum-elastic bougie
- Monitor capable of waveform capnography.

Airway and breathing

Check and open the upper airway as normal. Look, listen and feel for breathing at the stoma site for no more than 10 seconds.

If the patient is breathing, apply high-flow oxygen to the stoma site. If the patient is not breathing, making agonal gasps or there are no signs of life, start chest compressions and follow the BLS/ALS algorithms while continuing to troubleshoot the laryngectomy stoma, since this may be the cause of the cardiac arrest.

Laryngectomy stoma patency

Most patients will not have a tube in place, but you should remove any stoma cover (sometimes called a 'button') if in place. If a tracheostomy tube is in place and is of a double-cannula design, remove the inner cannula, but remember with some types of tubes the connector required for bag-mask ventilation is mounted on the inner cannula.

Pass a suction catheter through the stoma and into the trachea to check patency. It should pass easily into the trachea. If it does, the stoma is patent, so suction the trachea and attempt to ventilate the patient if they are not breathing. If this fails and there is a cuffed tracheostomy tube in place, deflate it and reassess the patient, preferably with capnography.

Next steps

If everything attempted thus far has failed to improve the patient's condition, remove any tracheostomy tubes, if present. Reassess the patient again and hopefully they will be breathing. If the patient is in cardiac arrest continue with BLS/ALS.

Attempt to ventilate the patient using a paediatric face-mask or SAD placed over the stoma. Don't rush to escalate your airway management if you can achieve effective ventilation with basic methods. If this fails, a suitable clinician will attempt to intubate the stoma with either a smaller diameter tracheostomy or endotracheal tube. They will need to use capnography as well as bilateral chest rise to confirm correct placement.

4 Choking in adults

4.1 Learning objectives

By the end of this lesson you will be able to:
- Define choking and list some common causes
- State the signs that an adult is choking
- Describe the procedure for managing the choking adult.

4.2 Introduction

Choking is a mechanical obstruction of the airway occurring anywhere between the mouth and carina (where the left and right bronchi split from the trachea). Common causes include [Walls, 2012]:

- Foreign bodies
- Blood
- Secretions
- Teeth
- Vomit.

It is not known how common choking is in adults. Death from choking is thankfully rare, mostly because choking episodes are witnessed [Nolan, 2010]. In England and Wales, around 370 people die each year as a result of a foreign body in the respiratory tract. Most of these are over 65 years of age [ONS, 2013].

4.3 Recognition

The signs of choking in an adult depend on the severity of the airway obstruction that has occurred. Typically, the episode will have occurred while eating, and if the patient is still conscious, they may clutch their neck (Figure 4.1).

In the case of a mild airway obstruction, if you ask the patient if they are choking, they will still be able to speak and confirm that this is the case. They will also be able to breathe and cough.

However, in cases of severe airway obstruction, the patient will be unable to speak, so may only be able to respond to you by nodding their head in response to your question about whether they are choking. Any attempts at coughing will be

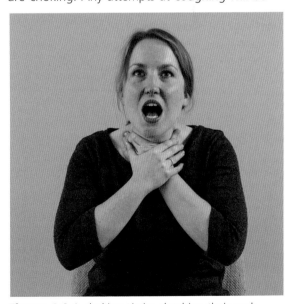

Figure 4.1 A choking victim clutching their neck

silent, and if this continues the patient will lose consciousness, possibly before your arrival [Nolan, 2012].

4.4 Management

Start by determining the severity of the obstruction. In adults, this is typically determined by the patient's response to the question "Are you choking?" A patient who can reply "Yes", i.e. can speak, cough and breathe, is classified as mild, whereas the patient who is clutching their throat, is unable to speak and who cannot breathe falls into the severe category.

Conscious and choking

If the patient is coughing, do not perform any interventions other than encouraging the patient to continue coughing.

If the obstruction is severe, administer up to five back blows, by standing just to the side and slightly behind the patient, leaning them forward, and then administering sharp blows between the shoulder blades with the heel of one hand.

If this fails, move on to abdominal thrusts. Position yourself behind the patient and place a clenched fist just under the xiphisternum. Grasp the fist with your other hand and pull sharply upwards and inwards up to five times.

Repeat the back blows/abdominal thrusts until the obstruction is relieved, or the patient becomes unconscious [Nolan, 2012].

Unconscious and choking

Lay the patient on their back and start chest compressions and ventilations at a rate of 30:2. If you are working with a paramedic, they may decide to attempt laryngoscopy in order to directly view the obstruction and clear it with forceps or suction (Figure 4.2).

Before each set of ventilations, check the mouth to see whether the chest compressions have expelled the foreign body, enabling you to remove it.

4.4.1 Adult choking management algorithm

Figure 4.3 shows the choking treatment algorithm, which summarises the explanation provided in the previous section.

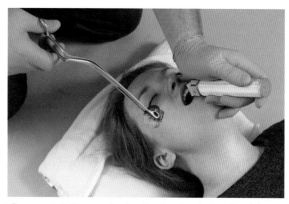

Figure 4.2 Removal of a foreign body by direct laryngoscopy

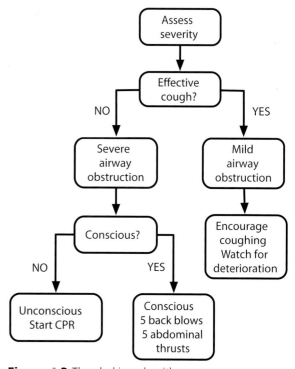

Figure 4.3 The choking algorithm

5 Choking in the paediatric patient

5.1 Learning objectives

By the end of this lesson you will be able to:
- Demonstrate how to manage a choking paediatric patient.

5.2 Introduction

It is estimated that around 20 children aged 0–14 years of age per 100,000 population will experience at least one food-related choking episode each year. It is more common in boys and children under 1 year of age [Chaplin, 2013]. Since most choking episodes involving infants and children are witnessed by an adult, intervention can commence straight away, as long as the adult knows the correct action to take [Maconochie, 2012].

5.3 **The paediatric airway**

Children's airways more readily obstruct than those of adults, and are particularly sensitive to soft tissue swelling. With a tracheal diameter of around 4mm in infants compared with 8mm in the adult, small amounts of swelling dramatically increase airflow resistance and the work of breathing required to maintain adequate ventilation.

The most dramatic differences are found in infants. By the age of 10–12 years, children have mostly adult anatomy, albeit smaller in size [Walls, 2012; Benger, 2009]. Other differences include [ALSG, 2010; Fuchs, 2012; AAP, 2013]:

- Infants have a large, prominent occiput, which results in neck flexion if they are laid supine on a flat surface. Use padding under the torso to maintain a neutral alignment
- The glottic opening is at the level of the 1st cervical vertebra (C1) in infants, descending to C3–C4 by the age of 5, resulting in a high, anterior larynx
- The epiglottis is horseshoe (or omega) shaped, floppy and proportionally larger than that of an adult
- The tongue is proportionally larger than that of adults, occupying more of the mouth
- Children possess a small cricothyroid membrane, and in children under 3–4 years of age it is virtually non-existent, making needle cricothyroidotomy very difficult
- The narrowest portion of the airway in children is at the level of the cricoid ring due to their funnel-shaped larynx compared to the more cylindrical shape of the adult larynx.

5.4 **Recognition**

Major choking episodes in children and infants usually occur during feeding or playing and are often witnessed by a carer. However, remember to ask about any recent history of playing with or eating small objects and consider choking in any child with a sudden onset of breathing problems.

The severity of the obstruction can be determined by the effectiveness of the patient's ability to cough. An effective cough is better than external manoeuvres, so an actively coughing child should be encouraged to continue to do so. Other signs of a mild obstruction include [Biarent, 2010]:

- Crying/verbal response to questions
- Long cough
- Able to take breaths before coughing
- Fully alert.

Contrast this with signs of a severe airway obstruction and an ineffective cough:

- Unable to verbalise
- Quiet/silent cough
- Unable to breathe
- Cyanosis
- Decreasing level of consciousness.

5.5 **Management**

The management of the choking paediatric patient depends on their ability to effectively cough and on whether they are conscious or unconscious (Figure 5.1) [Maconochie, 2012].

Conscious and choking

Infants

Start with back blows. If your patient is an infant, sit on a chair or kneel on the floor and place the infant across your lap in a prone (face down) position. Support their head with the thumb and fingers of one hand at the angle of their jaw, taking care not to compress the soft tissues. Administer up to five sharp blows between their scapulae with the heel of your other hand.

If these fail, turn the infant onto their back with their head downwards. Locate the landmarks for chest compression (i.e. one finger width above the xiphisternum) and administer up to five chest compressions, making them sharper and slower than those administered during cardiac arrest.

Children (over 1 year of age)

If the patient is a child, support them in a head-down position and administer up to five inter-scapular blows. If this does not clear the obstruction, administer abdominal thrusts by standing behind the child and leaning them forward. Place a clenched fist midway between the xiphisternum and belly button. Grasp the fist with your other hand and pull inwards and upwards, up to five times.

Frequently reassess and alternate between back blows and chest thrusts in the infant, and back blows and abdominal thrusts in the child.

Unconscious and choking

If a child or infant becomes, or is, unconscious, place them on their back with appropriate padding to maintain an open airway. Check the mouth for a visible obstruction and make a single attempt to remove it if a foreign body (FB) is visible.

Attempt to ventilate, but if this does not cause chest expansion try repositioning the head and try again. If after five attempts you still cannot ventilate the child, move on to chest compressions and alternate with further ventilations using a ratio of 15:2. Don't forget to check the airway for a dislodged FB after re-opening the airway prior to ventilating.

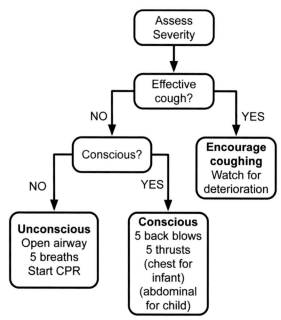

Figure 5.1 Management of choking in the paediatric patient

Chapter 10: **Breathing**

1 **Respiratory system physiology**

1.1 **Learning objectives**
By the end of this lesson you will be able to:
- Describe and explain the function of the respiratory system.

1.2 **Introduction**
In the AIRWAY ANATOMY lesson (chapter 9), you learnt about the structure (or anatomy) of the respiratory system, but it is important to understand the function (physiology) of the respiratory system. Functionally, the respiratory system is split in two portions [Tortora, 2008]:
- Conducting portion: This is made up of the interconnecting cavities and tubes starting at the mouth and nose and ending at the terminal bronchioles. These filter, warm and moisten the air and transfer it to the lungs and out again.
- Respiratory portion: This is made up of the tissues inside the lungs which exchange the gas. It consists of the respiratory bronchioles, alveolar ducts and sacs, and the alveoli. This is where gas exchange between the air and blood occurs.

These portions combined enable the respiratory system to perform its functions:
- Gas exchange: Imports oxygen, which is taken up into the blood and delivered to the body's cells. Expires the waste gas carbon dioxide
- Assists in the regulation of blood acidity levels
- Removes small amounts of heat and water
- Filters inspired air, produces vocal sounds and contains receptors providing a sense of smell.

1.3 **Respiration**
Respiration is the process of gas exchange in the body (mainly of oxygen and carbon dioxide). It consists of three steps [Tortora, 2008]:
- Pulmonary ventilation: The process of moving air into and out of the lungs. It is divided into inspiration (inhalation), when air is moved into the lungs, and expiration (exhalation), when air is moved out of the lungs [Pilbery, 2013]
- External respiration: The exchange of gases between the alveoli of the lungs and the blood inside the pulmonary capillaries
- Internal respiration: The exchange of gases between the blood in capillaries around the body and tissue cells.

1.4 **The lungs**
In order to understand ventilation and external respiration, we just need to cover a little more anatomy. Recall from the AIRWAY ANATOMY lesson that the lungs extend from the diaphragm to just above the clavicles. The left lung is smaller than the right due to the space taken up by the heart. It also has only two lobes, the upper and lower, whereas the right lung has three, the upper, lower and middle lobes [Tortora, 2008].

The lungs are divided into lobes by deep grooves known as fissures. Both lungs have an oblique fissure, but the right lung also has a horizontal fissure (Figures 1.1, 1.2 and 1.3).

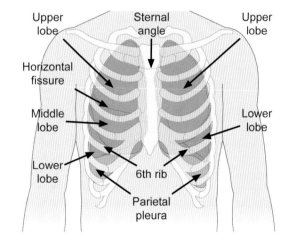

Figure 1.1 Anterior view of the lungs in relation to surface anatomy

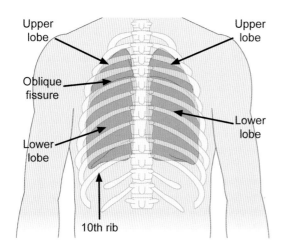

Figure 1.2 Posterior view of the lungs in relation to surface anatomy

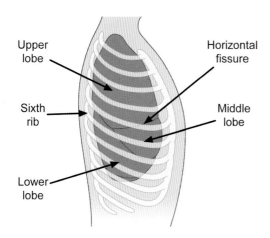

Figure 1.3 Lateral view of the right lung in relation to surface anatomy

1.4.1 **Lobes, lobules and alveoli**

Each lobe of the lung has its own secondary branch (bronchus), branching from the right and left primary bronchus (Figure 1.4).

These in turn divide into tertiary bronchi, each supplying a segment of lung called a bronchopulmonary segment. Within these are many much smaller components known as lobules, within which are contained 3–5 respiratory units, which is where the gas exchange occurs. Respiratory units (or acini) emerge from the terminal bronchioles and consist of several respiratory bronchioles, which

subdivide into alveolar ducts and, finally, the alveoli [Patel, 2008].

Alveoli

The alveoli are cup-shaped pouches with very thin walls that enable the exchange of oxygen and carbon dioxide with the pulmonary capillaries that surround them. There are around 140–150 million in each normal lung, creating a surface area for gaseous exchange in the region of two tennis courts [Patel, 2008]!

1.5 **Mechanics of breathing**

Air pressure

Air moves into and out of the lungs because ventilation changes the pressure inside the alveoli. This is achieved by changing the volume of the thoracic cavity (the contents of the body surrounded by the ribs and diaphragm). As the volume inside this cavity increases, the pressure inside decreases (a relationship known as Boyle's Law). This causes the lungs to expand, increasing their volume and so decreasing the alveolar pressure.

Since air moves from areas of high pressure to low pressure, once the pressure inside the alveoli drops below that outside the body, i.e. atmospheric pressure, air enters the lungs. At the end of inspiration, the volume of the thoracic cavity decreases, and the pressure rises; once it becomes higher than that of atmospheric pressure, air leaves the lungs [Patel, 2008].

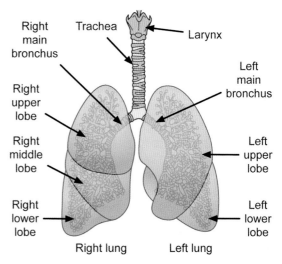

Figure 1.4 The lower respiratory tract showing the left and right bronchi

Inspiration

During normal, quiet respiration, most of the work of respiration is undertaken by the diaphragm. This is a dome-shaped muscle that seals the thoracic cavity from the abdomen. When it contracts, it flattens and descends, increasing the volume inside the thoracic cavity, and is responsible for about 75% of the air entering the lungs.

The remaining 25% of air entering the lungs is as a result of the external intercostal muscles contracting, which pulls the ribs upwards and outwards like a bucket handle [Tortora, 2008].

Expiration

During normal, quiet respiration, breathing out (expiration) is a passive process as no muscles are involved. This is because of elastic recoil, a property of the thoracic wall and the lungs to 'spring back' to their original position when they are stretched by the muscles of inspiration.

Forceful breathing

When exercising and in other instances when the body requires more oxygen, additional, accessory, muscles can be used to aid in inspiration and expiration (Figure 1.5). These can often be seen in use by patients with respiratory distress.

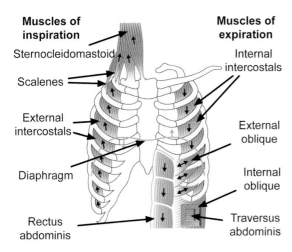

Figure 1.5 Muscles of inspiration and expiration

1.6 Gas exchange

You have already read that gas moves from areas of high pressure to low, and it turns out that this is the case even for a mixture of gases. Take room air, which you are breathing in. It is made up of the following (percentages are approximate) [Tortora, 2008]:

- Oxygen (O_2): 20.9%
- Nitrogen (N_2): 79%
- Carbon dioxide (CO_2): 0.04%
- Other gases/water vapour: 0.06%

The pressure each of the gases exerts to make up the pressure of air is known as the gas's partial pressure. For example, the partial pressure of oxygen (PO_2) in the air is 21 kiloPascals (kPa).

Each gas acts independently of the others, so in the alveoli, oxygen moves from an area of higher pressure (the alveoli) to an area of lower oxygen pressure (the pulmonary circulation), by a property known as diffusion.

Diffusion

Diffusion is a process by which molecules (such as oxygen and carbon dioxide) move around. It has two key characteristics [Patel, 2008]:

1. Diffusion occurs from areas of high concentration to areas of low concentration.
2. Diffusion continues until both areas have the same concentration of molecules.

Oxygen diffuses from the alveoli into the pulmonary circulation, whereas carbon dioxide has a higher partial pressure inside the pulmonary circulation so moves across into the alveoli, where it can be expired. In this way, oxygen is taken up by the body and the waste gas, carbon dioxide, is removed [Kapit, 2000].

1.7 Control of breathing

The muscles of respiration are dependent on the nervous system to tell them to contract and relax. This is achieved with two types of nervous system control [Kapit, 2000; Tortora, 2008]:

- Voluntary (or conscious) control: This originates in the cerebral cortex and is the way you can control your breathing by holding your breath or controlling the flow of air in order to play a wind instrument, for example. In addition, other centres in the brain, such as the hypothalamus and limbic system, can stimulate respiration, allowing laughing and crying to affect the breathing pattern
- Automatic control: These originate from groups of nerve cells (neurons) in the brain stem (mainly the pons and medulla). The neurons in the medulla are responsible for the basic rhythm of breathing and send impulses to the

inspiratory muscles via the phrenic and intercostal nerves. Expiratory neurons generally become active only during forceful breathing, such as when exercising.

The respiratory centres containing these inspiratory and expiratory neurons are influenced by sensory input from nerves around the body. For example, stretch receptors prevent the lungs from being overinflated and others are linked to receptors that can detect movement, stimulating the respiratory centres to increase ventilation during exercise.

Breathing is also regulated by the partial pressures of oxygen (PaO_2) and carbon dioxide ($PaCO_2$), and hydrogen ion concentration (pH) in the blood. $PaCO_2$ is the most important and has the most profound effect on respiration. Special sensory neurons called chemoreceptors are located close to the medulla (central chemoreceptors) and in the walls of the aortic and carotid arteries [Tortora, 2008].

NOTE: The extra 'a' in PaO_2 denotes the partial pressure of oxygen in arterial blood.

Chemical control

The central chemoreceptors are sensitive to $PaCO_2$, not PaO_2, and are responsible for 80% of the drive to breathe. They are also affected by drugs such as opiates (like morphine). Regulatory mechanisms are very sensitive and precise, keeping the $PaCO_2$ levels stable even when exercising. For example, once $PaCO_2$ levels begin to rise, ventilation is rapidly increased to expire more CO_2. Conversely, when the $PaCO_2$ level falls, ventilation is slowed, allowing the $PaCO_2$ level to increase.

The peripheral chemoreceptors are sensitive to PaO_2, $PaCO_2$, pH, blood flow and temperature. However, they are particularly sensitive to hypoxia, which causes PaO_2 to fall. Once this drops below 6.7 kPa ventilation is dramatically increased. When this was first discovered, it was suggested that if low levels of oxygen could increase ventilation, then giving too much might decrease ventilation. This is known as the hypoxic drive theory. In fact, when the PaO_2 rises above 8 kPa there is no significant reduction in ventilation, and when PaO_2 is above 13 kPa there is no further reduction in ventilation at all [Patel, 2008].

2 Using medical gases safely

2.1 Learning objectives

By the end of this lesson you will be able to:

- Describe dangers of using compressed gas
- Outline the safe use, storage and handling of medical gases
- State the guidelines for the use of oxygen therapy including:
  - Indications
  - Contra-indications
- Outline the safe use of entonox including:
  - The properties of entonox
  - Complications of environmental temperature with regards to entonox
  - The benefits of entonox therapy
  - Indications
  - Cautions and contra-indications

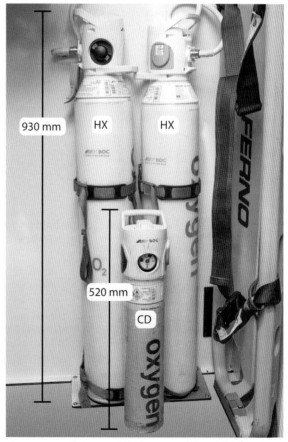

Figure 2.1 Oxygen cylinders – CD (portable) and HX (fitted to ambulance)

- Explain the use of facial barriers, the bag-valve-mask and mechanical ventilators.

2.2 Introduction

There are two main medical gases in use by ambulance services: oxygen and entonox. These gases are compressed into cylinders of varying sizes. Typically, you will have a small, portable cylinder for carrying into a patient's house or for transporting on the ambulance trolley, for example, and a larger, heavier cylinder which is fitted to the ambulance and is generally removed only when it is empty and needs replacing (Figure 2.1). **Note** that entonox is usually only provided as the smaller, portable cylinder.

2.3 Medical gas cylinder storage

Somewhere on your ambulance station is a medical gas cylinder store (Figure 2.2). It should meet all of the following requirements [DoH, 2006a]:

- On ground level, as close as possible to delivery point
- Clearly identifiable, so it can easily be located in an emergency
- Not close to any installation that may cause a fire risk (such as the fuel pump)
- Have a level floor, made of concrete or other non-combustible material
- Well ventilated
- Only containing medical gases
- Adequate means of securing large cylinders to prevent falling
- Clear and separate areas for full and empty cylinders
- Kept free from naked flames and marked with signage such as 'No Smoking'
- Not prone to excessively hot or cold temperatures
- Contain shelving to store smaller cylinders horizontally
- Be secure enough to prevent theft and misuse.

2.4 Anatomy of a medical gas cylinder

Integrated valve cylinders (Figure 2.3) are the most common type found in UK ambulance services and are covered in this section. You may find, however, that your service still uses the older style cylinders, which require a regulator

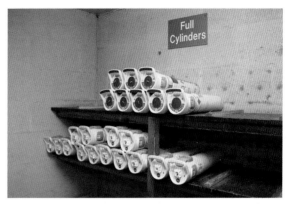

Figure 2.2 An ambulance station medical gas cylinder store

head to be fitted before they can be used, and you should seek guidance on their use.

Some of the important components of the cylinder are [BOC, 2013a]:

- Flow selector
  - Desired flow rate can be selected by rotating the dial
  - Positive 'click' between flow rates to ensure correct setting is chosen
- 'Live' contents gauge
  - Shows contents of cylinder, even when turned off
  - Green = full
  - Red = low/empty
- Handwheel
  - Simple on/off dial. No spanner required
  - Turn anti-clockwise to open
  - Turn clockwise to close
- Clear product identity
  - Name of gas is written on cylinder collar and body
- Flat base
  - Easier to handle
  - Improves stability
- Firtree
  - Attachment point for oxygen tubing
- Batch label
  - Located on guard or collar
  - Shows expiry date
  - Required when reporting cylinder defect

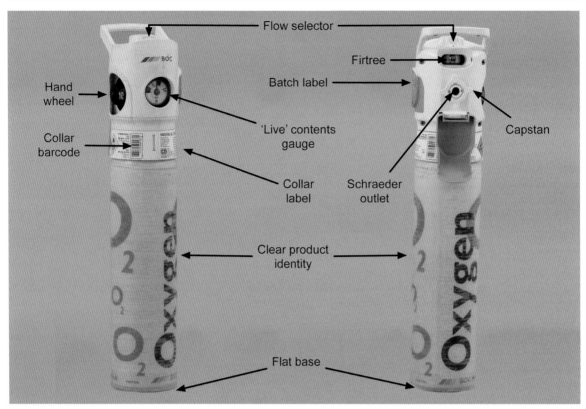

Flow selector

Firtree

Batch label

Hand wheel

Collar barcode

'Live' contents gauge

Capstan

Collar label

Schraeder outlet

Clear product identity

Flat base

Figure 2.3 CD-sized integrated valve oxygen cylinder

- Schrader outlet
  - Push-fit connector for other methods of administration/connection to artificial ventilators
  - Gas-specific to avoid inadvertent inappropriate administration
  - Out sleeve (capstan) can be twisted to release.

2.5 Safety first

Prior to using a medical gas, there are a number of safety checks required [BOC, 2013a]:

- Make sure your hands are clean. If you have used an alcohol-based hand rub, ensure that it has evaporated completely
- Check the cylinder to ensure it is clean and free from damage

- Ensure the cylinder is free from oil and grease, especially around the Schrader and firtree outlets
- Both oxygen and entonox are non-flammable, but strongly support combustion. Keep away from naked flames, sources of ignition and combustible materials.

If the medical gas is entonox, check that it has not been allowed to get too cold. Below ?6°C the nitrous oxide will separate from the gas mixture. To prevent this, it should be stored above 10°C for at least 24 hours prior to use. If this is not possible and the bottle is of a portable size (ED), warm the bottle to 10°C and then invert three times prior to use to mix the gases.

2.6 Preparing a new cylinder for use

Procedure

The following steps apply to both oxygen and entonox cylinders [BOC, 2013a; BOC, 2013b]:

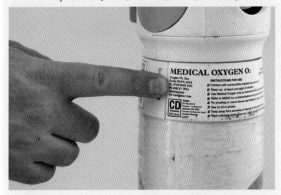

1. Ensure you have the correct medical gas by checking the cylinder label

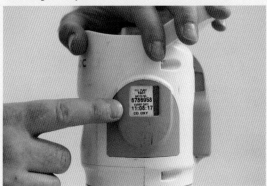

2. Check the expiry date on the batch label fitted to the cylinder

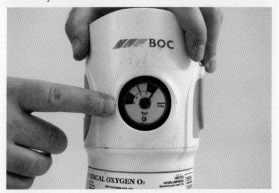

3. Make sure the contents gauge is in the green zone. This indicates that the cylinder is full

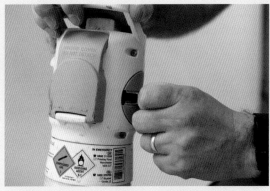

4. Remove the tamper-evident handwheel cover by pulling the tear ring

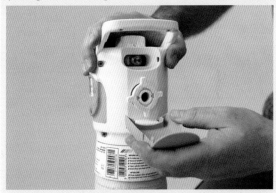

5. Remove the valve outlet cover. Pull the grey cover downwards. It stays attached to the cylinder

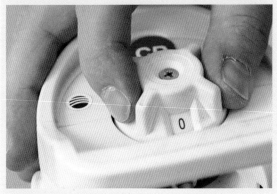

6. Ensure the flow selector on top of the cylinder is set to zero and the handwheel is turned off before connecting equipment

2.7 **Oxygen**

The two most common sizes of oxygen cylinder in the ambulance service are CD and HX size cylinders. Table 2.1 shows how long a CD-sized cylinder will supply oxygen for (in minutes) based on the flow rate and gauge level. Table 2.2 provides the same information for an HX-sized cylinder.

Table 2.1: CD-sized oxygen cylinder (460 litres)

Flow rate	Gauge level		
(l/min)	Full (100%)	Half (50%)	Low (25%)
15	30	15	7
10	46	23	11
4	115	57	28

Table 2.2: HX-sized oxygen cylinder (2300 litres)

Flow rate	Guage level		
(l/min)	Full (100%)	Half (50%)	Low (25%)
15	153	76	38
10	230	115	57
4	575	284	143

2.7.1 **Oxygen delivery devices**

The firtree connector (Figure 2.4) is used to connect oxygen tubing to the cylinder, which in turn can provide oxygen to a bag-valve-mask (BVM), oxygen-driven nebuliser, oxygen masks and nasal cannulae (Figure 2.5).

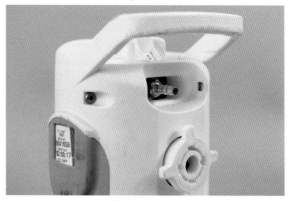

Figure 2.4 Oxygen firtree connector

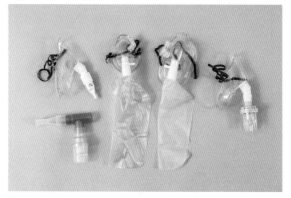

Figure 2.5 A variety of devices to administer oxygen to patients

NOTE: The masks and nasal cannulae all require the patient to be spontaneously breathing in order to work. If the patient is not breathing effectively, they require assisted and artificial ventilation.

Procedure for using the firtree

Follow the steps below to provide oxygen to the appropriate oxygen delivery device [BOC, 2013a]:

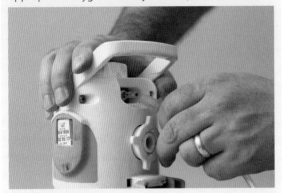

1. Attach tubing from mask or nasal cannula to the firtree outlet. Ensure the tubing is pushed on securely

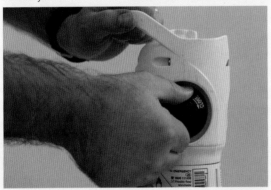

2. Slowly turn on the cylinder by rotating the hand wheel anticlockwise until it comes to a complete stop. Do not use excessive force

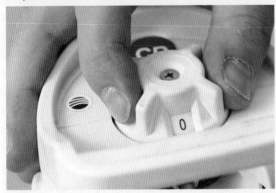

3. Set the prescribed flow by rotating the flow selector dial. Ensure that the correct flow rate number is clearly visible in the flow selector window. Check the gas is flowing

Supplemental oxygen delivery devices

Non-rebreathe mask

This mask is used when the patient requires a high concentration of oxygen. At 15 l/min, the mask can deliver up to 85% inspired oxygen. It consists of a mask and reservoir bag that is fitted with a one-way valve, ensuring that the patient can only inhale oxygen from it and not exhale into the bag. The bag must be inflated in order to ensure maximum inspired oxygen.

Medium concentration mask (Simple face mask)

This face mask has ports on either side to allow room air to be drawn inside. At 10 l/min, it will deliver around 40% oxygen, but this is variable depending on how well fitting the mask is.

Venturi mask

This mask also draws in (or entrains) room air, but allows for more accurate oxygen delivery than the medium concentration face mask. It comes with a variety of spigots, which are capable of delivering a variety of oxygen concentrations. The percentage oxygen and flow rate required are usually clearly marked on the spigot. They are particularly useful when providing oxygen to patients with chronic obstructive pulmonary disease (COPD).

Nasal cannulae

These deliver oxygen via two nasal prongs, which sit just inside the patient's nostrils. Oxygen flow rates are typically limited to 1–4 l/min as higher rates lead to irritation of the nasal lining. They are often used by patients on long-term oxygen therapy and may be preferred by patients who do not tolerate a face mask.

Nebuliser

This is used to deliver aerosolised drugs. The pressurised chamber when powered by oxygen turns the liquid drug inside (usually salbutamol or ipratropium) into a mist (i.e. aerosolises the drug), which is then inhaled by the patient. Some nebulisers (particularly if the patient has one at home) are powered using compressed room air.

Firesafe

You may notice a small device inserted into a patient's tubing if they are on home oxygen (Figure 2.6). This is a Firesafe, a cannula valve that is designed to cut the oxygen supply to the patient in the event of a fire. It will not affect the oxygen flow to the patient as long as it is inserted the correct way around (the arrow shows the direction of gas flow).

2.7.2 Assisted ventilation

Patients who are breathing inadequately, for example because they have a slow respiratory rate or an irregular pattern of respiration, and patients whose breathing is too shallow or who are not breathing at all, require assisted ventilation. Assisted ventilation can be provided with a pocket mask, BVM or oxygen-powered ventilation device.

Gastric distension

In contrast to the normal way we breathe (i.e. the negative pressure inside the chest cavity draws air into the chest), assisted and artificial ventilation requires the use of positive-pressure ventilation, actively blowing air into the lungs. This has some disadvantages as high inflation pressures can result in air going into the stomach instead of the lungs, leading to gastric distension and ultimately vomiting. This is more likely if:

• High inflation pressures are used

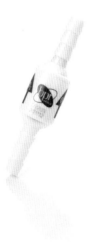

Figure 2.6 A Firesafe

• Ventilations are performed too fast
• The airway is partially obstructed.

A distended stomach is bad for the patient as vomit can rise up into the airway and be inhaled (aspirated). It also pushes the diaphragm, reducing the amount of space for lung expansion [Pilbery, 2013].

Mouth-to-mouth

The most basic ventilation device is your mouth and lungs, using mouth-to-mouth ventilation. However, healthcare professionals and members of the public are sometimes reluctant to perform mouth-to-mouth on people they do not know. In addition, there are risks relating to exposure to blood and other body fluids through direct contact with the patient's mouth and nose. In certain cases, direct mouth-to-mouth contact is not appropriate, such as in cases of poisoning [Nolan, 2010].

Procedure

Take the following steps to perform mouth-to-mouth ventilation [SJA, 2014]:

1. Place the patient on their back (supine)
2. Open the airway using a head tilt–chin lift, or jaw thrust if cervical spine injury suspected
3. Pinch the patient's nose to close the nostrils
4. Take a breath and seal your lips over the patient's mouth
5. Blow steadily for about one second, just enough to make the chest rise
6. While maintaining the head tilt–chin lift, take your mouth away from the patient and watch the chest fall
7. Repeat, aiming to provide a breath to an adult every 6 seconds.

NOTE: If the patient is not breathing and has no signs of life, commence chest compressions, not ventilations (you'll cover this in the CARDIAC ARREST lesson (chapter 21)).

Facial shields

To provide some protection for yourself, a face shield can be used, which provides a plastic barrier between you and the patient. They are also fitted with a filter which fits over the patient's mouth. As with mouth-to-mouth ventilation, this method does not allow for the administration of supplemental oxygen. The technique is the same for mouth-to-mouth ventilation.

Mouth-to-mask ventilation

Using a pocket mask to provide mouth-to-mask ventilation uses your lungs as before, but does not require direct contact with the patient's mouth. The one-way valve also prevents you coming into contact with blood and secretions from the patient's mouth. You use both hands to hold the mask to the patient's face, which makes it easier to get a good seal and deliver effective ventilations (Figure 2.7) [Pilbery, 2013].

Some pocket masks also have an oxygen port, allowing administration of supplemental oxygen. Even with pocket masks without an oxygen port, oxygen tubing can be placed under one side of the mask.

Procedure

Take the following steps to perform mouth-to-mask ventilation [Nolan, 2012]:

1. Place the patient supine with their head in the sniffing position (neck slightly flexed and head extended)
2. Apply the mask to the patient's face using the thumbs of both hands
3. Grip the jaw and perform a jaw thrust, while pressing down with the thumbs to make a tight seal
4. Blow gently for 1 second through the valve and watch the chest rise
5. Stop inflation and watch the chest fall
6. Repeat every 6 seconds or as instructed by the senior clinician

Leaks between the face and pocket mask can be reduced by increasing the jaw thrust, or changing finger position and pressure being applied. Oxygen, if available, should run at 10 l/min.

2.7.3 Bag-valve-mask ventilation

The bag-valve-mask (BVM) consists of a self-inflating bag, one-way valve and mask. Optionally, the mask can be removed and the bag-valve attached to other airway devices such as catheter mounts, supraglottic airway devices (SAD) and endotracheal tubes (see the ASSISTING THE PARAMEDIC: AIRWAY lesson in chapter 16).

When used without oxygen, it delivers room air (21% oxygen). This can be increased to 45% when high-flow oxygen is attached, but it should generally be used with a reservoir bag attached, as this can result in oxygen concentrations of around 85% (Figure 2.8) with oxygen supplied at 10 l/min [Nolan, 2012].

The BVM can be used by one person, but this requires considerable skill. Where possible, a two-person technique is generally recommended [Nolan, 2010].

Procedure – One-person ventilation

Take the following steps to perform BVM ventilation with one person [EEAST, 2014]:

1. Use appropriate personal protective equipment (PPE)
2. Choose the correct mask size, which should rest on the bridge of the nose to the chin
3. Prepare the BVM, by connecting the mask and high-flow oxygen. Ensure the reservoir bag is inflated
4. Position the mask onto the patient's face and ensure an adequate seal
5. Form a 'C' shape with the thumb and index finger and rest this on top of the mask; place the middle and ring fingers on the ridge of the jaw and the little finger behind the angle of the jaw (Figure 2.9)
6. Gently squeeze the bag just enough to see the chest rise.

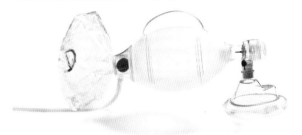

Figure 2.8 Bag-valve-mask with oxygen reservoir bag attached and inflated

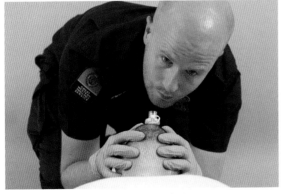

Figure 2.7 Mouth-to-mask ventilation

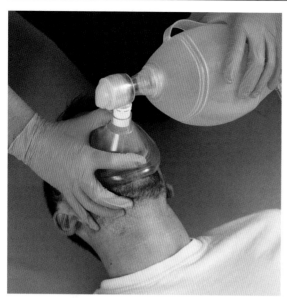

Figure 2.9 Correct hand position for one-person BVM use

Procedure – Two-person ventilation

This is the same as one-person, with the exception that another person holds the mask to the patient's face using the same method as for the pocket mask (Figure 2.10) [EEAST, 2014].

2.7.4 Mechanical ventilation

There are a wide variety of transport mechanical ventilators, so ensure that you are familiar with the one used by your ambulance service. One of the most commonly used ventilators in UK ambulance services is the Pneupac paraPAC ventilator (Figure 2.11); the instructions listed here apply to this ventilator, although the steps are likely to be similar with other ventilators.

Indications for the use of the ventilator will also depend on the service, but use will typically be restricted to patients who have a supraglottic device or endotracheal tube inserted, who are in respiratory or cardiac arrest and being transported to hospital [NEAS, 2014].

Procedure

Take the following steps to prepare a mechanical ventilator for use [EEAST, 2014]:

1. Connect to the gas supply and switch the main pneumatic switch to CMV/DEMAND
2. Allow the ventilator to complete a self-check for approximately 60 seconds
3. Ensure the pressure indicator shows O_2 (red – no supply, white – supply)
4. Set frequency and tidal volume (V_{TDEL}) controls for ADULT, CHILD or INFANT
5. Set air mix control to NO AIR MIX for respiratory arrest, CPR or in a contaminated atmosphere
6. Set relief pressure control to 40 cmH$_2$O and set the ventilation parameters to suit the patient
7. Temporarily occlude the patient connection to confirm the relief pressure and alarm function, and adjust if required
8. Connect the mask/ET tube in the correct manner
9. Check for air-tightness and adequate chest movement, and adjust the tidal volume as appropriate
10. Check the correctness of the indicated air pressure

- A high-pressure alarm may indicate an excessive tidal volume, incorrect airway position or kinked ET tube
- A low-pressure alarm may indicate a leakage or insufficient tidal volume

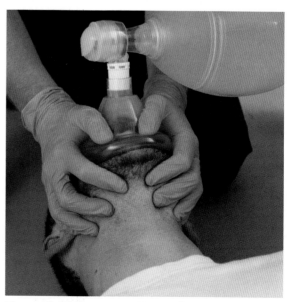

Figure 2.10 Two-person BVM technique

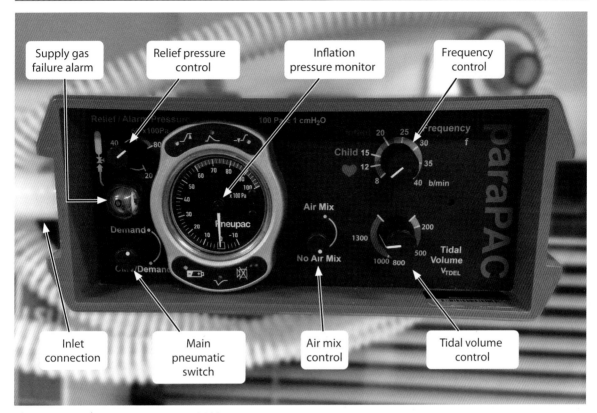

Figure 2.11 The Pneupac paraPac 200D

Schrader outlet

In order to connect a mechanical ventilator to the oxygen supply, you will need to use the Schrader outlet. In addition to being present on the integrated valve cylinders, there are usually several wall outlets on ambulances, though they may have a pressure-compensated flowmeter in place already (Figure 2.12). These flowmeters have a small ball inside a tube which rises or falls depending on the oxygen flow rate. Because they are affected by gravity, it is important that they remain upright.

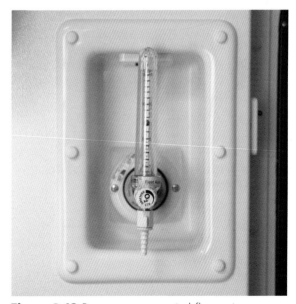

Figure 2.12 Pressure-compensated flowmeter attached to a Schrader outlet

Procedure

Take the following steps to prepare a pressure-compensated flowmeter for use [BOC, 2013a]:

1. Insert the oxygen probe into the Schrader outlet. Ensure the probe clicks securely into place

2. Slowly turn on the cylinder by rotating the handwheel anti-clockwise until it comes to a stop. Do not use excessive force

3. Check for leaks, which may be indicated by a hissing sound. If you suspect that you have a leak, turn off the cylinder and check the equipment is properly connected. Turn on the cylinder and re-check for leaks. If the leak continues, turn off and remove the cylinder from service. Report it using your ambulance service equipment defect procedure

2.7.5 Oxygen administration

The UK Ambulance Services Clinical Practice Guidelines [AACE, 2013] have divided oxygen administration for adults into four categories.

NOTE: Children are not included here. They should always receive high-concentration oxygen if they have a significant illness or injury. Follow the advice of your senior clinician.

Indications

- Critical illnesses requiring high levels of supplemental oxygen
- Serious illnesses requiring moderate levels of supplemental oxygen if the patient is hypoxaemic
- COPD and other conditions requiring controlled or low-dose oxygen therapy
- Conditions for which patients should be monitored closely but oxygen therapy is not required unless the patient is hypoxaemic.

Contra-indications (when not to administer the drug)

- Explosive environments.

Cautions

- Oxygen increases the fire hazard at the scene of an incident
- Defibrillation: Ensure pads are firmly applied to reduce spark hazard.

Side effects

- Non-humidified oxygen is drying and irritating to mucous membranes over a period of time
- In patients with COPD there is a risk that even moderately high doses of inspired oxygen can produce increased carbon dioxide levels, which may cause respiratory depression and this may lead to respiratory arrest.

Dosage and administration

- Measure oxygen saturation (SpO_2) in all patients using pulse oximetry
- For the administration of moderate levels of supplemental oxygen, nasal cannulae are recommended in preference to simple face masks as they offer a more flexible dose range
- Administer the initial oxygen dose until a reliable oxygen saturation reading is obtained
- If the desired oxygen saturation cannot be maintained with a simple face mask, change to a reservoir (non-rebreathe) mask
- For dosage and administration of supplemental oxygen, refer to Table 2.3 for patients with critical illnesses, Table 2.4 for serious illnesses and Table 2.5 for patients who need controlled or low-dose oxygen therapy
- For conditions where NO supplemental oxygen is required unless the patient is hypoxaemic, refer to Table 2.6.

Table 2.3: High levels of supplemental oxygen for adults with critical illnesses

Administer the initial oxygen dose until the vital signs are normal, then reduce oxygen dose and aim for target saturation within the range of **94–98%**

Condition	Initial dose	Method of Administration

• Cardiac arrest or resuscitation:
  • basic life support
  • advanced life support
  • foreign body airway obstruction
  • traumatic cardiac arrest
  • maternal resuscitation
• Carbon monoxide poisoning
	Maximum dose until vital signs are normal	Bag-valve-mask (BVM)

• Major trauma:
  • abdominal trauma
  • burns and scalds
  • electrocution
  • head trauma
  • limb trauma
  • neck and back trauma (spinal)
  • pelvic trauma
  • immersion
  • thoracic trauma
  • trauma in pregnancy
• Anaphylaxis
• Major pulmonary haemorrhage
• Sepsis e.g. meningococcal septicaemia
• Shock
	15 litres per minute	Non-rebreathe mask

• Active convulsion • Hypothermia	Administer 15 litres per minute until a reliable SpO_2 measurement can be obtained and then adjust oxygen flow to aim for target saturation within the range of 94–98%	Non-rebreathe mask

Table 2.4: Moderate levels of supplemental oxygen for adults with serious illnesses if the patient is hypoxaemic Administer the initial oxygen dose until a reliable SpO_2 measurement is available, then adjust oxygen flow to aim for target saturation within the range of **94–98%**

Condition	Initial dose	Method of administration
• Acute hypoxaemia (cause not yet diagnosed) • Deterioration of lung fibrosis or other interstitial lung disease • Acute asthma • Acute heart failure • Pneumonia • Lung cancer • Postoperative breathlessness • Pulmonary embolism • Pleural effusions • Pneumothorax • Severe anaemia • Sickle cell crisis	**SpO$_2$ < 85%** 10–15 l/min **SpO$_2$ 85–93%** 2–6 l/min **SpO$_2$ 85–93%** 5–10 l/min	Non-rebreathe mask Nasal cannulae Simple face mask

Table 2.5: Controlled or low dose supplemental oxygen for adults with COPD and other conditions requiring controlled or low-dose oxygen therapy Administer the initial oxygen dose until a reliable SpO_2 measurement is available, then adjust oxygen flow to aim for target saturation within the range of **88–92%** or pre-specified range of detailed on the patient's alert card

Condition	Initial dose	Method of administration
• Chronic obstructive pulmonary disease (COPD) • Exacerbation of cystic fibrosis	4 l/min Increase flow rate to 6 l/min if respiratory rate is >30 breaths/min (i.e. 50% above minimum specified for the mask)	28% Venturi mask (or patient's own)
• Chronic neuromuscular disorders • Chest wall disorders • Morbid obesity	4 l/min	28% Venturi mask (or patient's own)
NOTE: If the oxygen saturation remains below 88% change to simple face mask	5–10 l/min	Simple face mask
NOTE: Critical illness **AND** COPD or other risk factors for hypercapnia	As for Table 2.3	As for Table 2.3

Table 2.6: No supplemental oxygen required for adults with these conditions unless the patient is hypoxaemic but patients should be monitored closely if hypoxaemic
(SpO$_2$ < 94%) administer the initial oxygen dose, then adjust oxygen flow to aim for target saturation within the range of **94–98%**

Condition	Initial dose	Method of Administration

• Myocardial infarction and acute coronary syndromes
• Stroke
• Cardiac rhythm disturbance
• Non-traumatic chest pain/discomfort
• Implantable cardioverter defibrillator firing
• Pregnancy and obstetric emergencies:
  • birth imminent
  • haemorrhage during pregnancy
  • pregnancy-induced hypertension
  • vaginal bleeding
• Abdominal pain
• Headache
• Hyperventilation syndrome or dysfunctional breathing
• Most poisonings and drug overdoses (see Table 2.3 for carbon monoxide poisoning and special cases below for paraquat poisoning)
• Metabolic and renal disorders
• Acute and sub-acute neurological and muscular conditions producing muscle weakness (assess the need for assisted ventilation if SpO$_2$ <94%)
• Post convulsion
• Gastrointestinal bleeds
• Glycaemic emergencies
• Heat exhaustion/heat stroke
SPECIAL CASES
Poisoning with paraquat:
Patients with paraquat poisoning may be harmed by supplemental oxygen so avoid oxygen unless the patient is hypoxaemic.
Target saturation **88–92%**.
	SpO$_2$ < 85%
	10–15 l/min
	SpO$_2$ 85–93%
	2–6 l/min
	SpO$_2$ 85–93%
	5–10 l/min
		Non-rebreathe mask
		
		Nasal cannulae
		
		Simple face mask

2.7.6 **After use**

Procedure

Once you have finished administering oxygen to a patient, take the following steps [BOC, 2013a]:

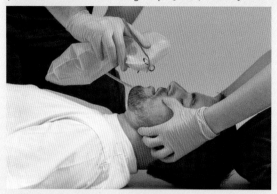

1. Remove the mask or nasal cannula from the patient

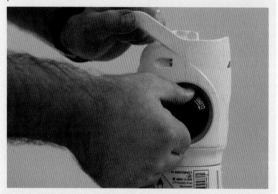

2. Turn off the cylinder by rotating the handwheel clockwise until it comes to a stop. Do not use excessive force

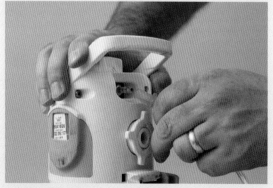

3a. Disconnect equipment. Remove the tubing by firmly pulling the tube while holding the cylinder handle

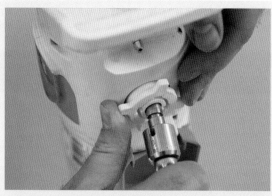

3b. If you have used the Schrader valve, release by twisting the capstan clockwise

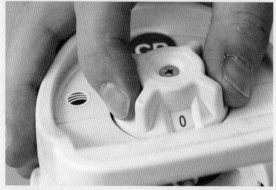

4. Turn the flow selector to zero

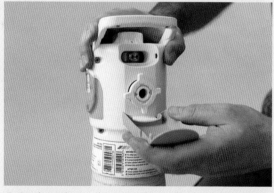

5. Replace the outlet cover by pulling up the hinged grey cover

Procedure continued →

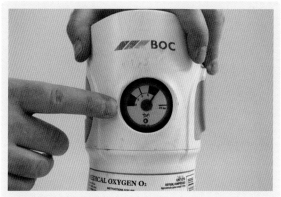

6. Check the cylinder gauge and replace if necessary

2.8 Entonox

Entonox is a combination of 50% nitrous oxide and 50% oxygen. The cylinders that contain entonox have a blue and white collar (Figure 2.13).

Procedure – Preparing entonox administration set

Take the following steps to prepare entonox for administration [BOC, 2013b]:

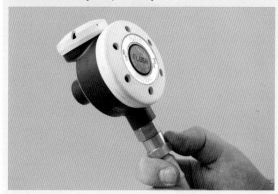

1. Ensure the demand valve is clean and ready for use

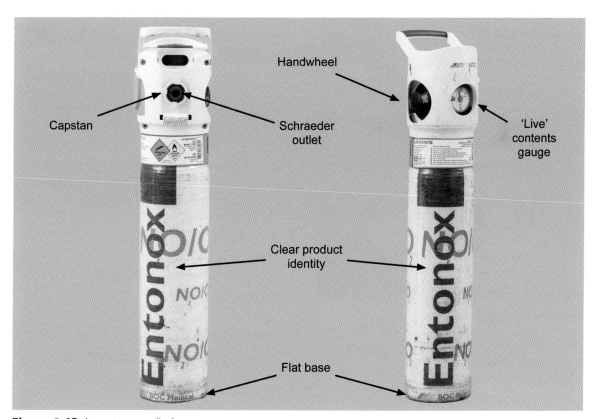

Figure 2.13 An entonox cylinder

Procedure continued →

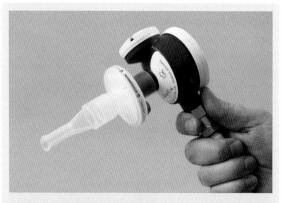

2. Fit a new microbial filter to the demand valve. They are single use

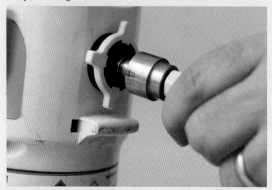

3. Insert the probe on the hose connected to the demand valve into the Schrader outlet on the entonox cylinder. Push firmly to ensure the probe clicks into place

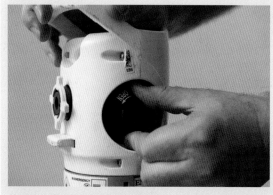

4. Slowly turn the cylinder on by rotating the handwheel anti-clockwise until fully open. Do not use excessive force

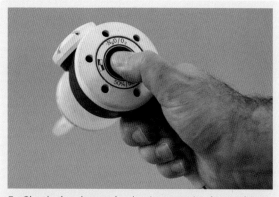

5. Check the demand valve is operative by pushing the 'test button'. You should hear the gas flowing

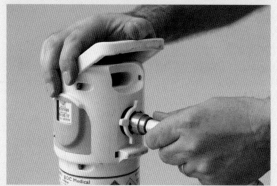

6. Check for leaks which maybe indicated by a hissing sound. If you suspect that you have a leak, turn off the cylinder and check the equipment is properly connected. Turn on the cylinder and re-check for leaks. If the leak continues, turn off and remove the cylinder from service. Report it using your ambulance service equipment defect procedure

2.8.1 **Entonox administration**
The UK Ambulance Services Clinical Practice Guidelines [AACE, 2013] for entonox administration are as follows:

Indications
• Moderate to severe pain
• Labour pains.

Actions
• Inhaled analgesic agent.

Contra-indications
• Severe head injuries with impaired consciousness
• Decompression sickness (the bends) where entonox can cause nitrogen bubbles within the bloodstream to expand, aggravating the

problem further. Consider anyone that has been diving within the previous 24 hours to be at risk

- Violently disturbed psychiatric patients.

Cautions

- Any patient at risk of having a pneumothorax, pneumomediastinum and/or a pneumoperitoneum e.g. polytrauma, penetrating torso injury.

Side effects

- Minimal side effects.

Dosage and administration
Adults:

- Entonox should be self-administered via a facemask or mouthpiece, after suitable instruction. It takes about 3–5 minutes to be effective, but it may be 5–10 minutes before maximum effect is achieved.

Children:

- Entonox is effective in children provided they are capable of following the administration instructions and can activate the demand valve.

Additional information

- Administration of entonox should be in conjunction with pain score monitoring.
- Entonox's advantages include:
  - Rapid analgesic effect with minimal side effects
  - No cardio-respiratory depression
  - Self-administered
  - Analgesic effect rapidly wears off
  - The 50% oxygen concentration is valuable in many medical and trauma conditions
- Entonox can be administered while preparing to deliver other analgesics.

2.8.2 After use

Procedure

Take the following steps once the patient has finished using the entonox [BOC, 2013b]:

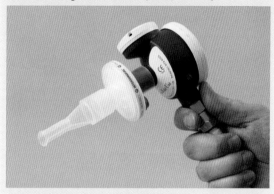

1. Remove the demand valve from the patient. Dispose of the filter and mouthpiece

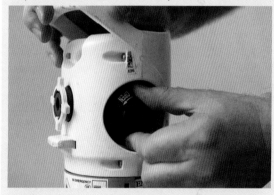

2. Turn off the cylinder by rotating the handwheel clockwise until it comes to a stop. Do not use excessive force

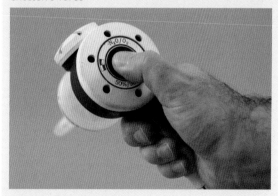

3. Vent any residual gas in the hose by pressing the test button on the demand valve. Keep pressing until the gas has stopped venting

Procedure continued →

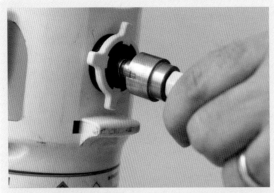

4. Disconnect the probe from the cylinder outlet. Holding the probe, twist the capstan and withdraw the probe from the Schrader outlet

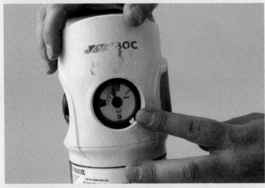

5. Replace the outlet cover by pulling up the hinged grey cover. Check the cylinder gauge and replace if empty

3 Assessment of breathing

3.1 Learning objectives

By the end of this lesson you will be able to:
- Record the following observations:
  - Respiratory rate
  - Oxygen saturations
  - Peak flow
  - Capnography
- Describe how to auscultate the chest.

3.2 Respiratory rate

A normal adult respiratory rate is 12–20 breaths per minute (breaths/min) [Nolan, 2012].

The respiratory rate is often overlooked as an important vital sign, but in adults, respiratory rates of 25 breaths/min or more are an indicator of serious illness and a warning that your patient may deteriorate quickly [Smith, 2011a; BTS,

2008]. Patients with a respiratory rate of less than 10 breaths/min or more than 30 breaths/min may need assisted ventilations, so inform your senior clinician immediately [AACE, 2013].

Measuring respiratory rate

How fast are you breathing now? Before considering this question, it is likely that you weren't even thinking about your respiratory rate. So it is with patients. Don't tell them that you are going to record their respiratory rate!

Ideally, you want to measure your patient's respiratory rate for a full minute using one of the following techniques [Gregory, 2010b]:
- Watching the chest rise and fall
- Counting the respiratory rate while listening to the chest with a stethoscope
- Using an oxygen mask with an integral respiratory rate indicator (Figure 3.1).

3.3 Oxygen saturations

Most oxygen is transported around the body bound to haemoglobin in the blood, as it travels from the lungs to the body's tissues. When haemoglobin has oxygen molecules attached, it is called oxyhaemoglobin. Oxygen saturation is the ratio of oxyhaemoglobin to the total amount of haemoglobin and is usually shown as a percentage [Tortora, 2008].

Oxygen saturations are measured in two ways: invasively and non-invasively. In hospital, it is common for patients to have an arterial blood gas sample taken, whereby a small amount of blood from an artery (often the radial) is taken and the arterial oxygen saturation measured (SaO_2). However, this is not practical to undertake

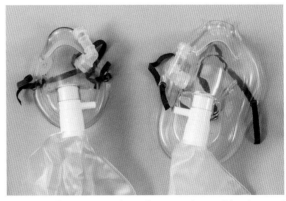

Figure 3.1 Non-rebreathe masks with integral respiratory rate indicator

outside of hospital, so oxygen saturations are measured non-invasively using a technique known as pulse oximetry (SpO$_2$) [Gregory, 2010b].

Pulse oximetry

Pulse oximetry works by shining red and infrared light through a part of the body that is relatively translucent and has an arterial pulse, such as a finger, toe or earlobe. The amount of light transmitted through the tissue depends on the amount of oxyhaemoglobin present; this enables the pulse oximeter to calculate the oxygen saturation and will also provide the pulse rate [Pilbery, 2013].

If you refer back to the oxygen guideline, you will see that the target oxygen saturation for most patients is 94–98%, and in a normal, healthy person oxygen saturations should be 95% and above [Pilbery, 2013].

3.3.1 Indications and limitations

Indications

Pulse oximetry is useful for [Gregory, 2010b; Walls, 2012]:

- Assessing severity of respiratory illness or injury
- Providing early warning of a patient who is deteriorating
- Providing feedback about the effectiveness of oxygen therapy
- Detecting pulses in limbs which have been fractured.

Limitations

Like any tool, the pulse oximeter can produce inaccurate results, particularly in the presence of the following [Pilbery, 2013; Walls, 2012]:

- Bright ambient light: Simple to solve with a towel over the probe
- Excessive patient motion: Such as shivering, convulsions or a bumpy ambulance ride
- Poor perfusion: Since the pulse oximeter requires an arterial pulse to work, conditions that result in poor peripheral perfusion can lead to problems. Examples include patients in shock, cardiac arrest and who are cold
- Nail varnish/polish: Some dark-coloured nail varnish can affect the accuracy of pulse oximeters, although this is not likely to be too serious. Finger probes can be rotated 90° if this is a worry, but if a reliable and consistent

reading is being obtained through nail varnish, then the reading is probably accurate [Chan, 2003; Hinkelbein, 2007].

- Low blood pressure: Pulse oximetry becomes more inaccurate as the systolic blood pressure drops below 80 mmHg
- Abnormal haemoglobin: Other molecules can attach themselves to haemoglobin and create an artificially high oxygen saturation reading. Carbon monoxide is probably the most well known, so don't be reassured by a high oxygen saturation in a patient who is a victim of smoke inhalation, for example
- Response time: Pulse oximetry is not instantaneous; typically, a reading can take up to 20 seconds depending upon the patient's physiological state. Probes closer to the heart (such as one sited on an earlobe) usually respond faster than probes on fingers and toes.

3.3.2 Recording oxygen saturations

Procedure

Take the following steps to record a patient's oxygen saturations [WHO, 2011]:

1. Turn the pulse oximeter on
2. Select the appropriate probe with particular attention to correct sizing and where it will go (usually the finger, toe or ear). If used on a finger or toe, make sure the area is clean. Consider removing nail varnish, or rotate the probe 90°
3. Connect the probe to the pulse oximeter
4. Position the probe carefully; make sure it fits easily without being too loose or too tight. If possible, avoid the arm being used for blood pressure monitoring as cuff inflation will interrupt the pulse oximeter signal
5. Allow several seconds for the pulse oximeter to detect the pulse and calculate the oxygen saturation
6. Look for the displayed pulse indicator that shows that the machine has detected a pulse. Without a pulse signal, any readings are not reliable
7. Once the unit has detected a good pulse, the oxygen saturation and pulse rate will be displayed
8. Like all machines, oximeters may occasionally give a false reading – if in doubt, rely on clinical judgement, rather than the machine
9. If in doubt, check the pulse oximeter is working properly by placing it on your own finger.

3.4 Peak flow

The measurement of the peak expiratory flow rate (PEFR), or peak flow, is common in patients with obstructive airways diseases such as asthma and chronic obstructive pulmonary disease (COPD). You should record an asthmatic patient's peak flow before and after treatment, assuming they are capable of undertaking the technique (Figure 3.2) [AACE, 2013].

3.4.1 Procedure

Procedure

Take the following steps to record a peak flow [CCI, 2011; Booker, 2007]:

1. Explain the procedure to the patient before starting and ask if they know what their normal or best peak flow value is. You can use the normal value chart (Figure 3.3), but a comparison with the patient's usual value is better.

2. Insert the mouthpiece into the meter (these are single patient use)

3. Ask the patient to hold the peak flow meter with their fingers clear of the scale and slot. Ensure that the holes at the end of the meter are not blocked

4. With the patient in a standing, or upright sitting, position, ask them to take a deep breath

5. Ask them to place the peak flow meter in their mouth and hold horizontally, closing their lips around the mouthpiece before blowing as hard and fast as they can. This should be a short, sharp 'huff'

6. Note the number on the scale indicated by the pointer

7. Return the pointer to zero and repeat steps 3–6 twice to obtain three readings

8. The patient's peak flow is the highest of the three readings.

Common errors in recording a peak flow measurement

- Failure to take a deep breath
- The patient holding their breath and not expiring into the flow meter straight away
- Blocking the mouthpiece with the teeth or tongue
- Air leaking around the mouthpiece due to blowing the cheeks out, loose-fitting teeth or facial palsy.

3.5 Capnography

In the RESPIRATORY SYSTEM PHYSIOLOGY lesson, you learnt that carbon dioxide (CO_2) is a waste gas that is expired. It is a normal byproduct of body metabolism, and the quantity expired is dependent on metabolism, venous return to the heart and the pulmonary circulation (carrying blood to, from and around the lungs). Expired CO_2 can provide an insight into all three of these.

Terminology

A number of terms are related to expired CO_2 monitoring, and these are sometimes used incorrectly, which can cause confusion. These are:

Capnography: The measurement of carbon dioxide in exhaled breath

Capnometry: A numerical measurement of exhaled carbon dioxide. Usually this is the amount of expired CO_2 at the end of expiration and is known as the end-tidal CO_2 ($EtCO_2$)

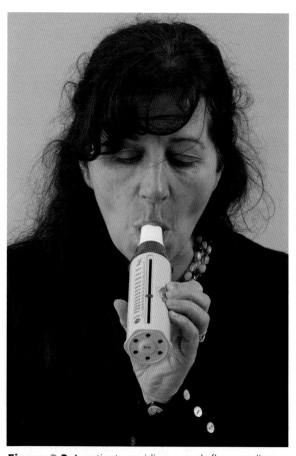

Figure 3.2 A patient providing a peak flow reading

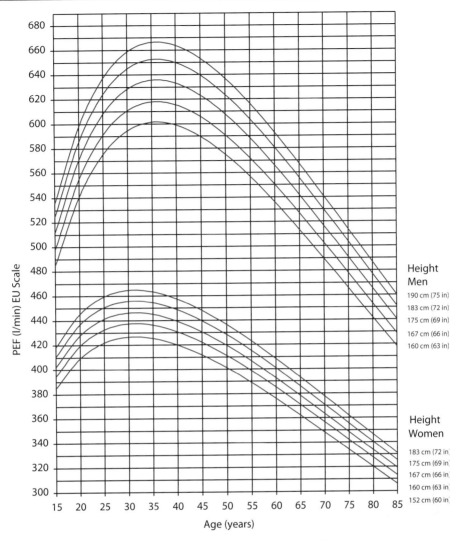

Adapted by Clement Clarke for use with EN13826 / EU scale peak flow meters
from Nunn AJ Gregg I, Br Med J 1989:298;1068–70

Figure 3.3 Normal adult peak flow values
Image reproduced by the kind permission of Clement Clarke International.

Capnogram: A wave form illustrating the measurement of carbon dioxide across time and with a height corresponding to the quantity of carbon dioxide exhaled.

Uses for capnography

The ability to measure $EtCO_2$ has a number of uses in the ambulance service including [Helm, 2003; Burton, 2006; Pokorná, 2010]:

- Preventing hyper- and hypo-ventilation of head-injured patients
- Giving early warning of respiratory distress or failure in patients who have received sedative

drugs (such as epileptic patients who have been given diazepam by paramedics)
- Indicating the correct positioning of an endotracheal tube or supraglottic airway device
- Indicating a return of spontaneous circulation (ROSC) of a patient who has been in cardiac arrest.

3.6 Auscultation

Auscultation is the technique of listening to the sounds inside the body, most commonly with the help of a stethoscope.

The stethoscope

In 1816, René-Théophile-Hyacinthe Laennec needed to examine the chest of a young woman. Since the technique of listening for breath sounds at the time consisted of placing your ear on the patient's chest, a practice then, as now, generally frowned upon if your patient is a young woman, he rolled up some paper into a tube and discovered that he could hear the woman's heart sounds much more clearly than by direct auscultation [Thadepalli, 2002].

With experimentation, he developed his discovery into a wooden cylinder, which he called a stethoscope. Many of the terms in use today in relation to breath sounds came from Laennec, including pectoriloquy, crepitation (now more commonly called crackles) and rub. Laennec's wooden stethoscope design continued to be used until the mid-19th century, when rubber tubing was developed. However, not until 1925 did the bell and diaphragm design, typically found in modern stethoscopes, come into use after being developed by Bowles and Sprague (Figure 3.4) [Roguin, 2006].

3.6.1 Breath sounds

There are broadly two types of breath sounds you will hear on auscultation: normal and added (or adventitious).

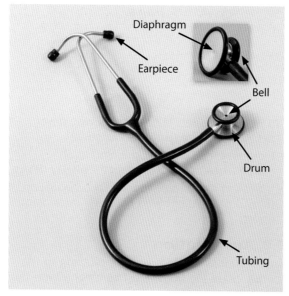

Figure 3.4 A stethoscope

Normal breath sounds

These sounds are caused by turbulent airflow in large airways and are loudest at the trachea at the start of inspiration, and quietest at the end of inspiration, as airflow decreases. If you auscultate elsewhere on the chest, the sound diminishes as it passes through the lung tissue and the chest wall itself [Macleod, 2005]. Normal breath sounds are often split into three sub-types:

- Vesicular: These are soft and low-pitched and can be heard throughout inspiration and the first third of expiration [Bickley, 2006]. They have been described as the sound of wind rustling through leaves [Talley, 2006]
- Bronchial: These breath sounds have a high-pitched and hollow or blowing quality, similar to the sound you hear by placing a stethoscope over the trachea. Bronchial breath sounds are similar in duration during both inspiration and expiration, with a gap in between as airflow slows prior to changing direction. These are typically heard over lung tissue that has been affected by pneumonia [Macleod, 2005]
- Bronchovesicular: This is one for the fence sitters, as these breath sounds are louder than vesicular, but quieter than bronchial sounds. Inspiratory and expiratory duration is typically the same, but unlike bronchial sounds, there may not be a gap between the two. These sounds are usually the result of fluid-filled or consolidated lung tissue [Bickley, 2006].

Added (adventitious) sounds

There are two types of added sounds: crackles and wheezes.

- Crackles: These are interrupted, non-musical sounds, formerly called rales or crepitations [Talley, 2006]. Usually, they are caused by the re-opening of collapsed alveoli and small bronchi. The timing and pitch of crackles can provide clues as to the cause. For example, early inspiratory crackles that are rather coarse in quality suggest small airways disease and are common in chronic obstructive pulmonary disease (COPD) [Piirilä, 1995]
  - Fine crackles that occur late in inspiration are typically caused by pulmonary fibrosis, whereas coarser crackles late in inspiration are more suggestive of left-sided heart failure

- Crackles can also be heard when air bubbles through secretions in the major bronchi, or the dilated bronchi of bronchiectasis. These are usually very coarse, may be heard without a stethoscope and will typically resolve or change location on coughing [Buss, 2010].
- Wheezes: These are continuous, musical sounds that are caused by air passing through partially obstructed bronchi and are normally only heard on expiration. They can be localised (e.g. in cancer of the lung) or diffuse, as is typical in asthma. Note that wheeze on inspiration is generally taken to be a significant sign of airway narrowing [Macleod, 2005]. Wheezes can be monophasic, that is at a single pitch (which used to be called rhonchi), or polyphonic, i.e. more musical, due to the sound being produced at different pitches
  - One type of loud monophasic (and usually) inspiratory wheeze that can be heard without a stethoscope is stridor. This is caused by laryngeal spasm and mucosal swelling, which causes vocal cord contraction and airway narrowing [Buss, 2010].

Absent sounds

Breath sounds are decreased or absent when airflow is limited. This can be due to low inspiratory airflow rates, which generate less turbulent flow required to produce sound. Air or fluid in the pleural space (due to a pneumothorax or pleural effusion, for example) can increase the acoustic impedance and filter or stop transmission of breath sounds to the chest wall. This also occurs at the chest wall itself, if there is an excessive amount of adipose tissue [Buss, 2010].

3.6.2 Auscultating the chest

Procedure

Ideally, you should expose the patient's chest to perform auscultation, but this will depend on whether you can ensure privacy and adequate environmental heating (such as a warm ambulance). Ensure that you inform the patient about what the procedure involves and obtain consent.
Then take the following steps [Gregory, 2010b]:

1. Ask the patient to take deep breaths in and out through their mouth
2. Place the diaphragm on the chest, starting above the clavicle. If the patient is very slim or has a hairy chest, use the bell instead

3. Listen during inspiration and expiration, before moving the stethoscope to another area of the chest
4. After each breath, move the stethoscope to the opposite side of the chest to compare each part of the lung fields. Listen to anterior (Figure 3.5), posterior (Figure 3.6) and lateral (Figure 3.7) aspects of the chest for normal and adventitious breath sounds.

Hints

It may be helpful to coach the patient to breathe using "in ... and out".

Avoid long periods of deep breathing as it may cause dizziness. Patients who are short of breath may not be able to comply with your instructions.

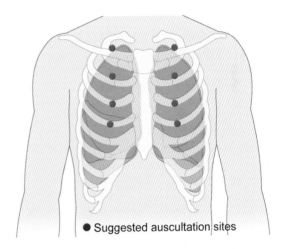

Figure 3.5 Auscultation sites of the chest: anterior

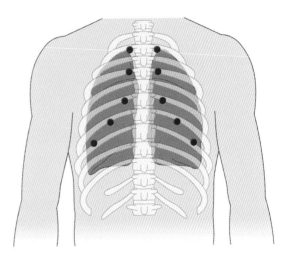

Figure 3.6 Auscultation sites of the chest: posterior

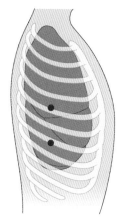

● Suggested auscultation sites

Figure 3.7 Auscultation sites of the chest: lateral

4 Common respiratory conditions

4.1 Learning objectives

By the end of this lesson you will be able to:
- Describe the following conditions of the respiratory system:
  - Asthma
  - Chronic obstructive pulmonary disease (COPD)
  - Pneumonia
  - Pulmonary embolism.

4.2 Asthma

Definition

Asthma is a condition characterised by intermittent, reversible, airway obstruction [Simon, 2010].

Pathophysiology

Asthma is caused by a chronic inflammation of the bronchi, making them narrower. The muscles around the bronchi become irritated and contract, causing sudden worsening of the symptoms. The inflammation can also cause the mucus glands to produce excessive sputum which further blocks the air passages.

The obstruction and subsequent wheezing are caused by three factors within the bronchial tree:
- Increased production of bronchial mucus
- Swelling of the bronchial tube mucosal lining cells
- Spasm and constriction of bronchial muscles.

These three factors combine to cause blockage and narrowing of the small airways in the lung. Because inspiration is an active process involving the muscles of respiration, the obstruction of the airways is overcome on breathing in. Expiration occurs with muscle relaxation, and is severely delayed by the narrowing of the airways in asthma. This generates the wheezing on expiration that is characteristic of this condition.

Medication

Asthma is managed with a variety of inhaled and tablet medications. Inhalers are divided into two broad categories: preventer and reliever.

Preventer

The preventer inhalers are normally anti-inflammatory drugs and these include steroids and other milder anti-inflammatories such as Tilade. The common steroid inhalers are beclomethasone (Becotide), budesonide (Pulmicort) and fluticasone (Flixotide). These drugs act on the lung over a period of time to reduce the inflammatory reaction that causes the asthma. Regular use of these inhalers often eradicates all symptoms of asthma and allows for a normal lifestyle.

Reliever

The reliever inhalers include salbutamol (Ventolin), terbutaline (Bricanyl), tiotropium (Spiriva) and ipratropium bromide (Atrovent). These inhalers work rapidly on the lung to relax the smooth muscle spasm when the patient feels wheezy or tight-chested. They are used in conjunction with preventer inhalers. Inhalers are often used through large plastic spacer devices (Figure 4.1). This allows the drug to spread into a larger volume and enables the patient to inhale it more effectively. In mild and moderate asthma attacks some patients may be treated with high doses of 'relievers' through a spacer device. This has been shown to be as effective as giving a salbutamol nebuliser [BTS, 2012].

4.2.1 Signs and symptoms

History

Patients will typically tell you about increasing shortness of breath with wheezing over the past 6–48 hours, with increasing inhaler use. The reliever inhalers may also be proving less effective than normal.

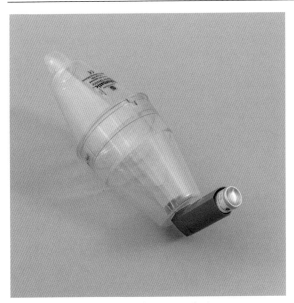

Figure 4.1 An inhaler with spacer device

Ask specifically about:

- Repeated attendances at ED for asthma care in the past year
- Previous admissions for asthma
- Previous near-fatal asthma, e.g. previously required ventilation/intensive care
- Heavy use of reliever inhalers
- Brittle asthma.

Signs and symptoms

The signs and symptoms of asthma are organised according to their severity [BTS, 2012].

Near-fatal asthma

- Patients requiring assisted ventilation with high inflation pressures.

Life-threatening asthma

Any one of the following in a patient with severe asthma:

- Altered level of consciousness
- Exhaustion
- Hypotension
- Cyanosis
- Silent chest
- Poor respiratory effort
- Peak flow less than 33% of best or predicted
- SpO_2 less than 92%.

Acute severe asthma

Any one of the following:

- Peak flow 33–50% of best or predicted
- Respiratory rate of 25 breaths/min or more
- Heart rate of 110 beats/min or more
- Inability to complete sentences in one breath.

Moderate asthma

- Increasing symptoms
- Peak flow over 50–75% of best or predicted
- No features of acute severe asthma.

4.2.2 Management

The management of asthma attacks is tailored to their severity.

Moderate asthma

- Move patient to a calm, quiet environment
- Encourage use of the patient's own inhaler, ideally via a spacer device. The correct technique is for the patient to take two puffs, followed by two puffs every two minutes up to 10 puffs
- If the peak flow is over 50–75% of best or predicted:
  - Oxygen-driven nebuliser with 5mg salbutamol
  - Oral steroids
  - If final on-scene peak flow is over 75% of best or predicted, your senior clinician may elect to leave the patient at home with a course of steroids, or refer the patient to their own GP or an advanced paramedic.

Severe asthma

- These patients will receive oxygen-powered nebulisers (which may be repeated) and steroids (usually intravenously).

Life-threatening asthma

- These patients will receive the same treatment as for severe asthma, but with the addition of intramuscular adrenaline.

Near-fatal asthma

- As respiration fails, patients may require assisted ventilation with a bag-valve-mask. Nebulisation can continue with the use of a T-piece, which keeps the nebuliser chamber vertical (Figure 4.2)

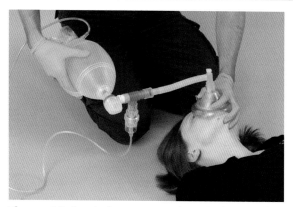

Figure 4.2 A nebuliser connected to a T-piece to allow nebulising of a supine patient

4.3 Chronic obstructive pulmonary disease

Definitions

Chronic obstructive pulmonary disease (COPD) is an umbrella term for a range of respiratory diseases that result in airflow obstruction. This obstruction is usually progressive and, unlike asthma, is not fully reversible and does not change markedly over several months [NICE, 2010].

It is estimated that there are around 3.7 million people with COPD in the United Kingdom (UK), but only 90,000 have been diagnosed. COPD kills about 30,000 people a year in the UK, making it the fifth biggest killer [BLF, 2007].

The two most important respiratory diseases related to COPD are chronic bronchitis and emphysema. Emphysema is a permanent enlargement of the air spaces below the terminal bronchioles as a result of the destruction of the alveolar walls. Chronic bronchitis, on the other hand, is defined clinically as a persistent cough with sputum production for at least 3 months of the year for two consecutive years [Patel, 2008].

Pathophysiology
COPD

The most important causative factor in chronic bronchitis and emphysema is smoking, although only 15% of smokers develop COPD [Patel, 2008]. The general effects of smoking in COPD are:

• Inflammation resulting from activation of inflammatory cells, which release substances that trigger an immune system response. This activates enzymes that can damage lung tissue, although normally these are kept in check. However, in COPD, so many enzymes are produced that they overwhelm the neutralising mechanism, and lung tissue is digested and destroyed. This is thought to be particularly important in the development of emphysema

• Inflammation as a direct result of inhaling oxidants in the cigarette smoke (you may have heard of free radicals) which damage the cells directly

• Both of these mechanisms lead to alveolar destruction and production of excess mucus, which is made worse by the impairment of the respiratory cilia, hair-like projections that line the airways and move debris and mucus upwards and out of the respiratory tract [Tortora, 2008].

Chronic bronchitis

Cigarette smoking, occupational exposure and/or recurrent bronchial infections leads to inflammation that narrows the airways, and increase in mucus secretions coupled with inhibition of the cilia, which leads to accumulation of secretions and bronchoconstriction due to irritant receptor activation, which also causes the chronic productive cough [Patel, 2008].

Emphysema

In emphysema, the walls of the alveoli are destroyed by enzymes called proteases. These are usually kept under control by another group of enzymes imaginatively called anti-proteases. Once the balance is upset (due to smoking, for example) destruction of the alveoli occurs, leading to a collapse of the airways, resulting in obstruction. In addition, as the walls of the alveoli are destroyed, bullae (small, blister-like air pockets) form on the lung. If these bullae form, air can directly enter the pleural cavity, causing a pneumothorax and collapse of the lung on the affected side [Patel, 2008].

4.3.1 Oxygen and COPD

Research studies and audits suggest that over-oxygenation increases mortality and morbidity, but careful pre-hospital titration of oxygen administration to patients with COPD can significantly reduce mortality [Austin, 2010].

The most significant effect of hyperoxia (excessive oxygen) on the respiratory system is hypercapnic respiratory failure in vulnerable populations (such as patients with severe COPD). This can occur even with a partial pressure of arterial oxygen (PaO_2) within normal or near-normal values. It is thought that there are a number of mechanisms that are responsible [O'Driscoll, 2008].

Hypercapnia in exacerbation of COPD is not universal. Some patients have repeated hypercapnic respiratory failure, whereas others may not. Even in COPD patients with chronic respiratory failure, not all will develop high partial pressures of carbon dioxide and acidosis during acute exacerbations.

4.3.2 Signs and symptoms

Patients will usually call for an ambulance during an exacerbation of COPD. Their clinical presentation will depend on which of the two diseases (chronic bronchitis or emphysema) is more dominant. In reality, most patients will have elements of both, but Table 4.1 shows the two ends of the spectrum of illness.

Table 4.1: Chronic bronchitis vs emphysema

	Chronic bronchitis	Emphysema
Also known as	Blue bloater	Pink puffer
Hyperinflated chest	Yes	Yes
Body size	Obese	Thin
Cyanosis	Yes, centrally	No
Blood levels of CO_2	High	Low

Features of an acute exacerbation of COPD include [AACE, 2013]:

- Increased dyspnoea
- Increased sputum production/purulence (containing pus)
- Increased cough
- Upper airway symptoms, such as cold and sore throat
- Increased wheeze

- Reduced exercise tolerance
- Fluid retention
- Increased fatigue
- Acute confusion.

Features that warn of a severe episode of COPD include [AACE, 2013]:

- Marked dyspnoea
- Tachypnoea
- Purse-lip breathing
- Use of accessory muscles
- New-onset cyanosis
- New-onset peripheral oedema
- Marked reduction in activities of daily living.

Despite the lists above, it is not always clear that the patient with difficulty breathing has COPD and only 35% of patients will tell you that they have COPD [Durrington, 2005]. Therefore you should consider this as a possibility for any patient who meets the following criteria [NICE, 2010]:

- Over 35 years of age
- Smoker (or ex-smoker)
- Have any of:
  - Exertional breathlessness
  - Chronic cough
  - Regular sputum production
  - Wheeze
- Have no clinical features of asthma.

4.3.3 Management

The management of the patient with COPD depends on the presence of any time-critical features:

- Major ABCD problems
- Extreme breathing difficulty (compared to normal)
- Cyanosis (although peripheral cyanosis can be normal)
- Exhaustion
- Hypoxia unresponsive to oxygen (in COPD patients hypoxia is considered to be an SpO_2 below 88%).

These patients require a blue-light transfer to the nearest emergency department and may also require suction, airway management and assisted ventilation. Follow the advice of your senior clinician [AACE, 2013].

For patients with no time-critical features, you should ask if they have a treatment plan and follow this, if available. Treatments typically include [AACE, 2013]:

- Oxygen: Target range of 88–92%. Venturi masks are a good choice for delivering accurate percentages of oxygen, although nasal cannulae may be better tolerated by patients. If you are using a Venturi mask and the patient's respiratory rate is greater than 30 breaths/min, remember to increase the recommended flow rate by 50%. So if the flow rate should be set at 4 l/min, then increase this to 6 l/min
- Bronchodilators: Salbutamol and ipratropium (once only). If the nebuliser is powered by oxygen, nebulisation should be limited to six minutes
- Patients may need taking to hospital, but depending on how well they respond to treatment, they may be suitable for referral to their GP, respiratory team or advanced paramedic.

4.4 Pneumonia

Definition

Pneumonia is an infection of the terminal bronchioles and alveoli (lung parenchyma) [Patel, 2008]. It is more common in the elderly and during the winter months [Simon, 2010].

It is often classified in three main ways, although the first is the most commonly used [Dunn, 2005; Osler, 2012]:

- Setting: i.e. hospital or community acquired pneumonia
- Anatomy: Lobar, if the infection is localised to a lobe of the lung, or bronchopneumonia if the infection is more widespread
- Organism: Bacterial, viral, fungal.

Risk factors for community acquired pneumonia (CAP)

These are factors that undermine the lung's natural defences and so increase the risk of pneumonia [Patel, 2008]:

- Excessive alcohol
- Cigarette smoking
- Chronic heart and lung diseases
- Bronchial obstruction
- Immunosuppression (e.g. due to chemotherapy for cancer)
- Drug abuse.

Pathophysiology

This inflammatory process is typically due to a bacterial or viral infection, which has usually entered the lungs having been inhaled from the environment or nasopharynx. Normally, these organisms should be destroyed by the body's lung defences, but if they survive and multiply, infection results. This leads to a build up of fluid and blood cells (red and white) in the alveoli, known as consolidation [Porth, 2003].

4.4.1 Signs and symptoms

When taking a history, the following symptoms are suggestive of pneumonia [Johnson, 2012]:

- Fever with or without rigors
- Cough (often productive with green, blood-stained or rusty-coloured sputum)
- Pleuritic chest pain
- Muscle or joint pain

When examining a patient you may notice the following signs:

- High temperature (pyrexia)
- Increased respiratory rate (tachypnoea)
- Increased heart rate (tachycardia)
- Chest sounds such as those shown in Figure 4.3.

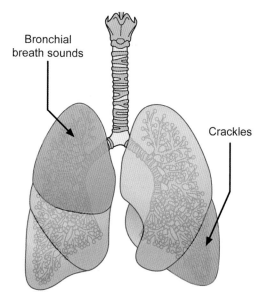

Bronchial breath sounds

Crackles

Figure 4.3 Breath sounds in the patient with pneumonia

4.4.2 **Management**

Not all patients with pneumonia need to go to hospital. Patients who score a zero on the CRB-65 severity score may be able to be managed at home [BTS, 2010].

CRB-65 severity score

Patients score one point for each of the following:

- Confusion
- Respiratory rate of 30 breaths/min or greater
- Blood pressure (BP): Systolic BP less than 90 mmHg or diastolic BP 60 mmHg or lower
- Age: 65 years of age or older.

You must also consider their social circumstances and home support provision if these patients are to be left at home.

Depending on local arrangements, your senior clinician may refer patients to their own GP for antibiotics or to an advanced practitioner in the ambulance service.

Advice

If patients are to remain at home, they should be advised not to smoke, to rest and to drink plenty of fluids. Pleuritic pain can be managed with simple analgesia such as paracetamol.

Transport

Any patient who scores 3 or more on the CRB-65 severity score should go to hospital. Treatment is supportive and patients should be given oxygen if their SpO_2 is below 94% [AACE, 2013].

4.5 **Pulmonary embolism**

Definitions

An embolus is a blood-borne substance (including air) that is transported from one part of the circulation to another, lodging in a vessel which is too small to allow the embolus to pass. When the embolus lodges in the pulmonary vessels, it is termed a pulmonary embolism (PE) [Patel, 2008]. Deep vein thrombosis (DVT) and pulmonary embolism represent the spectrum of one disease known as venous thromboembolism (VTE) [Tapson, 2008]. Although an embolus can consist of air, fat, or amniotic fluid, for example, the most common is a clot from a DVT [Porth, 2003; Torbicki, 2008].

Risk factors

The risk factors for developing a venous thromboembolism are well known and can help to identify patients who may have a PE [Torbicki, 2008]:

- High risk
  - Fracture (hip or leg)
  - Major general surgery
  - Major trauma
  - Spinal cord injury
- Moderate risk
  - Chronic heart or respiratory failure
  - Chemotherapy
  - Hormone replacement therapy
  - Cancer
  - Oral contraceptive therapy
  - Paralytic stroke
  - Post-partum
  - Previous VTE
  - Thrombophillia
- Low risk
  - Bed rest for more than 3 days
  - Immobility due to sitting (e.g. prolonged car or air travel)
  - Increasing age
  - Obesity
  - Pregnancy
  - Varicose veins.

Pathophysiology

Thrombi (blood clots) most often form in the deep veins of the calf (hence the name, deep vein thrombosis!) and can grow to lengths of 30–50cm [Tapson, 2008]. The proximal end of the thrombus can extend into the popliteal vein, where the risk of embolisation is greater. Once the thrombus (or a portion) breaks off, it becomes an embolus, travelling up the femoral vein and into the iliac veins. From there it is free to ascend via the inferior vena cava to the heart. It continues into the right atrium, the ventricle and finally into the lungs via the pulmonary trunk and left and right pulmonary arteries (the only arteries to carry deoxygenated blood), which divide and sub-divide until they form capillaries around the alveoli.

In healthy patients, an obstruction of up to 25% of the pulmonary arterial bed will only cause mild respiratory symptoms, such as shortness of breath. Once this increases to 30–50% there will also be cardiovascular compromise, including cardiac arrest. Patients with pre-existing respiratory and/or cardiovascular disease will be symptomatic at much lower percentages [Torbicki, 2008; Wood, 2002].

4.5.1 Signs and symptoms

Common signs and symptoms of PE include difficulty breathing (dyspnoea) and rapid breathing (tachypnoea). Pleuritic chest pain is the most common symptom [AACE, 2013].

Other signs and symptoms include:

- Signs
  - Respiratory rate greater than 20 breaths/min
  - Pulse rate greater than 100 beats/min
  - Pulse oximeter reading (SpO_2) less than 92% in air
  - Signs of a deep vein thrombosis (DVT), which includes pain, swelling and/or tenderness on only one leg, often in the calf [Simon, 2010].
- Symptoms
  - Cough
  - Haemoptysis (blood from the respiratory tract, usually coughed up)
  - Syncope (faint).

4.5.2 Management

Patients with suspected PE need swift transport to hospital. Treatment is mainly supportive of the ABCs (airway, breathing and circulation). Place the patient in a position of comfort (often sitting up, unless they have low blood pressure), provide oxygen if required, to maintain the SpO_2 in the range 94–98%, and be prepared for cardiac arrest [AACE, 2013].

Chapter 11: **Circulation**

1 **Cardiovascular system anatomy and physiology**

1.1 **Learning objectives**

By the end of this lesson, you will be able to:

- State the functions of the cardiovascular system
- Describe the anatomy and function of the heart
- State the components of the electrical pathway of the heart
- Explain the difference between arteries and veins
- Describe the stages of the cardiac cycle.

1.2 **Introduction**

At the most basic level, the cardiovascular system is composed of blood vessels that transport blood around the body thanks to the work of a pump, the heart [Pilbery, 2013]. The heart is actually two pumps (the ventricles), each with its own reservoir (the atria), which normally serve two different circulations. The right side of the heart pumps blood to the pulmonary circulation, which travels around the lungs enabling the blood to take up oxygen and give up carbon dioxide. This blood then returns to the left side of the heart, where it is pumped into the systemic circulation to be transported all around the body via the largest artery in the body, the aorta. Both these pumps operate simultaneously and, thanks to valves in the heart, in one direction.

The main functions of the cardiovascular system are [Evans, 2012]:

- Transport of nutrients, such as oxygen, glucose (sugar), fatty acids and water
- Removal of waste products from metabolic processes, such as carbon dioxide, urea and creatine
- Hormonal control, by secreting hormones to their target organs (and secreting some of its own)
- Regulation of temperature by controlling heat distribution between the core and skin of the body

- Reproduction, by producing penile erection and providing nutrition for the unborn fetus
- Host defence, by transporting immune cells and other mediators.

1.3 **Heart**

The heart is relatively small, considering the work it has to do; it is only about the size of your fist. It sits within the mediastinum, a region in the thoracic cavity that extends from the sternum to the vertebral column, and sits between the lungs. About two-thirds of the heart sits to the left of the body's midline. It is cone-shaped, with the pointed apex orientated anteriorly (to the front), inferiorly (downwards) and to the left, and the flat base directed posteriorly (to the back), superiorly (upwards) and to the right [Tortora, 2008].

1.3.1 **Pericardium and heart wall**

The pericardium is a fibrous sac that surrounds and protects the heart, keeping it fixed within the mediastinum, but allowing for the vigorous contractions required to move blood around the pulmonary and systemic circulations [Tortora, 2008]. The outer, parietal, layer is fixed to the fibrous pericardium, whereas the inner, visceral, layer (also called the epicardium) forms the outer layer of the heart wall.

The wall of the heart is made up of three layers:

- Epicardium: Also known as the visceral layer of the pericardium
- Myocardium: The heart muscle, which makes up most of the bulk of the heart and is responsible for the pumping action that moves blood around the body
- Endocardium: The smooth inner layer which also covers the valves of the heart and is continuous with the innermost lining (endothelium) of the blood vessels attached to the heart.

1.3.2 **Chambers of the heart**

The heart has four chambers. The two superior chambers are called atria and the two inferior chambers, the ventricles (Figure 1.1) [Tortora, 2008; Kapit, 2001; Evans, 2012].

Right atrium

The right atrium receives deoxygenated blood from the body, via large veins called the superior and inferior vena cavae, and from the coronary (heart) circulation via the coronary sinus.

It is separated from the left atrium by a thin partition known as the interatrial septum, and from the right ventricle by the tricuspid valve, so called because it is made up of three cusps. This valve is also sometimes referred to as the right atrioventricular valve.

Right ventricle

The right ventricle makes up most of the anterior surface of the heart and receives blood from the right atrium via the tricuspid valve. To prevent this valve from everting (turning inside out like an umbrella in strong winds!) during contraction of the ventricles, the valve is anchored by tendon-like cords known as the chordae tendineae, which connect to papillary muscles. Like the atria, the ventricles are separated by a partition, known as the interventricular septum.

Blood leaves the ventricle via the pulmonary valve, where it enters the pulmonary trunk, which splits into the left and right pulmonary arteries. As you will discover later in the lesson, these arteries are unusual because they transport deoxygenated blood.

Left atrium

The left atrium makes up the majority of the base of the heart. Blood enters the atrium from the lungs via four pulmonary veins and exits through the bicuspid (two cusps) valve. This is also known as the mitral valve (because of the valve's resemblance to a bishop's mitre or hat) and the left atrioventricular valve.

Left ventricle

This forms the apex of the heart and also contains the chordae tendineae and papillary muscle assembly to secure the mitral valve. Blood exits via the aortic valve where it travels up the ascending aorta. Some blood leaves here and enters the coronary arteries to provide oxygen and nutrients to the heart itself. The remaining blood is transported throughout the body.

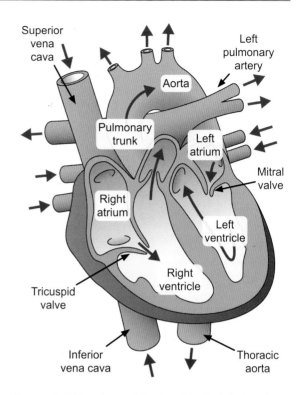

Figure 1.1 Chambers of the heart and related anatomy

1.3.3 Electrical conduction pathway

In order to ensure an effective pumping action of the heart, there is a network of specialised auto-rhythmic (self-excitable) muscle cell fibres that trigger co-ordinated muscle contraction (Figure 1.2), forcing blood around the heart chambers in the direction dictated by the heart valves.

Sino-atrial node

The sino-atrial (SA) node is the main pacemaker of the heart and in textbooks is typically shown as a small area of tissue at the junction of the superior vena cava (SVC) with the right atrium. However, electrophysiology studies have shown that the pacemaker site can spontaneously move down the terminal crest of the right atrium, giving rise to the phenomenon of the wandering pacemaker and suggesting that there is a much larger area of pacemaker cells [Boyett, 2009].

The SA node is usually supplied by the sino-atrial artery, which branches off the right coronary artery about 50% of the time (it branches off the

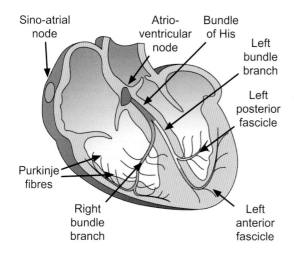

Figure 1.2 The electrical conduction pathway of the heart

left circumflex artery the other 50%) [Smithuis, 2008]. Electrical impulses travel from the SA node to the atrioventricular (AV) node and also cross the interatrial septum via a set of specialised cells known as Bachmann bundles.

Atrioventricular node and Bundle of His

The AV node is found in the right atrial wall, close to the opening of the coronary sinus and septal leaflet of the tricuspid valve. Its primary function is to delay the electrical impulse from the SA node long enough for the atria to depolarise, allowing time for atrial muscle contraction to squeeze additional blood into the ventricles (known as the atrial kick). Between the AV node and bundle branches is the Bundle of His, which originates in the wall of the right atrium and straddles the interventricular septum. In normal physiology, this is the only way electrical impulses can pass between the atria and ventricles [Garcia, 2004].

Left bundle branch

The left bundle branch starts at the end of the His, travelling through the interventricular septum, providing fibres which innervate the left ventricle and left side of the interventricular septum. It splits into two fascicles: anterior and posterior. The left posterior fascicle is a fan-like structure that provides innervation to the posterior and inferior left ventricle via the

Purkinje system. Being so widely distributed, it is hard to completely block. The left anterior fascicle, on the other hand, is a single strand, innervating the anterior and superior portions of the left ventricle [Garcia, 2015].

Right bundle branch

The right bundle branch also originates from the Bundle of His and sprouts fibres that innervate the right ventricle and right face of the interventricular septum, stimulating the Purkinje fibres. These fibres (named after a Czech physiologist, Jan Purkinje) consist of individual cells located just under the endocardium, and directly innervate myocardial cells causing them to depolarise [Boyett, 2009].

1.3.4 Coronary arteries

The heart requires its own blood supply in order to function properly. There are two main arteries that serve the heart, the right and left coronary arteries, which originate at the base of the ascending aorta (Figure 1.3).

Right coronary artery

The right coronary artery (RCA) runs down the right side of the heart in the coronary sulcus (depression) between the right atrium and ventricle. Most people (around 80%) are right dominant; the RCA gives rise to the posterior descending artery (PDA). In around 8%, this artery arises from the left circumflex (C_x) artery (termed left dominance), with the remainder

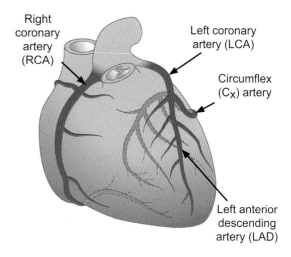

Figure 1.3 Coronary artery anatomy

being served by both arteries [Goldberg, 2007]. The PDA serves the inferior wall of the left ventricle as well as the inferior part of the septum.

Left coronary artery

The left coronary artery (LCA) passes behind the pulmonary trunk and splits almost immediately into two branches, the anterior interventricular branch (often referred to as the left anterior descending artery, LAD) and the circumflex artery (C_x). The LAD descends obliquely towards the apex of the heart in the anterior interventricular sulcus, supplying the anterior part of the septum and anterior wall of the left ventricle via one or two diagonal branches [Drake, 2005].

1.4 Blood

Blood is a connective tissue consisting of a liquid (plasma) and cells performing a range of essential functions for the body [Tortora, 2008; Munden, 2002]:

- Plasma makes up around 55% of blood and carries antibodies (an important part of the immune system), and nutrients to the body's tissues, and removes waste products.
- The formed elements make up the remaining 45% and consist of red and white blood cells and platelets
    - Red blood cells (erythrocytes) carry oxygen to the tissues and remove carbon dioxide
    - White blood cells (leukocytes) are an important part of the immune and inflammatory processes
    - Platelets (thrombocytes) along with clotting factors are an essential component of normal blood clotting, particularly in cases of bleeding (haemorrhage).

1.5 Blood vessels

There are five main types of blood vessels in the body. The largest are the elastic arteries that leave the heart before subdividing into medium-sized muscular arteries. These further subdivide into even smaller arteries known as arterioles. These are important vessels as they control blood flow into the capillaries, thin-walled vessels that allow for the exchange of substances between the blood and tissues. The capillaries unite to

form small veins, known as venules, which subsequently merge to form larger and larger veins that return blood to the heart [Tortora, 2008].

Vessel structure

Most blood vessels (except capillaries) are made up of three layers or tunics (Figure 1.4). The internal layer (tunica intima or interna) consists of a smooth inner layer (the endothelium), a basement membrane and, in medium-sized arteries, a layer of elastic tissue that helps to maintain blood pressure. Ordinarily, the endothelial layer is the only one that comes into contact with blood in the lumen of the artery [Kapit, 2001].

The medium-sized veins have one-way valves formed from the endothelial layer. These are designed to prevent blood flow from travelling in the wrong direction (i.e. away from the heart). They resist gravity-induced pooling, particularly in the lower limbs (i.e. the legs).

The next layer is the tunica media. This is made up of smooth muscle and elastic fibres, and is most developed in the medium-sized arteries and least developed in the veins. In the aorta and other large arteries there is a higher proportion of elastic fibres, making the walls highly compliant and able to stretch easily without tearing when subjected to pressure changes. This is advantageous, because as blood is ejected from the heart, the walls of the aorta stretch,

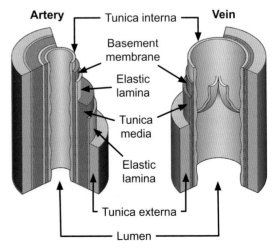

Figure 1.4 The structure of blood vessels

acting as a pressure reservoir which can ensure blood flow continues, even when the ventricles are relaxed [Tortora, 2008].

The final layer is the tunica externa, which is constructed mostly from elastic and collagen fibres, but is also home to the vasa vasorum (the blood supply to the arteries) and nervi vasorum (motor nerves) [Kapit, 2001].

1.5.1 Arteries

Figure 1.5 shows the main arteries that branch from the aorta. Don't worry about memorising them all now, you are going to revisit a number of these in future lessons.

1.5.2 Veins

Figure 1.6 shows the main veins that are drained by the superior and inferior vena cavae. It's not necessary to remember them all!

1.6 Cardiac cycle

During a single cardiac cycle, both the atria and ventricles take it in turns to contract and relax, forcing blood from an area of high pressure (due to the contracted muscle) to low pressure. The cycle is short, just 0.8 seconds in a person with an average heart rate of 75 beats/min [Tortora, 2008; Garcia, 2015; Kapit, 2000].

Atrial systole

This takes about 0.1 seconds. It starts with the sino-atrial (SA) node generating an action potential (electrical signal) when it depolarises (its voltage changes from negative to positive). This in turn causes the depolarisation of the atrial cardiac muscle cells, which contract (atrial systole). Blood is forced out of the atria, through the atrioventricular (AV) valves and into the ventricles, topping them up.

During this period, the electrical impulses from the SA node reach the AV node, pause to allow

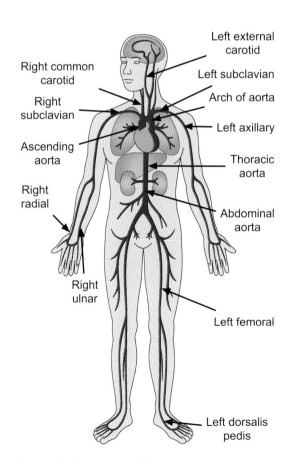

Figure 1.5 The aorta and its branches

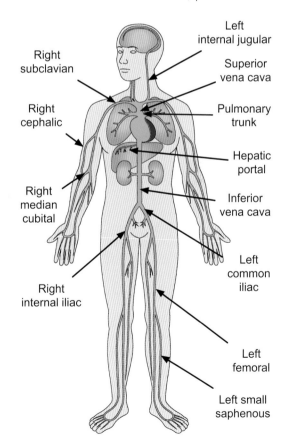

Figure 1.6 Veins of the body

for atrial muscle contraction and then continue down the Bundle of His, the bundle branches and into the Purkinje fibres, leading to ventricular depolarisation.

Ventricular systole

This lasts about 0.3 seconds, and during this time the atrial muscle relaxes (atrial diastole). Ventricular depolarisation causes the ventricular muscles to contract, and as the pressure inside the ventricles increases, the AV valves close and there is a brief period where all four valves of the heart are shut. This is known as isovolumetric contraction and lasts 0.05 seconds.

Contraction of the ventricles continues and eventually overcomes the pressure in the pulmonary and systemic circulations, causing the pulmonary and aortic valves (collectively known as the semilunar valves) to open. Blood is ejected into the pulmonary trunk and ascending aorta.

Meanwhile, the cardiac cells reset their voltage from positive (depolarised) to negative, a process known as repolarisation.

Relaxation period

This is the longest period in a cardiac cycle (around 0.4 seconds) and now both the atria and the ventricles are relaxed. This period is the most shortened when heart rate increases.

Ventricular repolarisation leads to relaxation of the ventricles (ventricular diastole), and as the pressure inside the ventricles falls, the semilunar valves close. As with systole, there is a brief period where all four valves are closed (isovolumetric relaxation). The pressure continues to fall, leading to the AV valves reopening and passive filling of the ventricles begins. By the end of diastole, the ventricles will be 75% full, just in time for another action potential from the SA node to start the process all over again.

2 Assessment of circulation

2.1 Learning objectives

By the end of this lesson you will be able to:
- Describe how to accurately measure the following:
  - Pulse
  - Capillary refill time
  - Blood pressure
- Explain how to prepare a patient and acquire a 3- and 12-lead ECG.

2.2 Introduction

If you are asked to assess a patient's pulse, or obtain a manual blood pressure, you have been given a big responsibility, since only you will know how fast, regular and strong the pulse feels, or when you can hear the Korotkoff sounds in your stethoscope as the blood pressure cuff is deflated.

Treatment decisions are made on the basis of clinical observations, so make sure you record observations accurately.

2.3 Pulse

The alternating expansion and recoil of the elastic arteries after ventricular systole creates a pressure wave, called a pulse, that can be felt in any artery that lies near the surface of the body and which can be compressed against a bone or other firm structure [Tortora, 2008].

Pulses are assessed for two main reasons [Gregory, 2010b]:
- To determine the patient's cardiovascular status
- To provide reassurance and gain a bond with patients who may be anxious.

Pulse locations

Pulses are palpable all over the body, but you should be able to confidently locate the radial, brachial and carotid pulses (Figure 2.1). The other sites are useful for specific conditions, for example, checking that a patient with a leg fracture has a dorsalis pedis pulse.

Radial pulse

The radial artery can be palpated at the wrist, on the radial side (thumb side) of the palmar (inner) aspect of the forearm. It is lateral to the long flexor tendons of the forearm (Figure 2.2) [Allan, 2004].

Brachial pulse

There are two locations for measuring this pulse. The first is in the mid-arm and can be found medially in the cleft between the biceps and triceps muscles (Figure 2.3). However, this is where a blood pressure cuff is usually placed, so in that instance you can also palpate the pulse in the crease of the elbow (antecubital fossa, Figure 2.4). The pulse can be palpated just medial to the biceps tendon [Drake, 2005].

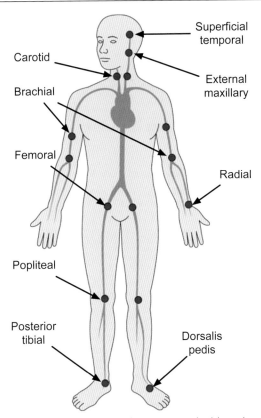

Figure 2.1 The location of common palpable pulses

Carotid

Superficial temporal

Brachial

External maxillary

Femoral

Radial

Popliteal

Posterior tibial

Dorsalis pedis

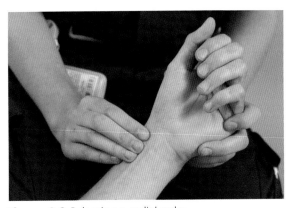

Figure 2.2 Palpating a radial pulse

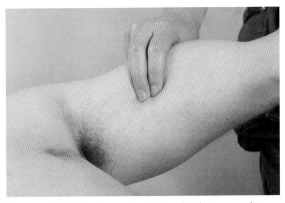

Figure 2.3 Palpating a brachial pulse between the biceps and triceps muscles

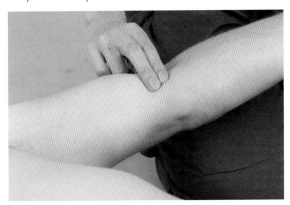

Figure 2.4 Palpating a brachial pulse in the crease of the elbow

Carotid pulse

The carotid artery can be palpated between the larynx and the sternocleidomastoid muscle. Gently press to feel the pulse (Figure 2.5) [Gregory, 2010b].

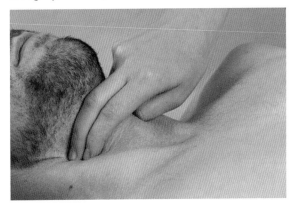

Figure 2.5 Palpating a carotid pulse

2.3.1 Assessment

When you assess a patient's pulse, you are looking for four things:

- Rate
- Rhythm
- Volume
- Character.

Rate

The normal pulse rate for an adult is 60–100 beats/min [Allan, 2004]. If the pulse rate is less than 60 beats/min this is termed bradycardia, and if greater than 100 beats/min, tachycardia [Talley, 2006; Douglas, 2005].

Causes of bradycardia include:

- Sleep
- Athletic training
- Hypothyroidism
- Medications such as beta-blockers
- Hypothermia
- Some types of arrhythmia (abnormal electrical activity within the heart).

Causes of tachycardia include:

- Exercise
- Pain
- Excitement/anxiety
- Hyperthyroidism
- Fever
- Some types of stimulant drugs such as caffeine and cocaine
- Some arrhythmias.

Rhythm

In healthy patients, the rhythm should be regular. However, in certain arrhythmias this regularity can be interrupted. Try to identify whether the irregularity is regular, i.e. seems to occur in a pattern, or the beats are apparently completely random, i.e. irregularly irregular [Gregory, 2010b].

Volume and character

The volume reflects the strength of the pulse. A high volume is typically noted during times when the cardiac output is high, such as during exercise, stress, heat and pregnancy. On the other hand, a low volume pulse can be due to heart failure or peripheral vascular disease. A weak (also described as 'thready') pulse is most often seen in patients who are suffering from a decreased blood volume (hypovolaemia, or shock) [Douglas, 2005].

The character of the pulse is slightly different as you need to picture how the pulse changes during the cardiac cycle. This is tricky to master and will require practice.

2.3.2 Recording a pulse

Procedure

Take the following steps to record a pulse [Gregory, 2010b]:

1. Explain the procedure and obtain consent from the patient
2. Place your index, middle and ring fingers along the artery and press gently. Avoid using the thumb as it has its own pulse. Don't push too hard, or you will occlude the artery. As a general rule, palpate the radial pulse first in conscious patients, and the carotid pulse first in unconscious patients
3. In pulses with a regular rhythm, count for 15 seconds and then multiply by 4. If the pulse is very fast or slow and/or irregular then count for a full 60 seconds.
4. Record the pulse rate on the patient record.

2.4 Capillary refill time

Capillary refill time (CRT) is defined as the time taken for a distal capillary bed to regain its colour after pressure has been applied to cause blanching [Pickard, 2011]. It was introduced during World War 2 to estimate the degree of shock in battlefield survivors. In 1981, an upper limit of 2 seconds was arbitrarily chosen as the acceptable upper limit; this has become the acceptable normal value and is published widely [King, 2014].

This presents a problem, because subsequent research has generally determined that it is not a good indicator of the degree of hypovolaemia in seriously ill and injured adult patients, and should not be used [Lewin, 2008].

It does have a place in assessment of children, although it should not be taken in isolation: i.e. take into account the other aspects of patient assessment that you will undertake, such as pulse rate, respiratory rate, work of breathing, level of consciousness etc. [King, 2014].

Because the usefulness of CRT is uncertain, you will need to follow your ambulance service guidance about when to use CRT and in which age group.

2.4.1 Assessment

Be aware of the following external factors that can affect the accuracy of capillary refill time (CRT) measurement in children and neonates [King, 2014]:

- Temperature: Children in cool environments will have a prolonged CRT, even when they are completely healthy. There is no evidence that CRT is affected by a child's body temperature, such as when they are feverish due to an illness
- Ambient light: Assessing CRT in poor light leads to errors. Ensure you are somewhere well lit
- Site: CRT is longer in neonates if the heel is used. One study demonstrated that fingertip and sternum CRTs are different in children [Crook, 2013]. Current paediatric guidelines advocate only using the sternum to assess CRT in children [Maconochie, 2012]
- Pressure application: It is not known how long pressure should be applied prior to assessing CRT, but current paediatric guidelines suggest pressing on the sternum for 5 seconds [Maconochie, 2012]
- Observer: When different people (observers) measure CRT at the same time, on the same child, they end up with different results! As a rule of thumb, try to ensure that the same clinician assesses CRT each time.

2.4.2 Recording the capillary refill time

Procedure

Follow these steps to obtain a capillary refill time (CRT) [Gregory, 2010b; King, 2014]:

1. Ensure the environment is warm and well lit
2. Explain the procedure to the parent, and to the child if they are able to understand
3. Apply pressure to the sternum for 5 seconds to compress blood from the tissues. Only apply enough pressure to cause blanching of the skin
4. Release the pressure and count how long it takes for the colour of the skin to return to that of the surrounding tissues. This is the CRT
5. Document your findings
6. Consider this result in the light of other assessment of the child's cardiovascular status.

2.5 Blood pressure

Blood pressure (BP) is the measurement of the pressure by the blood on the walls of a blood vessel. It is highest in the aorta and large systemic arteries and lowest in the large veins [Tortora, 2008].

A BP that you record consists of two measurements [Gregory, 2010b]:

- Systolic blood pressure: The BP during the systole phase of the cardiac cycle, when the ventricles contract and blood is forced out of the heart. This is the highest reading of blood pressure
- Diastolic blood pressure: The BP during the diastole phase of the cardiac cycle, when the ventricles are relaxed. This is the lowest reading of blood pressure.

It is usually measured in millimetres of mercury (mmHg) and recorded as the systolic value over the diastolic, for example 120/80 mmHg.

2.5.1 Assessment

Blood pressure (BP) values

The normal range for adult BP is a systolic value of 120–129 mmHg and/or diastolic of 80–84 mmHg. Hypertension (high BP) is defined as a systolic value of 140 mmHg or higher and/or a diastolic of 90 mmHg or higher [Mancia, 2013].

Hypotension is usually defined as a systolic blood pressure of less than 90 mmHg and this is the threshold for treatment with intravenous fluids in the current ambulance service clinical practice guidelines [AACE, 2013]. However, there is evidence to suggest that, in trauma, a systolic value of 110 mmHg should be the cut-off point for treatment [Eastridge, 2007; Hasler, 2011; Hasler, 2012] and even higher values are advocated for the elderly patient [Oyetunji, 2011].

Measurement of BP

Blood pressure can be measured directly, by inserting a sensor into a patient's artery, or indirectly using a cuff, which is applied to a patient's arm. The advantage of direct measurement is that it is accurate and continuous; it is typically used in hospital intensive care units. This method is not practicable outside of hospital and so non-invasive methods are used.

Non-invasive blood pressure (NIBP) measurement

There are two methods of NIBP used by the ambulance service [Gregory, 2010b]:

- Auscultatory: This method uses a stethoscope and an aneroid sphygmomanometer, a device consisting of an inflatable cuff and an aneroid manometer to measure the pressure on a dial (Figure 2.6)

- Automated: This consists of an inflatable cuff with a sensor inside that detects the oscillations generated by turbulent blood flow and calculates systolic and diastolic values using an algorithm.

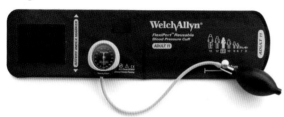

Figure 2.6 An aneroid sphygmomanometer
Image reproduced by the kind permission of Welch Allyn

Korotkoff sounds

When using the auscultatory method of measuring BP, you will place a stethoscope over the patient's brachial artery and listen for turbulent blood flow, known as the Korotkoff sounds, after a Russian surgeon, Nikolai Korotkoff, who first described them in 1905 [Talley, 2006].

The sounds are split into five phases [O'Brien, 2003]:

1. The first appearance of faint, repetitive, clear tapping sounds that gradually increase in intensity for at least two consecutive beats is the systolic blood pressure. This corresponds to the restoration of blood flow, and is confirmed by the presence of a palpable pulse

2. A brief period may follow during which the sounds soften and acquire a swishing quality. In some patients, sounds may disappear altogether for a short time.

3. The return of sharper sounds, which become crisper, to regain or even exceed the intensity of phase 1 sounds.

4. The distinct, abrupt muffling of sounds, which become soft and blowing in quality.

5. The point at which all sounds finally disappear completely is the diastolic pressure.

Note that in some groups of patients, the phase 4 sounds may be heard until the BP measurement reaches 0 mmHg. In these cases, the onset of phase 4 is taken to be the diastolic BP measurement [O'Brien, 2003].

2.5.2 Blood pressure measurement

Manual blood pressure measurement procedure

Take the following steps to manually record a blood pressure: [Mancia, 2013; Kauffman, 2014; Gregory, 2010b; O'Brien, 2003]

1. Ideally, allow the patient to sit for 3–5 minutes before measuring, and obtain consent

2. Ask about any medical conditions that might prevent a BP being recorded on a particular arm, e.g. mastectomy or arterio-venous shunts in dialysis patients

3. Ensure the arm is free of restrictive clothing and bare the arm. Do not apply a cuff over clothes

4. Palpate the brachial artery. This can be found by placing the pads of the index and middle fingers of one hand on the biceps tendon and then move medially and press deeply. If you have trouble locating the brachial pulse, ask the patient to extend their arm, which will bring the artery into a more superficial position. Once it is located, ask the patient to relax their arm so that their wrist rests on their thigh

5. Ask the patient to remain still and not talk during the BP measurement

6. Select the appropriate cuff size. A standard bladder is 12–13 cm wide and is 35 cm long, but have smaller and larger sizes available

7. Ensure the cuff is at heart level and wrap snugly around the patient's upper arm and clear of the antecubital fossa, so that the cuff will not touch the stethoscope

8. Place the artery marker on the cuff over the patient's brachial artery

9. Palpate the brachial artery and inflate the cuff until the pulse disappears. Continue to inflate 30 mmHg above this point

10. Slowly deflate the cuff and note when the pulse returns. This gives an estimation of the systolic blood pressure

11. Wait 30 seconds and then place the diaphragm of the stethoscope over the brachial artery

12. Rapidly inflate the cuff 30 mmHg above your estimation of the systolic blood pressure

Procedure continued →

13. Deflate at a rate of 2–3 mmHg per pulse beat
14. Note the pressure at which you first hear the Korotkoff sounds (systolic BP), the point at which they become muffled (Phase 4) and then disappear (Phase 5). The disappearance of sounds is usually taken to be the diastolic blood pressure
15. Document the blood pressure, including which arm the measurement was taken from.

Automated blood pressure measurement procedure

Follow the manufacturer's instructions for the measurement of an automated blood pressure. The steps below apply to recording a BP using a LifePak 15 monitor/defibrillator [Physio-Control, 2009]:

1. Press ON
2. Select the appropriately sized cuff and apply it snugly to the arm
3. Connect the tubing to the cuff and to the NIBP port on the monitor
4. Change the initial inflation pressure, if necessary
5. Position the arm in a relaxed and supported position at approximately the same level as the patient's heart. Inform the patient that the cuff will inflate and cause a 'big squeeze' around the arm and that the patient's fingers may tingle
6. Press NIBP to start the measurement, and check that the patient's arm is not moving. When the measurement is complete, the blood pressure measurements are displayed.

2.6 **Electrocardiograms**

The electrical signals that are responsible for the muscle contraction and relaxation during the cardiac cycle can be recorded on an electrocardiogram (ECG, Figure 2.7). They are useful for determining cardiac rhythm disturbances (arrhythmias) and detecting myocardial injury, such as occurs during a heart attack (myocardial infarction).

As the heart's muscle cells depolarise and repolarise during the cardiac cycle, a potential difference (voltage) is generated, which can be detected on the surface of the body. Each cell generates its own electrical impulse, which has a strength and direction. The sum of all of these vectors is known as the heart's electrical axis and this is recorded on the ECG.

Recording the ECG is achieved with the use of electrodes that are placed in specific locations on the body, to capture the electrical activity of the heart. They are often compared to cameras placed around the heart to build up a 3-dimensional picture. In reality, we do not refer to these electrical views as cameras, but as leads, which are not to be confused with the physical leads that the electrodes are attached to. To record a 12-lead ECG, for example, you will only actually place 9 or 10 physical leads on the patient.

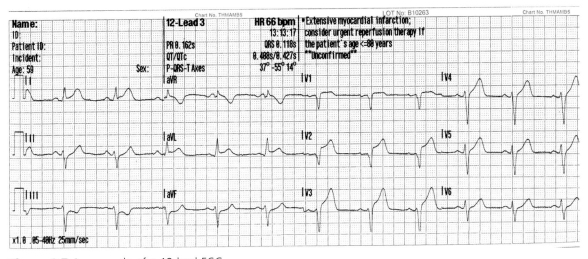

Figure 2.7 An example of a 12-lead ECG

The ECG complex

An ECG complex is made up of a series of waves (a deflection from the baseline), segments and intervals which represent electrical events in the heart (Figure 2.8) [Garcia, 2015]:

- P wave: Atrial depolarisation
- PR segment: This is the part of the complex between the end of the P wave and the start of the QRS wave. It should be along the baseline (the line from one TP segment to the next)
- PR interval: This is the time period from the start of the P wave to the start of the QRS wave. It should be 0.12–20 seconds (3 to 5 small squares)
- QRS complex: This represenst ventricular depolarisation and is typically made up of a Q, R and S wave. It should be less than 0.12 seconds or 3 small squares in duration
- ST segment: This is the part of the complex between the end of the QRS wave and the start of the T wave. The point at which the QRS wave ends and the ST segment begins is known as the J point. The ST segment should be on the baseline
- T wave: This wave represents ventricular repolarisation and is the first deflection (positive or negative) that occurs after the ST segment. It should begin in the same direction as the QRS complex.

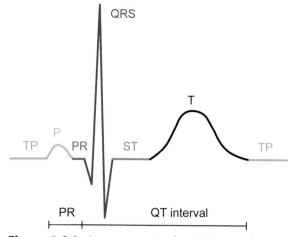

Figure 2.8 Basic components of an ECG complex

2.6.1 Assessment

You will not be expected to interpret an ECG, but it should be recorded so that accurate interpretation is possible by the clinician.

ECG paper

ECGs are recorded on standardised graph paper which is moved past a heated stylus at a standard speed of 25 mm per second. On the vertical axis, the standard calibration amplitude is 10 mm/mV. This is shown by a calibration box which is printed at the beginning of each line of the ECG (Figure 2.9A) and should be 10mm tall. It is possible to change both of these settings, so always check your ECG. If standard calibration is used, the horizontal measurement of each large square is 0.2 seconds (Figure 2.9B) and each small square represents 0.04 seconds (Figure 2.9C).

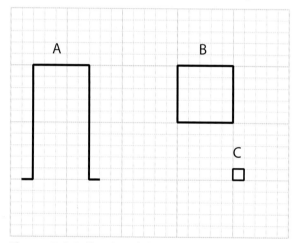

Figure 2.9 Calibration of the ECG and standard square durations

Artefact

The quality of the ECG can be affected by a range of factors. Electrical interference, poor electrode contact, damaged ECG cables, muscle tremors, shivering, hiccups and deep respiration can all lead to artefact or a 'wandering' baseline (Figure 2.10).

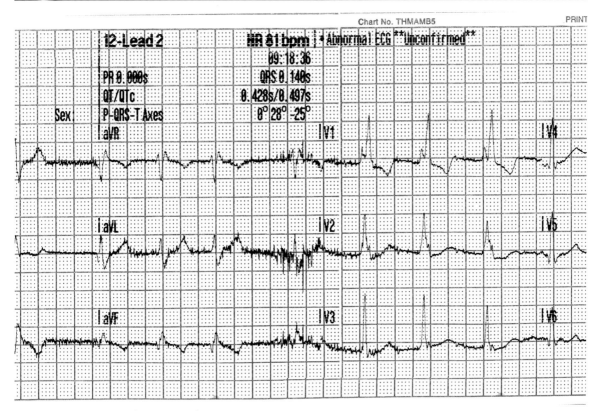

Chart No. THMAMB5

PRINT

12-Lead 2   HR 81 bpm   Abnormal ECG **unconfirmed**

09:18:36

PR 0.000s   QRS 0.140s

QT/QTc   0.428s/0.497s

Sex   P-QRS-T Axes   0° 28° -25°

Figure 2.10 An ECG showing artefact

2.6.2 Recording an ECG

Procedure

Take the following steps to record a 3- and 12-lead ECG: [Pilbery, 2013; Physio-Control, 2009]

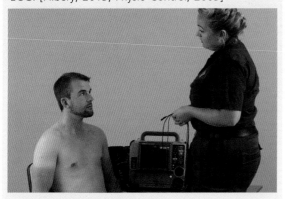

1. Explain the procedure to the patient. Removing their top without explanation can give them the wrong idea about your intentions

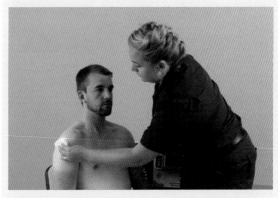

2. Prepare the skin. This will include shaving any hair at the electrode sites, cleaning oily skin with an alcohol wipe, and gently scraping the skin to remove the surface layer of dead skin cells. Patients who are sweating profusely can be a problem, but an alcohol wipe and/or gauze swabs should help. All of these will improve electrical conduction

Procedure continued →

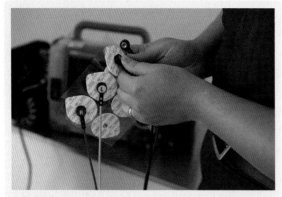

3. Check your electrodes are in date and then attach them to the leads prior to applying them to the patient's skin. When you apply the electrodes flat to the skin, smooth the tape outward and avoid pressing the centre of the electrode. Also, avoid placing electrodes over tendons and major muscle masses

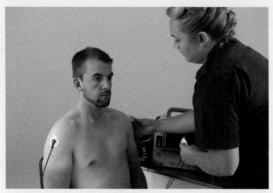

4. Apply the limb leads. Although traditionally placed on the wrists, limb leads can be placed anywhere on the limbs, and in cases of either patient and/or vehicular movement, a more proximal location may reduce artefact [Physio-Control, 2009]. Place the leads as follows:
- Red: Right wrist/arm
- Yellow: Left wrist/arm
- Green: Left ankle/leg
- Black: Right ankle/leg

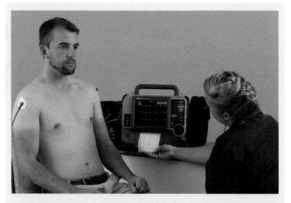

5. Turn on the monitor and record a 3-lead ECG. Label it with the patient's name and date of birth

12-lead ECG only:

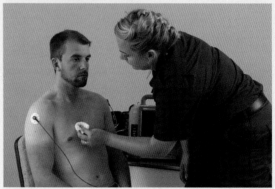

6. Prepare the chest skin as in step 2 and attach electrodes to the chest leads

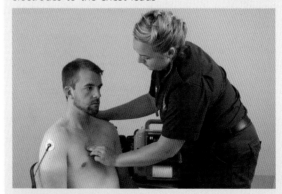

7. Move your finger downwards crossing the manubrium until you feel a small horizontal ridge. This is the sternal angle or Angle of Louis, where the manubrium and body of the sternum join

Procedure continued →

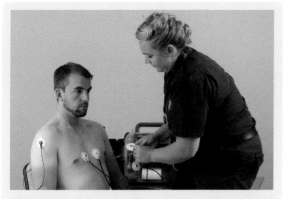

8. Slide your finger laterally and slightly downwards into the second intercostal space and move down two more intercostal spaces to locate the fourth intercostal space. Place lead V1 just to the left of the sternal border, and V2 just to the right

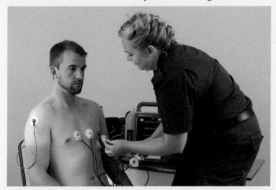

9. Move into the fifth intercostal space and laterally to the mid-clavicular line. This is the location of V4. Place V3 midway between V2 and V4

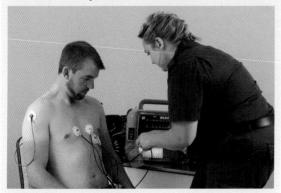

10. Place lead V6 level with V4, and in the mid-axillary line. V5 should be placed level with, and midway between, V4 and V6 in the anterior axillary line [Kligfield, 2007]

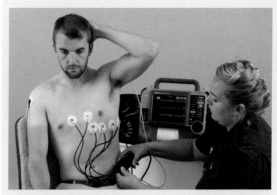

11. Connect the cables to the monitor

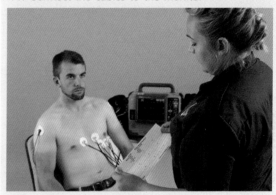

12. Press the 12-lead ECG Analyse button and record a 12-lead ECG. Review the 12-lead ECG to check it is of sufficient quality for diagnostic purposes

Breasts

Female breasts can make things a bit tricky in terms of placing leads V4–V6. Current guidance provided by two monitor/defibrillator manufacturers states that these leads should be placed **under** breast tissue. While there is some evidence to suggest that signal reduction by placing electrodes over breast tissue may not be significant, and the procedure has the benefit of ensuring correct anatomical placement of the chest leads, this is not strong enough at present to change the common practice of placing V4–V6 under the breast [Crawford, 2008; BCS, 2010].

3 Common cardiovascular conditions

3.1 Learning objectives

By the end of this lesson you will be able to:

- Describe the following conditions of the cardiovascular system:
  - Coronary artery disease
  - Stable angina
  - Acute coronary syndromes
  - Heart failure
- Explain the types, causes and stages of shock.

3.2 Introduction

Many of the cardiovascular conditions you are going to learn about in this lesson are most commonly caused by the consequences of coronary artery disease (CAD), which worldwide is the most common cause of death, with around seven million people dying each year [Steg, 2012].

Shock is a clinical state in which the delivery of oxygenated blood (and other nutrients such as glucose) to the body's tissue is not adequate to meet metabolic demand [Maconochie, 2012].

The types of shock vary between textbooks, but five types that will be covered in this lesson are:

- Hypovolaemic shock
- Distributive shock
- Cardiogenic shock
- Obstructive shock
- Dissociative shock.

3.3 Coronary artery disease

Coronary artery disease (CAD, sometimes called ischaemic heart disease) is almost always caused by atherosclerosis of the coronary arteries. This is a systemic, lipid (fat) driven immune/inflammatory disease of the medium and large arteries. Over time (usually decades), atherosclerosis causes the formation of plaques: collections of lipids and cholesterol that accumulate in the intimal layer of arteries, some of which attract macrophages (a type of white blood cell). The macrophages secrete protein-dissolving enzymes and engulf the lipids, leaving behind a lipid-rich 'necrotic core' [Falk, 2003].

The interface between the plaque and the lumen of the artery is known as the fibrous cap. If it becomes thickened it can cause narrowing of the artery lumen (stenosis), which if significant, leads to cardiac ischaemia, particularly when myocardial oxygen demand rises, such as when the patient exercises. This can lead to stable or extertional angina. If the plaque ruptures, the artery can become occluded (blocked), leading to an acute coronary syndrome [Aaronson, 2004].

3.4 Stable angina

Angina is a pain or discomfort usually felt across or in the centre of the chest as a tightness or indigestion-like ache. This can radiate to one or both arms, the neck, back or epigastrium (the portion of the abdomen between the diaphragm and umbilicus or belly-button). It can be accompanied by belching, which may be wrongly assumed to be due to indigestion [Nolan, 2012].

To be classed as stable it should consist of [Montalescot, 2013]:

- Classic chest discomfort as described above
- Provoked by exertion or emotional stress
- Relieved by rest and/or nitrates (drugs that dilate the vessels) within minutes.

Stable angina is caused by significant stenosis (>70%) of at least one coronary artery due to coronary artery disease (CAD). This causes narrowing of the artery, which at rest still allows sufficient oxygenated blood to the myocardium. However, during exercise or stress, coronary oxygen demand increases. This demand can be met by increasing blood flow through increasing the diameter of the arteries. However, this is not possible in stenosed vessels and the resulting imbalance of oxygen supply and demand leads to myocardial ischaemia [Aaronson, 2004].

3.5 Heart failure

Heart failure is an abnormality of cardiac structure or function, leading to failure of the heart to deliver oxygen at a sufficient rate to meet cell and tissue metabolic needs, despite normal filling pressures [McMurray, 2012].

Patients who have been suffering from heart failure for some time are classed as having chronic heart failure. If their signs and symptoms have not changed in the past month, then it is considered to be stable. On the other hand, if there is an acute deterioration in these patients, they are considered to be suffering from acute decompensated heart failure (often just called acute heart failure, AHF) [Allen, 2007].

Although the most common cause of AHF is sudden worsening of chronic heart failure, about 20–30% of cases are a new onset heart failure, with a small percentage due to malignant hypertensive crisis (blood pressure that is high enough to damage the body's organs) or cardiogenic shock. Up to 25% of cases are caused by an acute coronary syndrome, although these are normally considered separately from 'typical' AHF because of the differing presentation, pathophysiology and treatment [Howlett, 2011].

Anatomy and physiology

Recall from the CARDIOVASCULAR SYSTEM ANATOMY AND PHYSIOLOGY lesson that the heart is essentially two pumps in one, with the right side moving deoxygenated blood from the venous to the pulmonary circuit and returning it to the left side, which pumps the oxygenated blood into the arterial circulation. Cardiac output (CO) is the volume of blood ejected from the ventricles every minute and is a product of heart rate and stroke volume. Heart rate is regulated by the autonomic nervous system, and the stroke volume is dependent on three key factors [Tortora, 2008]:

- Preload
- Contractility
- Afterload.

Preload

This is the volume of blood stretching the resting heart muscle at the end of diastole [Porth, 2003], and is largely determined by central venous pressure (CVP) and the compliance of the ventricular walls [Aaronson, 2004].

Contractility

The forcefulness of muscle contraction is known as its contractility; it can be increased by sympathetic nervous system innervation, and the stretching of heart muscle fibres, due to increases in end-diastolic pressures. In a similar way to stretching a rubber band, as heart muscle fibres are stretched by increasing blood volume, they contract with greater force, a characteristic known as the Frank–Starling mechanism [Porth, 2003]. This is an important method the heart

utilises to balance left and right ventricular volumes during normal physiological events, such as breathing and change of posture. It also plays an important compensatory role in heart failure [Aaronson, 2004].

Afterload

The final component of stroke volume is afterload. This is the pressure exerted by the systemic circulation that the left ventricle needs to overcome in order to eject blood from the heart [Tortora, 2008].

Pathophysiology

Heart failure usually begins with left ventricular dysfunction caused by myocardial injury (such as myocardial infarction, MI). This causes ventricular enlargement and dilation and impaired contractility. Untreated, this typically gets worse over time and the ventricle becomes less efficient at pumping blood around the systemic circulation. In the long term, this leads to a spiral of increased, but less efficient, cardiac energy expenditure and reduced myocardial perfusion. As a result, the heart becomes increasingly dependent on the sympathetic nervous system to maintain cardiac output [Magner, 2004].

As cardiac reserve (the difference between maximum and resting cardiac output) is consumed by declining heart muscle function, eventually the patient will suffer an episode of acute decompensation. Declining cardiac output on the left side of the heart (left heart failure) causes increased end-diastolic and pulmonary venous pressures as blood backs up into the pulmonary circulation. Fluid begins to accumulate in the lung tissue and this, coupled with the increasing volumes of blood in lung vessels, makes them stiffer and less compliant, causing difficulty in breathing (dyspnoea). In the early stages, this may only occur on lying flat (orthopnoea) and is one of the causes of sudden night-time waking with shortness of breath (paroxysmal nocturnal dyspnoea, PND). Large increases in pulmonary capillary pressure can force fluid into the alveoli, causing pulmonary oedema, severe dyspnoea, decreased gaseous exchange and hypoxaemia [Aaronson, 2004].

Right heart failure has a number of causes, including chronic obstructive pulmonary disease (COPD), pulmonary embolism, heart valve disease, and left heart failure. As central venous pressure increases, fluid accumulates in the peripheral tissues, causing pitting oedema in the ankles initially, but rising to the knees and sacrum in severe cases. Other signs of this fluid accumulation can also be seen in the abdomen [Porth, 2003].

3.6 Acute coronary syndrome

Acute coronary syndrome (ACS) represents a spectrum of three dangerous conditions, all of which constitute medical emergencies and result from a sudden decrease in coronary artery blood flow [Aaronson, 2004]. These three conditions, in order of increasing severity, are:

• Unstable angina (UA)
• Non-ST-segment elevation myocardial infarction (NSTEMI)
• ST-segment elevation myocardial infarction (STEMI).

Since the treatment of UA and NSTEMI is similar, they are usually considered together. The ST-segment in NSTEMI and STEMI refers to the portion of an ECG complex which may change (STEMI) or not (NSTEMI) during a myocardial infarction (heart attack).

Pathophysiology

The steps that lead to an ACS consist of [Aaronson, 2004]:

1. Rupture of the fibrous cap leads to platelet aggregation (clumping together)
2. Intraplaque thrombus (blood clot) expands the plaque and can occlude the artery if large enough
3. Intraluminal thrombus resulting in partial or complete occlusion of the artery
4. Release of vasoconstricting substances associated with platelet aggregation, which makes the vessel constrict and narrow
5. Endothelial damage promotes further vasoconstriction.

Assessment

The most common presentation of ACS is chest pain felt just under the sternum (sub-sternal) that may be described as heavy, squeezing, crushing or tight, that has lasted for more than 15 minutes and has not been relieved by GTN. The pain radiates to the left arm in about 40% of

patients although it can also radiate to the right arm/shoulder or both left and right arms [Body, 2010]. In addition, it can also radiate to the neck, jaw, upper back or epigastrium. The pain can be confused with indigestion and patients may even have tried antacid medication to relieve the discomfort. Pain is not typically altered by deep breathing or coughing. The patient may have other symptoms, such as [AACE, 2013]:

• Nausea and vomiting
• Marked sweating (diaphoresis)
• Pale, clammy skin
• Shortness of breath
• A feeling of impending doom.

Note that up to 5% of patients do not have chest pain [Valensi, 2011]. These are more likely to be women, and have diabetes or a history of heart failure [Canto, 2012].

Management

Patients with ACS require a 12-lead ECG as soon as possible. If this shows a STEMI, then they will receive either mechanical reopening of their arteries, if a receiving hospital capable of performing primary percutaneous coronary intervention (pPCI) can be reached within 2 hours, or chemical reopening of their arteries (thrombolysis), which can be undertaken by paramedics in some ambulance services. Even if the ECG is completely normal, patients with UA/NSTEMI may still require prompt restoration of coronary blood supply and should be treated as an emergency.

Other treatment will include [AACE, 2013]:

• Correction of major ABC problems
• Administration of aspirin, GTN, clopidogrel as per local and national clinical practice guidelines
• Oxygen, if the patient has oxygen saturations of less than 94% on air
• Rapid transport to an appropriate hospital.

3.7 Shock

Shock is a clinical state in which the delivery of oxygenated blood (and other nutrients such as glucose) to the body's tissue is not adequate to meet metabolic demand [Maconochie, 2012].

The types of shock vary between textbooks, but five types are included here:

- Hypovolaemic shock
- Distributive shock
- Cardiogenic shock
- Obstructive shock
- Dissociative shock.

Hypovolaemic shock

This is an acute loss of circulating blood volume either from dehydration (loss of fluids and electrolytes) or from bleeding (haemorrhage) externally or internally. Shock due to blood loss (haemorrhagic shock) has been classified into four classes (stages) [NAEMT, 2014]:

- Class 1: The body is able to cope with losses and there are no obvious clinical signs
- Class 2: This is the compensated stage. Blood loss is more significant, but the body has mechanisms to maintain blood pressure despite the reduction in blood volume
- Class 3: This is the decompensated stage. Despite the compensatory mechanisms, blood loss is now too severe to maintain blood pressure. These patients require blood and urgent surgical intervention to stop the bleeding
- Class 4: The irreversible stage. Even if the circulation is restored, the patient is still likely to die.

Note that the original stages of shock described by the advanced trauma life support (ATLS) and pre-hospital trauma life support (PHTLS) courses included blood loss estimates and clinical observations (such as heart and respiratory rate, blood pressure and level of consciousness) which would indicate the stage of shock the patient was experiencing [ATLS, 2008; NAEMT, 2014]. These have been shown by numerous studies to be inaccurate and so are not included here [Guly, 2010; Mutschler, 2013; Mutschler, 2014]. You will however, still find them in many textbooks.

Signs of hypovolaemic shock

The classic signs of hypovolaemic shock include [AACE, 2013]:

- Pallor
- Cool peripheries
- Anxiety and abnormal behaviour
- Increased heart and respiratory rates.

Note that these may not appear until 1000–1500 ml of blood has been lost, and even later in some patient groups such as pregnant women, patients on medication such as beta-blockers, and fit individuals.

Distributive shock

This type of shock is caused by widespread dilation of the peripheral vascular system because of dilation of the arterioles and/or venules. This in effect creates a larger container for the same blood volume, leading to decreased tissue perfusion. In addition, in causes such as anaphylaxis and sepsis, the vessels become 'leaky', allowing fluid to escape into the tissues and so becoming removed from the general circulation [Pilbery, 2013].

Common causes of distributive shock include:

- Anaphylaxis
- Sepsis
- Nervous system related cause such as spinal cord injury.

Cardiogenic shock

This is due to a primary cardiac problem when the heart is unable to circulate sufficient blood to meet the body's metabolic needs. This is most common following a myocardial infarction, but can also be caused by acute heart failure or arrhythmia [Pilbery, 2013].

Obstructive shock

This is an uncommon cause of shock and is due to an obstruction of blood flow to/from the heart. It can be caused by a tension pneumothorax, cardiac tamponade or a massive pulmonary embolism [Evans, 2012].

Dissociative shock

This occurs when the oxygen-carrying capacity of the blood is affected because of inadequate numbers of red blood cells available to carry sufficient oxygen (anaemia) or when competing molecules take up space on the red blood cells that would normally be used to carry oxygen, such as in cases of carbon monoxide poisoning [Maconochie, 2012].

Chapter 12: **Disability**

1 **Nervous system anatomy and physiology**

1.1 **Learning objectives**

By the end of this lesson you will be able to:

- State the functions of the nervous system
- Describe the anatomy and physiology of the nervous system.

1.2 **Introduction**

The nervous system performs three main functions in order to carry out a complex range of tasks including controlling body movements, regulating heart rate, creating memories and producing speech [Tortora, 2008; Briar, 2003]:

- Sensory function (perception): Receptors located around the body detect internal stimuli, such as a change in blood pressure, and external stimuli, such as a bad odour, and transmit this via afferent nerves through the cranial and spinal nerves and into the brain and spinal cord

- Information transfer and processing: Nerve cells (neurons) have special projections (axons) that allow the conduction of electrical impulses. These can be delivered to other neurons, and/or modified by or integrated with other impulses to create a complex web that can process sensory information received from afferent neurons

- Motor function: This is the nervous system's response to the processing stage and is communicated via efferent nerves, which carry electrical impulses from the brain via cranial or spinal nerves. This enables the brain to control the body as well as control ventilation and circulation.

1.3 **Anatomy and physiology**

The nervous system (Figure 1.1) consists of the brain and spinal cord (generally referred to as the central nervous system, CNS) and a network of peripheral nerves either originating from the brain (as 12 pairs of cranial nerves) or the spinal cord (as 31 pairs of spinal nerves). Together with

small collections of neurons known as ganglia, these form the peripheral nervous system (PNS).

The PNS consists of two divisions. The first is the sensory, or afferent, division, which is composed of large numbers of sensory receptors in the skin.

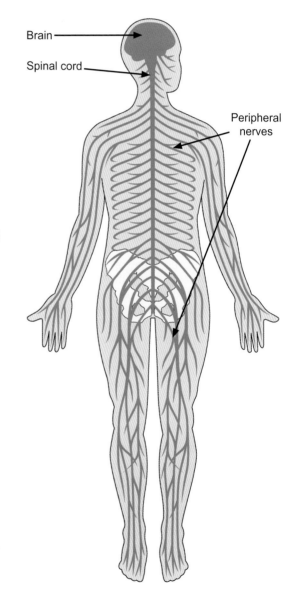

Brain

Spinal cord

Peripheral nerves

Figure 1.1 The nervous system

Their nerve impulses are conveyed by somatic sensory fibres, as well as internally around the body (impulses from which are transmitted by visceral sensory fibres), and an extensive network of neurons around the gastrointestinal tract, collectively known as the enteric plexus, which helps regulate digestion. The other division of the PNS is the motor, or efferent, division. This is split into the somatic nervous system and the autonomic nervous system [Marieb, 2013; Tortora, 2008].

1.4 Brain

The portion of the central nervous system that is contained within the skull is known as the brain. The brain occupies 80% of the cranial vault, with the remaining 20% made up of cerebral blood (12%) and cerebral spinal fluid (8%). It has a wide range of functions as well as serving as the centre for intellect, emotions, behaviour and memory. The brain is generally divided into four major sections (Figure 1.2) [Tortora, 2008]:

- Brain stem
- Cerebellum
- Diencephalon
- Cerebrum.

Brain stem

The brain stem consists of the medulla oblongata, pons and midbrain. Their functions include:

- Medulla oblongata
  - Relays sensory and motor input between other parts of the brain and spinal cord
  - Together with pons and midbrain, controls level of consciousness
  - Contains centres to manage heart rate, blood pressure and breathing
  - Contains origins of a number of cranial nerves
- Pons
  - Relays nervous impulses from one side of the cerebellum to the other and between medulla and midbrain
  - Contains origins of a number of cranial nerves
  - Contains centres to regulate breathing
- Midbrain
  - Relays motor output from the cerebral cortex and sensory input from the spinal cord to the thalamus
  - Controls and co-ordinates movement
  - Contains origins of two cranial nerves.

Cerebellum

This part of the brain is responsible for co-ordinating complex and skilled movements and regulates posture and balance.

Diencephalon

- Thalamus
  - Relays sensory input to the cerebral cortex
  - Provides perception of touch, pressure, pain and temperature
- Hypothalamus
  - Controls and integrates autonomic nervous system activity
  - Regulates behavioural patterns and circadian rhythms
  - Controls body temperature
  - Regulates eating and drinking behaviour.

Cerebrum

The cerebrum allows you to read, write and speak. Various regions are responsible for a range of other functions:

- Sensory areas are involved in perception of sensory information
- Motor areas control muscular movements
- Association areas are responsible for complex functions such as memory, personality and intelligence.

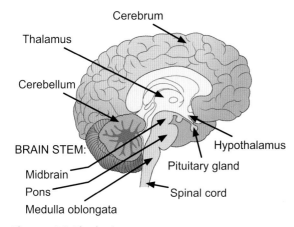

Figure 1.2 The brain

The cerebrum is split into two hemispheres and consists of an outer rim of grey matter and an internal region of white matter. The outer rim of grey matter contains the cerebral cortex which, although thin, contains billions of neurons. Each hemisphere can also be further divided into four lobes: frontal, parietal, occipital and temporal.

Meninges

In addition to the skull, the brain is protected by the meninges. There are three of them [Tortora, 2008]:

- Dura: Tough outer layer consisting of connective tissue
- Arachnoid: Middle layer. The sub-arachnoid space (between arachnoid and pia layers) is filled with cerebrospinal fluid
- Pia: Delicate inner layer containing small blood vessels which supply oxygen and nutrients to the brain.

Cerebrospinal fluid

Cerebrospinal fluid (CSF) is a clear, colourless liquid, which protects the brain and spinal cord from physical and chemical injury. It also carries oxygen, glucose and other nutrients that are essential for normal brain function, as well as removing waste products [Tortora, 2008].

1.4.1 Autoregulation

The brain accounts for only 2% of total body weight, yet consumes 25% of the body's glucose. It has no storage mechanism for oxygen or glucose, so needs a continuous supply of blood, which it achieves by the process of autoregulation. This is the intrinsic ability of the brain to constrict or dilate its blood vessels in order to maintain a stable blood flow, which remains constant, as long as the mean arterial pressure (MAP) stays between 50 and 150 mmHg [Mittal, 2009].

Mean arterial pressure

The MAP can be calculated from the systolic and diastolic blood pressure values using the following formula:

Diastolic blood pressure + 1/3 (systolic blood pressure – diastolic blood pressure)

Fortunately, most automatic blood pressure machines will calculate this value for you.

Cerebral blood flow is reliant on the cerebral perfusion pressure (CPP), which is the pressure gradient that causes cerebral blood flow. This must be above 60 mmHg in order to perfuse the brain, and is related to MAP and intracranial pressure (ICP) by the following equation [Marieb, 2013]:

$$CPP = MAP - ICP$$

1.5 Spinal cord

Recall from the lesson on MUSCULOSKELETAL ANATOMY AND PHYSIOLOGY (chapter 6) that the vertebral column consists of 33 vertebrae: 7 cervical, 12 thoracic, 5 lumbar, 5 sacral and 4 coccygeal. Part of their function is to provide physical protection for the spinal cord, which the vertebrae encapsulate. Additional protection is provided by vertebral ligaments, meninges and the cerebrospinal fluid (CSF) [Tortora, 2008]. Rather confusingly, there are 31 pairs of spinal nerves; 8 cervical, 12 thoracic, 5 lumbar, 5 sacral and 1 coccygeal.

The spinal cord is almost cylindrical in shape, although slightly squashed in the anterior–posterior dimension. Its average diameter is just 12 mm, and in adults it extends from the medulla oblongata to the superior border of the second lumbar vertebra (L2), i.e. it does not extend the full length of the vertebral column. Instead, it tapers to form a cone-like structure called the conus medullaris [Tortora, 2008]. Nerves that originate distal to the conus medullaris form the cauda equina (meaning horse's tail). These nerves have a dorsal root containing afferent fibres which transmit sensation, and a ventral root containing efferent motor fibres [Gitelman, 2008].

1.6 Somatic nervous system

The somatic nervous system is also sometimes known as the voluntary nervous system, since it allows the person to consciously control their skeletal muscles thanks to somatic nerve fibres, which conduct impulses from the central nervous system to skeletal muscles [Marieb, 2013]. However, the somatic nervous system also includes an involuntary component, reflexes. These are primarily a protective mechanism, for instance removing your hand when you touch something hot [Tortora, 2008].

1.7 **Autonomic nervous system**

The autonomic nervous system (ANS) is divided into three parts. These are the sympathetic, parasympathetic and enteric nervous systems. They are called autonomic because it was originally believed that they functioned completely independently from the central nervous system (CNS). However, it is now known that the hypothalamus and brain stem regulate ANS activity [Tortora, 2008]. The enteric division is an extensive network of neurons which reside within the walls of the gastrointestinal (GI) tract, pancreas and gall bladder. It has a sensory nervous function enabling the monitoring of the mechanical state of the alimentary canal and the chemical status of the stomach and intestines. In addition, it can output motor signals to modify the motility and secretions of the gut, as well as controlling the diameter of local blood vessels [Briar, 2003].

The sympathetic and parasympathetic divisions of the ANS are often thought of as being at either end of a see-saw. This is true in some organs such as the heart, but in reality this is rather a simplistic view. Some parts of the body receive inputs from only one division, whereas in others, the effects of the sympathetic and parasympathetic divisions are similar. However, their actions are carefully controlled and co-ordinated by the hypothalamus.

1.7.1 **Sympathetic division**

This is often referred to as the fight-or-flight division as its actions prepare the body to respond to stress, facilitating sudden strenuous exercise and increased vigilance. In addition, it helps control blood pressure, thermoregulation, and gut and urogenital function.

1.7.2 **Parasympathetic division**

The parasympathetic division is often referred to as the rest-and-digest division. Actions of the parasympathetic division include antagonising some effects of the sympathetic division, for example heart rate, gut motility and bronchiole diameter, and controlling many body functions in non-stress states such as GI secretion to aid digestion, micturition and defecation. Another important difference between the sympathetic and parasympathetic divisions is their structure. Parasympathetic neurons are clustered at either end of the spinal cord.

2 **Assessment of disability**

2.1 **Learning objectives**

By the end of this lesson you will be able to:
- Describe how to undertake and record the following:
  - Glasgow Coma Scale score
  - Pupillary response
  - Face, arm, speech test.

2.2 **Introduction**

A complete assessment of the nervous system is involved and requires a number of tests, which is beyond the scope of the SW. However, there are several useful and simple tests that you can perform, which will uncover the presence of serious neurological problems in your patient and help determine the most appropriate management for them. You have already met one of them, AVPU, in the PATIENT ASSESSMENT PROCESS lesson and will learn about a more thorough way to record a patient's level of consciousness using the Glasgow Coma Scale.

2.3 **Glasgow Coma Scale**

The Glasgow Coma Scale (GCS) was developed in 1974 as a way of objectively testing the level of consciousness in brain-injured patients and to improve communication between healthcare professionals [Teasdale, 1974]. It was originally a 14-point score, but the division of limb flexion into withdrawal and abnormal flexion led to the 15-point score familiar today (Table 2.1) [Teasdale, 1976]. Although designed for in-hospital use, it is now routinely used by the ambulance service and is an important marker for the early management of traumatic brain injury (TBI) [Bazarian, 2003].

The main use for the GCS is to indicate the level of injury or illness, enabling triage and intervention priorities to be established, and then to monitor trends in consciousness over time. In addition, GCS (in theory) provides an objective way of recording and communicating the patient's level of consciousness between healthcare professionals, when handing over care [Middleton, 2012].

Scores should ideally be given as their separate components, i.e. eyes, verbal and motor. The motor component, in particular, is of interest to neurosurgeons as it is most predictive of outcome

Table 2.1: The Glasgow Coma Scale

Component	Level of response	Score
Eye opening	Spontaneous	4
	To speech	3
	To pain	2
	None	1
Best verbal response	Orientated	5
	Confused	4
	Inappropriate words	3
	Incomprehensible sounds	2
	None	1
Best motor response	Obeys commands	6
	Localises	5
	Withdraws	4
	Abnormal flexion	3
	Extension	2
	None	1

in severe head injuries [Middleton, 2012]. The exact order doesn't matter, although eyes, verbal, motor has been advocated, as the top scores increase incrementally, i.e. eyes = 4, verbal = 5 and motor = 6. This also corresponds to the patient assessment sequence you will follow [Zuercher, 2009].

In the initial patient assessment phase, you will likely utilise a basic level of consciousness scoring system such as AVPU. The associated GCS scores for each part of the AVPU score equate to the following [Anne Kelly, 2004]:

- Alert: 15
- Verbal: 13
- Pain: 8
- Unresponsive: 3.

This is not a substitute for calculating the full GCS score, though, particularly as it is the component scores that are most important.Total GCS scores of less than 8 mostly reflect changes in the motor component of the score, since eye opening and best verbal response will be 1 in this case. Scores of 9–15 tend to be more dependent on eye and verbal components [Middleton, 2012].

2.3.1 Recording an accurate GCS

As you approach the patient, and as part of your global assessment (the general impression), take note of local injuries to the eyes, mouth and limbs, the presence of endotracheal (ET) or tracheostomy tubes, and prior administration of sedative or paralytic drugs, as all of these can affect the accuracy of the GCS. Alcohol consumption does not appear to cause clinically significant reductions in GCS in patients with TBI [Stuke, 2007], even if patients are twice the legal drink-drive limit [Lange, 2010]. As a result, reductions in GCS in the presence of a head injury should not just be attributed to the alcohol.

Painful stimuli

The aim of a pain stimulus is to assess the level of consciousness and depth of coma, but not to cause long-term pain or damage, which could be considered battery [Waterhouse, 2009]! There are two basic types of pain stimulus to use when assessing GCS; peripheral and central. Use a central pain stimulus first because if the patient opens their eyes and moves their arms in response to this, there is no need to test the peripheral pain response.

The preferred central pain stimulus is the trapezius pinch (Figure 2.1) [Middleton, 2012]. It can be tricky to apply sufficient pressure on the trapezius muscle in larger or obese patients and there is some concern about the spinal accessory nerve (which you are stimulating with a trapezius pinch), because it has only a small sensory component compared with its motor function, which increases the risk of a spinal reflex action when you pinch it [Tortora, 2008]. However, this will only lead to elevation or shrugging of the shoulders and not arm flexion, making it a good alternative if you are not confident in applying supra-orbital pressure.

Some common sense is required in deciding which central stimulus to use. A patient with a spinal injury that affects the arms should not have a trapezius pinch applied.

A peripheral pain stimulus is used to test for eye opening. Start with a touch or gentle shake before inflicting pain. Apply pressure with a pen over the lateral aspect of the distal interphalangeal joint of the index finger. Do not apply direct pressure over the nail bed as this can damage the capillary bed and may result in loss of the nail [Waterhouse, 2009].

2.3.2 Eye opening

If the eyes are open, give the patient a score of 4 and move on to the verbal component. If the patient opens their eyes to spoken or shouted speech (and not necessarily just the command to open their eyes), score a 3. If the patient responds to painful stimuli by opening their eyes, give them a 2, and award a 1 if they fail to respond at all.

2.3.3 Best verbal response

- Orientated patients score 5 and are required to be orientated to person, place, time and the event/situation
- Confused patients score 4 and can converse, but responses to your questions will reveal disorientation and misunderstanding [Iacono, 2005]
- Inappropriate words score 3 and consist of clear and understandable speech (often swearing or random words). However, it is not possible to hold a conversation with the patient. Repetition of a word or phrase (perseveration) is also awarded a 3
- Incomprehensible sounds score 2 and consist of moaning and groaning, but no recognisable words. Stroke patients with dysphasia may fall into this category but this is due to a different cause than patients with a moderate or severe TBI who lack sufficient cognition to speak. Make sure you document the difference [Iacono, 2005]
- No verbal response scores a 1 and should be given to patients who make no sound. Follow local guidance about documenting verbal GCS scores for patients who have an ET tube in situ (sometimes denoted as 1T) or who have been pharmacologically sedated or paralysed [Matis, 2008].

2.3.4 Best motor response

- A patient who obeys commands scores 6. Asking the patient to squeeze your fingers is not advocated as comatose patients may exhibit a grasp reflex. In addition, shouting at or touching the patient can also elicit reflex motor responses [Iacono, 2005]

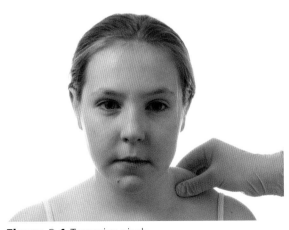

Figure 2.1 Trapezius pinch

- Localisation in response to pain scores a 5 and requires the patient to identify the location of a painful stimulus and attempt to remove it. In the case of a trapezius pinch, you should expect the opposite arm to cross the midline in an attempt to remove the source of the pain (i.e. you!) [Matis, 2008]. In response to supra-orbital pressure, a hand raised above the clavicle would score a 5
- Withdrawal to pain scores 4. This is a normal flexor response where the patient rapidly withdraws their arm and/or abducts the ipsilateral (same side) shoulder [Middleton, 2012]. A peripheral pain stimulus may be required to elicit this accurately
- Abnormal flexion in response to pain scores 3. This is also sometimes called a decorticate response, and consists of adduction and flexion of the arms, flexion of the wrists and fingers, and internal rotation of the legs with plantar flexion of the feet (Figure 2.2)
- Extension to pain (also called a decerebrate response) scores 2. In contrast to abnormal flexion, the arms go into rigid extension alongside the body with pronation of the forearms, and the same leg posture as for abnormal flexion (Figure 2.3) [Iacono, 2005]. Because of the need to record the 'best' score, in the event that there is abnormal flexion on one side of the body and extension on the other, the patient should receive a score of 3 not 2
- No response to pain scores 1. Only score the patient a 1 if they are flaccid and make no movement in response to your painful stimulus.

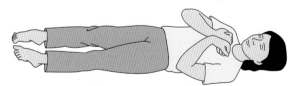

Figure 2.2 Abnormal flexion response

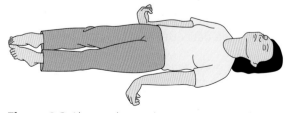

Figure 2.3 Abnormal extension response

2.4 Pupillary response

Before switching on your pen torch to check the patient's pupils, have a look at the pupils' relative size to determine whether they are unequal. This is known as anisocoria and is a normal finding in around 20% of the population [Kaeser, 2010]. Look for changes in shape (e.g. oval in acute angle-closure glaucoma, asymmetrical in a penetrating injury).

Pupillary reactions

There are three tests relating to pupillary reactions that you can perform [James, 2011]:

- Direct response to light: Light directly shone on the eye for three seconds should cause a prompt constriction of the pupil. Failure to do so is known as an afferent pupillary defect and indicates severe optic nerve pathology (transected nerve). There will also be failure of the opposite pupil to constrict. If there is no pupillary reaction but the opposite pupil does constrict, consider a traumatic iris paresis

- Swinging light test: This identifies the presence of a relative afferent pupillary defect (RAPD). Shine the light from one eye to the other in rapid succession. Stimulation of the normal eye should elicit a brisk constriction of both pupils, but when the light is shone on the diseased eye, both pupils dilate. The dilation due to withdrawing the light from the normal eye outweighs the weak constriction produced by shining light on the diseased eye

- Light-near dissociation: If the reactions to light are normal, you can go on to test for the accommodation reflex. Ask the patient to look to a faraway object. Hold an object such as a pen or watch just out of vision and tell the patient that as soon as they see it, they should focus straight on it. As they gaze to the distance, hold your object above the level of their eyes, making sure that your arm is not in the way. Then, drop it into their line of view and observe the pupillary reactions as they look at it. There should be a brisk constriction. Failure to do so is known as light-near dissociation.

If all these pupillary tests are normal, the patient can be said to have Pupils Equally Reacting to Light and Accommodation (PERLA).

2.5 Face, arm, speech test

With the advent of clot-busting drugs (thrombolytics) for the management of acute stroke, the need for prompt recognition of stroke by ambulance personnel has never been greater. A simple tool that can be used to identify a patient suffering from a stroke is the Newcastle face, arm, speech test (FAST) [NAO, 2010].

The FAST consists of three components [Harbison, 2003]:

- Facial palsy: Ask the patient to smile or show their teeth. Look for new lack of symmetry. This is positive if there is an unequal smile, grimace or obvious facial asymmetry

- Arm weakness: Lift the patient's arms together to 90° (45° if they are lying on their back) with the palms uppermost (Figure 2.4). Ask them to close their eyes and hold that position for 5 seconds. Look for one arm drifting or falling rapidly

- Speech impairment: During the course of a conversation (if the patient can speak), look for new speech disturbance. This may require asking someone who knows the patient. Specifically, look for slurred speech and word-finding difficulties. Ask the patient to identify common objects (such as keys, a cup, chair and pen). If the patient has a severe visual disturbance, place the object in the patient's hands and ask them to name it.

The presence of one or more of these signs constitutes a positive FAST (Figure 2.5).

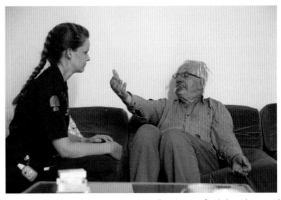

Figure 2.5 A positive FAST, due to a facial palsy and arm weakness

3 Disorders of the nervous system

3.1 Learning objectives

By the end of this lesson you will be able to:

- Describe the following conditions of the nervous system:
  - Epilepsy
  - Stroke
  - Meningococcal disease
  - Tetraplegia/Quadriplegia
  - Paraplegia
  - Hemiplegia
  - Monoplegia
- List a number of common and uncommon causes of coma.

3.2 Introduction

In this lesson, you will learn about a range of nervous system disorders. The nervous system is extremely complex and you will learn about only a few of the many disease processes. However, it is important to be able to recognise patients with epilepsy, stroke, meningococcal disease and coma. Timely and appropriate management can result in better outcome: in some cases, literally the difference between life and death, and/or life-altering disability.

3.3 Epilepsy

Epilepsy is not a single condition, but a term used to describe a tendency to have recurrent, unprovoked convulsions (also called seizures and

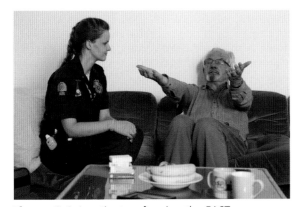

Figure 2.4 A patient performing the FAST

fits). It is the commonest of the serious neurological conditions [Smithson, 2012].

Convulsions result from the synchronised and excessive activation of neurons in the cerebral cortex. How this presents clinically depends on where this activity starts and how far and fast it spreads through the brain [Briar, 2003]. Convulsions are divided into two broad categories:

- Partial (focal) convulsions: As the name suggests, these originate from a specific area of the cortex, typically the temporal or frontal lobes. They are split into two sub-types [Smithson, 2012; Briar, 2003]:
  - Simple partial: Patients remain conscious but may complain of 'butterflies' in their stomach, fear, illusions and hallucinations. These are usually brief
  - Complex partial: Complex refers to an altered level of consciousness and is characterised by the patient chewing, lip-smacking and fiddling with their hands. These usually resolve within a few minutes
- Generalised convulsions: These convulsions are also divided into two sub-types:
  - Tonic-clonic: These convulsions consist of two phases. In the tonic phase, the patient goes stiff (and may cry out), falls (if standing) and bites their tongue as the jaw clenches. This is followed by the clonic phase, characterised by regular jerking movements, which start in the upper limbs. These eventually slow and stop, which may herald the onset of incontinence. Patients typically experience a post-ictal period following a tonic-clonic convulsion, where they may be sleepy and confused. This usually resolves within 20 minutes
  - Absence convulsions: These typically begin in childhood and adolescence and consist of 'day-dreaming', with a few seconds of staring into space, eyelid fluttering, swallowing and head flopping.

3.3.1 Febrile convulsions

Patients with febrile convulsions are not considered to be epileptic, since the convulsion is provoked by a sudden increase in temperature. The most commonly affected age group is from 6 months to 6 years. They are not associated

with an increased risk of developing epilepsy in later life [Lissauer, 2007].

3.3.2 Status epilepticus

Status epilepticus has traditionally been defined as a generalised convulsion lasting for more than 30 minutes, or a series of convulsions, where the patient does not become fully conscious between convulsions, lasting more than 30 minutes [ILAE, 1993]. However, it has been suggested that shortened timescales should be used since most convulsions last less than 5 minutes and those that last more than 5 minutes generally require therapeutic intervention, because they will not stop on their own [Brophy, 2012]. In addition, prolonged convulsions generally become resistant to the drugs typically administered for convulsions, and there is evidence from animal studies that brain injury can occur in under 30 minutes [Meldrum, 1973].

In adults and children, common causes of status epilepticus are withdrawal from or sub-therapeutic doses of anti-epileptic drugs. In children, the most common cause is febrile illness, whereas in adults, stroke is the most common cause [Chin, 2004; Neligan, 2010]. Approximately 16–38% of children diagnosed with status epilepticus are known epileptics. In adults, this figure increases to 42–50%.

3.4 Stroke

Stroke is a syndrome consisting of rapidly developing (usually seconds or minutes) symptoms and/or signs of focal central nervous system (CNS) function. The symptoms last more than 24 hours or lead to death. A transient ischaemic attack is essentially the same thing as a stroke, with the exception of the duration of symptoms, which last less than 24 hours and are not caused by a haemorrhage [Ginsberg, 2004]. Stroke is the third most common cause of death in England; around 110,000 strokes occur in England every year, a quarter of them in people under 65 years of age [NAO, 2005].

3.4.1 Anatomy and physiology

The brain cannot store oxygen or glucose and so is dependent on a constant supply of blood, which is provided by two pairs of vessels, the vertebral and internal carotid arteries (Figure 3.1). These arteries are interconnected in the cranial

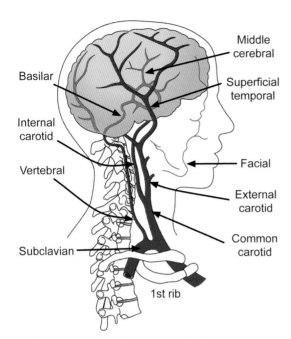

Note: all arteries shown are right sided except for the basilar artery

Figure 3.1 Arteries supplying the brain

cavity to produce an arterial circle (the Circle of Willis), which provides an alternative pathway for blood flow should one of the vessels become occluded [Drake, 2005].

3.4.2 Risk factors

Non-modifiable risk factors for stroke include age, sex, race and family or previous medical history of stroke, transient ischaemic attacks or myocardial infarction. The chance of having a stroke roughly doubles each decade after the age of 55 years, and although it is more common in men, over half of all stroke deaths occur in women. People of South Asian, African or African-Caribbean origin are more likely to suffer from a stroke [O'Donnell, 2010]. Modifiable risk factors include hypertension, smoking, atrial fibrillation, diabetes, diet, physical activity, alcohol consumption, blood cholesterol and obesity [Rodgers, 2004].

3.4.3 Types of stroke

Strokes can be classified as either ischaemic or vascular in origin. Ischaemic strokes are the most common and are caused by atherosclerosis or an embolus from the heart, for example. They are

responsible for around 80% of all new strokes [O'Donnell, 2010; EROS, 2009]. Less common are strokes of vascular origin, caused by haemorrhage. Time is brain, and with each passing minute 1.9 million neurons, 14 billion synapses and 12km (7.5 miles) of myelinated fibres are destroyed. This equates to the premature 'ageing' of the brain to the tune of 3.6 years for each hour without reperfusion treatment [Saver, 2006].

3.5 Meningococcal disease

Meningococcal disease is an umbrella term for a systemic bacterial infection caused by *Neisseria meningitidis* (meningococcus). It presents as meningitis (inflammation of the meninges), septicaemia (which you will learn more about in the SESPIS lesson) or a combination of both [PHE, 2014a].

Although uncommon, of those affected around 10% will die (increasing to 50% in patients with septicaemia without meningitis), and over 10% of those who survive will suffer long-term effects, such as convulsions. It is most common in children under 4 years of age, with a smaller peak in incidence in teenagers aged 15–19 years [PHE, 2014b].

3.5.1 Pathophysiology

Meningococci inhabit the nasopharynx in around 10% of the population, although it is less common in infants (under 5%) and most common in 19-year-olds (over 23%). If the meningococci manage to penetrate the protective mucosa of the nasal passages and enter the bloodstream they rapidly multiply, doubling in number every 30 minutes.

In some people, meningococci cross the blood–brain barrier, where the bacteria are free to multiply inside the cerebrospinal fluid. This leads to inflammation and swelling in the meninges and brain tissue, raising intracranial pressure, which can result in nervous system damage and even death. Surprisingly, patients with meningococcal meningitis do better than those who go on to develop septicaemia. This is thought to be because the body's immune response has prevented the bacteria from causing an overwhelming sepsis [Ninis, 2010].

3.5.2 **Signs and symptoms**

A major issue in the recognition of meningococcal disease is the non-specific nature of the signs and symptoms in the initial stages of the disease. These include [NICE, 2010a]:

- Fever
- Nausea/vomiting
- Lethargy
- Irritable/unsettled
- Ill appearance
- Refusing food/drink
- Headache
- Muscle ache/joint pain
- Respiratory signs and symptoms.

However, the diagnosis window is short. Many children will have non-specific signs and symptoms in the first 4–6 hours, but can be close to death after 24 hours [Thompson, 2006]. Children who are showing the following 'classic' signs and symptoms of meningitis or septicaemia are more likely to have the severe disease (Table 3.1) [NICE, 2010a].

3.5.3 **Sepsis and shock**

The first specific clinical signs to appear are likely to be those of sepsis and shock and include leg pain, abnormal skin colour, cold hands and feet and, in older children, thirst. Parents of younger children may also report drowsiness and difficulty in breathing (described as rapid or laboured) [Thompson, 2006]. Don't forget to enquire about how much urine a child has been passing or if they have had a wet nappy recently. Oliguria (low output of urine) is an early sign of shock [Ninis, 2010].

3.5.4 **Fever**

Many children with septicaemia will become acutely ill with a fever. This can be complicated by a trivial viral illness that precedes this, but look for a sudden change in the history. Remember that not all children with meningococcal disease have fever, and you should not dismiss a fever responsive to antipyretics (such as paracetamol and ibuprofen) as of viral origin [Ninis, 2010]. Rather counter-intuitively, infants can actually develop hypothermia in sepsis [Wells 2001].

3.5.5 **Rash**

The classic sign is a petechial non-blanching rash (Figure 3.2). However, only 10% of children presenting with the rash will have meningococcal disease. The remainder will have a viral infection. On the other hand, febrile and ill children with a purpuric rash (a non-blanching rash of greater than 2 mm in diameter) are very likely to have meningococcal disease [Wells, 2001]. Care needs to be taken with blanching rashes, such as a maculopapular rash, as up to 30% of children may initially present with this, although careful examination will generally yield some non-blanching elements (Figure 3.3) [Hart, 2006]. On dark skin, you may have to check the soles of the feet, palms of the hand, abdomen or conjunctivae and palate. You must fully undress the child and be thorough in your search. Petechial rashes may not be widespread initially and can be easily missed.

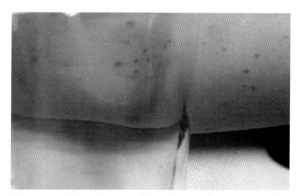

Figure 3.2 Petechial non-blanching rash. Note how this does not blanch under the pressure of a glass
Courtesy Meningitis Research Foundation www.meningitis.org

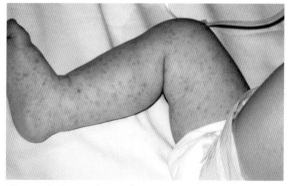

Figure 3.3 Maculopapular rash with scanty petechiae
Courtesy Meningitis Research Foundation www.meningitis.org

Table 3.1: Signs and symptoms of bacterial meningitis and meningococcal septicaemia

Signs and symptoms	Bacterial meningitis	Meningococcal disease	Meningococcal septicaemia	Notes
Common non-specific signs and symptoms				
Fever	YES	YES	YES	Not always present, especially in neonates
Vomiting/ nausea	YES	YES	YES	
Lethargy	YES	YES	YES	
Irritable/ unsettled	YES	YES	YES	
Ill appearance	YES	YES	YES	
Refusing food/ drink	YES	YES	YES	
Headache	YES	YES	YES	
Muscle ache/ joint pain	YES	YES	YES	
Respiratory symptoms/signs of breathing difficulty	YES	YES	YES	
Less common non-specific signs and symptoms				
Chills/shivering	YES	YES	Not Known	
Diarrhoea, abdominal pain/distension	YES	YES	Not Known	
Sore throat/ cold-like symptoms or other ear, nose and throat signs and symptoms	YES	YES	Not Known	
More specific signs and symptoms				

Table 3.1 (Continued):

Signs and symptoms	Bacterial meningitis	Meningococcal disease	Meningococcal septicaemia	Notes
Non-blanching rash	YES	YES	YES	Be aware that a rash may be less visible in darker skin tones – check soles of feet, palms of hands and conjunctivae
Stiff neck	YES	YES	Not Known	
Altered mental state	YES	YES	YES	Includes confusion, delirium and drowsiness, and impaired consciousness
Capillary refill time more than 2 seconds	Not Known	YES	YES	
Shock	YES	YES	YES	
Hypotension	Not Known	YES	YES	
Leg pain	Not Known	YES	YES	
Cold hands/feet	Not Known	YES	YES	
Back rigidity	YES	YES	Not Known	
Bulging fontanelle	YES	YES	Not Known	Only relevant in children aged under 2 years
Photophobia	YES	YES	NO	
Unconsciousness	YES	YES	YES	
Focal neurological deficit including cranial nerve involvement and abnormal pupils	YES	YES	NO	
Convulsions	YES	YES	NO	

3.5.6 **Meningism**

The signs of meningococcal meningitis are shown in Table 3.1, but remember that the picture can be complicated by concurrent septicaemia in the child, making it difficult to differentiate an altered mental state due to sepsis-induced hypoperfusion from one caused by raised intracranial pressure.

In younger children (particularly those under 2 years of age), there is less likely to be neck stiffness or photophobia. Babies with meningitis sometimes have a full or bulging fontanelle due to raised intracranial pressure, and become more distressed when handled than when left alone [Ninis, 2010].

3.6 **Paralysis**

In medical terminology, paralysis is typically represented by the suffix -plegia. This is not to be confused with paresis, which is used to refer to muscle weakness, or incomplete loss of muscle function [Porth, 2003]. Four common terms that you will hear used are [Macleod, 2005]:

- Monoplegia: Paralysis in a single limb
- Hemiplegia: Paralysis of both limbs on the same side of the body
- Quadriplegia (also tetraplegia): Paralysis of all four limbs
- Paraplegia: Paralysis of both the lower limbs.

3.7 **Coma**

Coma is the absence of consciousness and is often referred to as a loss of consciousness (LOC). This presents as a completely unaware patient unresponsive to external stimuli, with only eye opening to pain and no eye tracking or fixation, and limb withdrawal to a noxious stimulus (usually pain) at best (often with reflex motor movements) [Wijdicks, 2010].

Full consciousness is an awake state in which one is aware of oneself and the environment, including the ability to perceive and interpret stimuli and to interact and communicate with others in the absence of motor deficits [Young, 2014].

Common causes of coma include:

- Stroke – ischaemic and haemorrhagic
- Cardiac arrest
- Alcohol abuse
- Substance abuse and overdose
- Carbon monoxide poisoning
- Sepsis
- Bacterial meningitis
- Syncope (faint)
- Convulsions
- Traumatic brain injury
- Hyper/hypoglycaemia.

Uncommon causes of coma include:

- Subarachnoid haemorrhage
- Brain abscess or tumour
- Burns
- Hypo/hyperthermia.

It may not always be possible to determine the cause of coma and the management of the patient may just be supportive. However, for reversible causes, such as hypoglycaemia, convulsions and overdose, it is important to recognise these conditions as the patient can then receive the appropriate treatment out-of-hospital [AACE, 2013].

Chapter 13: Exposure/Environment

1 Extremes of temperature

1.1 Learning objectives
By the end of this lesson you will be able to:
- State the normal temperature range for an adult
- Explain the terms 'hypothermia' and 'heat-related illness'
- Describe the appropriate management for a patient with signs of hypothermia and heat-related illness.

1.2 Introduction
Despite being exposed to a wide range of environmental temperatures, the human body maintains a stable temperature of around 37°C and is maintained in the range 35.8–38.2°C. Normal fluctuations of about 1°C occur over a 24-hour period, with highest temperatures recorded in the afternoon and early evening, and lowest temperatures in early morning [Marieb, 2013].

Thermoregulation is primarily the job of the hypothalamus, which receives sensory information from peripheral and central thermoreceptors. This is necessary because the different body regions have differing temperatures [Tortora, 2008]:
- Core: Consisting of organs within the skull, thorax and abdomen
- Shell: The skin.

By controlling the flow of blood to the shell, the hypothalamus can control the amount of heat generated and lost.

Heat-promoting mechanisms
When the external temperature falls, the heat-promoting centre is activated. This maintains core body temperature by [Marieb, 2013]:
- Constricting peripheral cutaneous blood vessels
- Causing shivering – involuntary contractions of skeletal muscle, which generates heat
- Increasing the body's metabolic rate.

In addition, there are a number of behavioural changes that can be promoted:

- Putting on warmer clothes
- Drinking hot fluids
- Increasing physical activity.

Heat-loss mechanisms
Most heat loss occurs via the skin by dilation of cutaneous blood vessels and/or enhanced sweating, allowing for heat loss to occur by [Marieb, 2013]:
- Radiation: Infrared waves (thermal energy)
- Conduction: Direct contact with cooler objects (such as cold water)
- Convection: Since warm air expands and rises, warm air around the body is constantly replaced with cooler air, which absorbs the heat. This process can be enhanced by moving air more rapidly across the body surface, for example by the use of a fan
- Evaporation: As water absorbs heat from the body, it becomes energetic enough to escape the body as a gas, called water vapour.

1.3 Hypothermia
Hypothermia is defined as a core body temperature of less than 35°C. It is classified into three categories, based on temperature [AACE, 2013]:
- Mild: 32–35°C
- Moderate: 28–32°C
- Severe: Less than 28°C.

However, without a low-reading thermometer, it can be difficult to record accurate core body temperatures. Therefore, it is important to suspect that hypothermia might be a factor in the following [AACE, 2013]:
- Older patients (over 80 years of age)
- Children
- Some medical conditions: For example, hypothyroidism and stroke
- Intoxicated patients: Alcohol and/or recreational drugs
- Drowning
- Patients suffering from exhaustion
- Injured and immobile patients
- Decreased level of consciousness.

As patients succumb to hypothermia, they move through five stages [Durrer, 2003]:

1. Conscious and shivering
2. Decreased level of consciousness and not shivering
3. Unconscious
4. Not breathing
5. Death due to irreversible hypothermia.

1.3.1 Management

The mainstay of treatment is to prevent further heat loss. In the mildly hypothermic patient, this is likely to be enough, but severely hypothermic patients will require active rewarming, which realistically can only be performed in hospital [Nolan, 2012]. Adopt the following principles when managing a patient with hypothermia [AACE, 2013]:

- If using a foil blanket, ensure that you wrap the patient in a fabric blanket first
- Give the patient hot drinks if they are conscious, but NOT alcohol
- Do not rub the patient's skin – as with alcohol, this leads to peripheral vasodilation, which worsens hypothermia
- Avoid rough handling as it can cause arrhythmias and cardiac arrest
- If intravenous fluids are required, ensure they are warmed prior to administration
- Patients with a decreased level of consciousness should not be encouraged to walk, but managed horizontally.

1.4 Heat-related illness

Heat-related illnesses can occur as a result of external factors such as the sun, or internal factors such as drugs and exercise. It presents on a continuum, with heat stress the least serious heat-related illness, through to multi-organ dysfunction and even death at the other extreme [AACE, 2013]:

- Heat stress
- Heat exhaustion
- Heat stroke
- Multi-organ dysfunction.

Heat stress

This is a mild form of heat-related illness and is characterised by [Soar, 2010]:

- Normal temperature or mild temperature elevation
- Heat oedema: Swelling of feet and ankles
- Heat syncope: Vasodilation causes hypotension
- Heat cramps: Depletion of salts leads to muscle cramps.

Heat exhaustion

This is a more severe form of heat-related illness, with symptoms mostly as a result of fluid loss and electrolyte imbalances [Soar, 2010]:

- Systemic reaction to prolonged heat exposure (hours to days)
- Core body temperature over 37°C and less than 40°C
- Headache, dizziness, nausea and vomiting, tachycardia, hypotension, sweating, muscle pain, weakness and cramps
- Can progress quickly to heat stroke.

Heat stroke

Heat stroke is a systemic inflammatory response to a core body temperature of 40.6°C or more, and is associated with altered level of consciousness and organ dysfunction [Soar, 2010]. It comes in two types: non-exertional heat stroke, which is caused by high external temperatures and/or high humidity; and exertional heat stroke, which is caused by excess heat production. Non-exertional heat stroke tends to occur in the elderly, very young and chronically ill, whereas extertional heat stroke is more typical in active groups such as athletes, manual workers and military recruits [AACE, 2013].

Clinical features include [Soar, 2010]:

- Core body temperature 40.6°C or more
- Hot dry skin (although sweating is present in around half of all cases)
- Early signs and symptoms: Extreme fatigue, headache, fainting, facial flushing, vomiting and diarrhoea
- Arrhythmias and hypotension
- Respiratory distress
- Liver and kidney failure.

1.4.1 Management

Heat stress and exhaustion

The management of patients with heat-related illness broadly consists of cooling the patient and replacing lost fluid and electrolytes. For patients with signs and symptoms of heat stress consider the following [Lipman, 2013]:

- Remove the patient from the heat source
- Passively cool – move the patient into the shade or an air-conditioned ambulance. Loosen or remove tight-fitting clothing
- Provide oral isotonic fluid replacement
- Elevate oedematous extremities.

If the patient has developed heat exhaustion, similar management principles apply, except that depending on the patient's level of consciousness, fluid rehydration may have to be intravenous. In addition, cooling should be active, using conductive, evaporative and convective methods. Cold-water immersion is ideal for the ambulant, co-operative patient, but may not be practical otherwise. Alternatives include removing the patient's clothes and spraying or dousing the patient with water. Air movement can be augmented by fanning the patient [Lipman, 2013].

Heat stroke

While supporting the patient's airway, breathing, circulation and disability, begin rapidly cooling the patient while en route to hospital [Soar, 2010]. Ice water immersion is useful, but not practical, so consider the same techniques as for heat exhaustion to cool the patient. Ice packs are useful if they cover the body, not just the neck, axillae and groin, but should not be applied directly to the skin [Lipman, 2013]. Rehydration is safest intravenously as an altered level of consciousness increases the chance of aspiration [Soar, 2010].

2 Drowning

2.1 Learning objectives

By the end of this lesson, you will be able to:

- Explain the pathophysiology and management of drowning.

2.2 Introduction

The definition of drowning has been complicated in the past and so in 2002 (at the World Congress on Drowning, held in Amsterdam) a single definition was agreed. As a result, drowning is now defined as a process resulting in primary respiratory impairment from submersion/immersion in a liquid [Idris, 2003]. Whether the victim lives or dies after this process is not important, they have still drowned. If they do not survive, then they have fatally drowned [Szpilman, 2012].

2.3 Pathophysiology

When a drowning victim is unable to keep water (the most common liquid in drowning incidents) from their mouth, it is spat out or swallowed. If still conscious, victims will then attempt to hold their breath, but this is likely to continue for less than a minute, depending on levels of panic and the temperature of the water. Once the inspiratory drive is too high to resist, the victim will take a breath and water will be aspirated into the airways [Szpilman, 2012]. Laryngospasm may occur, but this is rapidly terminated by cerebral hypoxia, and active ventilation, with aspiration of water, will resume. It was once thought that laryngospasm might be responsible for drowning victims who were found not to have aspirated (so called dry-drowning). The theory was that the victim died due to hypoxic cardiac arrest because of laryngospasm or breath-holding [Layon, 2009]. However, autopsy studies have concluded that this is unlikely, as water does not passively seep into the lungs [Modell, 1999; Piette, 2006]. To drown therefore requires active ventilation while the victim is submerged (i.e. under the water and still alive).

Whether due to laryngospasm or breath-holding, with no gas exchange the victim becomes increasingly hypoxaemic, hypercarbic and acidotic. Unless they are rescued, the victim will succumb to hypoxaemia, leading to loss of consciousness and apnoea [Layon, 2009]. The cardiac rhythm deteriorates, usually following a sequence of tachyarrhythmias, bradyarrhythmias, pulseless electrical activity (PEA) and asystole [Szpilman, 2012].

Immersion in cold water (10°C or less) produces large and rapid reductions in skin temperature, which in turn leads to cold shock. This term refers to a collection of physiological responses including an inspiratory gasp (which can result in drowning if the victim's airway is submerged), hyperventilation, hypocapnia, tachycardia, peripheral vasoconstriction and hypertension [Datta, 2006]. Cold shock is thought to be caused by stimulation of cutaneous cold thermoreceptors, which result in an excessive sympathetic nervous system response. The magnitude of the cold shock response is reduced by the victims' clothing, their habituation to cold (regular winter swimming in just your Speedos, for example) and orientation on immersion [Shattock, 2012].

If the victim is fully submerged in cold water, the diving response may be activated. This is caused by cooling of the cold thermoreceptors on the face, which are innervated by the trigeminal nerve. This results in a profound sinus bradycardia due to parasympathetic nervous system stimulation of the heart, an expiratory apnoea due to inhibition of central respiratory neurons, and sympathetic nervous system mediated vasoconstriction of the trunk and limbs. A similar response is also possible by stimulation of vagal receptors in the pharynx and larynx [Angell-James, 1975].

It has been suggested that this simultaneous stimulation of both sympathetic and parasympathetic pathways of the autonomic nervous system results in an 'autonomic conflict', leading to life-threatening arrhythmias that may result in death in susceptible individuals (Figure 2.1) [Shattock, 2012].

Although the tonicity of the water (for example sea water versus fresh water) was once thought to be important, the effect on the lungs is ultimately the same, although with a different osmotic gradient. The fragile alveolar-capillary membranes are disrupted, leading to increased permeability and movement of fluid, plasma and electrolytes [Orlowski, 1989]. Clinically, this leads to significant amounts of blood-stained pulmonary oedema and decreasing gaseous exchange of oxygen and carbon dioxide. Following drowning, the presence of additional fluid in the lungs and the loss of surfactant lead to increasing areas of the lungs becoming regions of low, or no, ventilation and perfusion (pulmonary shunting), and there is widespread

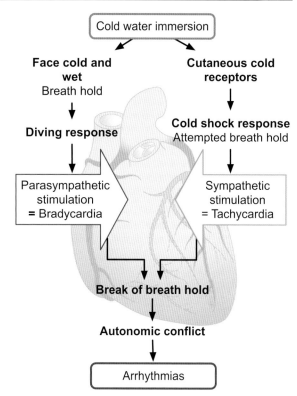

Figure 2.1 Autonomic conflict

atelectasis and bronchospasm [Layon, 2009]. Similarly, the haemodynamic and cardiovascular effects seen in drowning are not related to tonicity either, but primarily are a consequence of anoxia [Orlowski, 1989].

2.4 Management

Try to avoid getting wet. You should only go into the water to rescue a drowning victim as a last resort and only if you are adequately trained and equipped. Many victims who are drowning can help themselves with firm coaching, or will have already been rescued by bystanders or professional rescuers, who can have a dramatic impact on the victim's outcome. On beaches with a lifeguard, for example, less than 6% of victims will require hospital treatment and only around 0.5% will require cardiopulmonary resuscitation (CPR) [NWSF, 2012]. This is in stark contrast to the 30% of victims requiring CPR when rescued by untrained bystanders [Venema, 2010].

If you need to rescue the victim, remember to 'call, reach, throw, wade and row'. As previously mentioned, encourage victims to self-rescue first.

Next, try to reach them with an object such as a pole, tree branch or even items of clothing. Consider throwing something that is buoyant, ideally a rescue ring with a lifeline attached. Wading into the water is the next possibility as long as someone on the shore has hold of you, the water is shallow enough to stand in and the victim is within reach. Alternatively, use a boat, if available.

Resuscitation is limited while in the water and should consist of ventilations only. Chest compressions are futile in deep water, so wait until the patient is on a firm surface, such as the shore or the deck of a boat [Szpilman, 2004]. The incidence of spinal injuries is very low (around 0.5%) and spinal immobilisation delays effective resuscitation, so only do this when there is a clear mechanism of injury that could cause spinal injury (such as diving into shallow water or water ski-ing) [Watson, 2001; Soar, 2010].

Get the victim out of the water as soon as possible and place them supine (on their back), with head and torso at the same level, and check for breathing. If they are breathing but unconscious, provide high-flow oxygen via non-rebreathing mask as per clinical guidelines and place them in the recovery position. They are at high risk of gastric regurgitation, so ensure that you have suction available [AACE, 2013].

Victims of prolonged immersion in water (typically 30 minutes or more, but less as water temperature decreases) may also suffer the added complication of circum-rescue collapse [Golden, 1997]. This is due to the increased hydrostatic pressure from the water on the victim's legs and torso increasing venous return and cardiac output. Central baroreceptors mistake this for hypervolaemia resulting in increased diuresis. In addition, peripheral vasoconstriction will occur as the water is cold relative to the body, which magnifies this response [Lord, 2005]. Once the victim is removed from the water, the hydrostatic pressure is lost, exacerbating the hypovolaemia. This can also be compounded by hypothermia and physical effort [if the victim attempts to remove him- or herself from the water, for example]. The sudden drop in venous return can reduce coronary perfusion enough to induce cardiac arrest. For this reason, it is advised to remove victims horizontally from the water if possible [Szpilman, 2012].

Hypothermia is likely to occur and wet clothes should be cut off to minimise movement. Hypothermic patients are at risk of cardiac arrhythmias, including ventricular fibrillation, even with minor movement [Althaus, 1982]. Get the patient covered with blankets and in a warm ambulance as soon as possible.

Chapter 14: **Medical Emergencies**

1 **Anaphylaxis**

1.1 **Learning objectives**

By the end of this lesson you will be able to:

- Explain the term anaphylaxis and its common causes

- Describe signs and symptoms that a patient with anaphylaxis may present with

- State the management of anaphylaxis including the administration of adrenaline using the patient's own auto-injector.

1.2 **Introduction**

Anaphylaxis is a serious allergic reaction that is rapid in onset and may cause death [Sampson, 2006]. Its hallmark is rapidly developing life-threatening airway/breathing/circulation (or any combination of the three) problem(s) and it is usually associated with skin and mucosal changes [Soar, 2008].

The exact incidence of anaphylaxis is unknown as many episodes are not reported, but it is thought that around 1 in 1,333 of the population have an anaphylactic reaction at some point in their lives [Soar, 2008]. Approximately 3,000 people a year are admitted to hospital in England [DoH, 2006b] (600–700 in Scotland [SG, 2009]) with anaphylaxis, and it is estimated that there are 10–20 deaths per year in England and Wales [DoH, 2006b].

The most common causes (triggers) are food, medication and insect stings [Lee, 2011]. In children, food is the most common cause of allergy, whereas in adults, it is medication [Capps, 2010]. Death is unlikely more than 6 hours after exposure to a trigger, but cardiac arrest can occur in minutes, particularly if the trigger is medication that has been administered intravenously. Envenomation typically causes cardiac arrest within 15 minutes, and food takes a little longer on average, at around 30 minutes [Pumphrey, 2000].

1.3 **Signs and symptoms**

Anaphylaxis is highly likely when any one of the following criteria are fulfilled [Sampson, 2006]:

1. Acute onset of an illness (minutes to several hours) with involvement of the skin and/or mucosal tissue (e.g. generalised urticaria, pruritus or flushing, and swollen lips-tongue-uvula, also known as angioedema) and at least one of the following:

   - Respiratory compromise (e.g. difficulty breathing, bronchospasm, stridor)

   - Reduced blood pressure or associated symptoms of end-organ dysfunction (e.g. collapse)

2. Two or more of the following that occur rapidly after exposure to a likely allergen for that patient (minutes to several hours):

   - Involvement of the skin/mucosal tissue

   - Respiratory compromise

   - Reduced blood pressure or associated symptoms

   - Persistent gastrointestinal symptoms (e.g. crampy abdominal pain, nausea, vomiting, diarrhoea)

3. Rapid onset of reduced BP after exposure to a known allergen for that patient (minutes to several hours):

   - Infants and children: low systolic BP

   - Adults: systolic BP of less than 90 mmHg.

NOTE: Up to 20% of anaphylaxis cases do not have skin and/or mucosal changes, particularly reactions that occur intra-operatively in adults and food/insect sting induced reactions in children. Patients with severe anaphylaxis resulting in significant hypotension may not exhibit any cutaneous symptoms until their blood pressure is restored [Lee, 2011].

1.4 **Management**

Having conducted your standard ABCDE assessment and determined that your patient is likely to be suffering from anaphylaxis, you should identify the trigger and remove it if possible (e.g. stop any drug infusions, remove bee stings). However, if this is not possible, then do not delay treatment. If you suspect food-induced anaphylaxis, encouraging the patient to vomit is NOT recommended [Soar, 2008].

Patients with A or B problems are likely to be more comfortable sitting up, whereas those with C problems are best managed recumbent with or without legs raised. It is important not to make patients sit or stand if they feel faint as this can cause cardiac arrest!

Administer high-flow oxygen at 15 litres per minute and, if local guidelines allow, administer intramuscular (IM) adrenaline as soon as possible (Figure 1.1) [BTS, 2008; AACE, 2013]. Patients who still have a pulse should not have adrenaline administered intravenously (IV), except by those who do this in normal clinical practice (e.g. critical care paramedics, anaesthetists). The preferred route is IM into the anterolateral thigh as there is a greater margin of safety, it is quick to administer (versus gaining IV access) and the peak plasma concentration is higher when adrenaline is administered in the thigh compared to the deltoid [Simons, 2001]. In the event of a cardiac arrest, however, the patient should receive their adrenaline IV [Soar, 2008]. Doses of adrenaline can be repeated every 5 minutes depending on patient condition.

Once IV access has been obtained, the senior clinician is likely to administer fluid and consider other second line treatments, such as antihistamines and hydrocortisone. In addition, you may be asked to set up a nebuliser to administer bronchodilators such as salbutamol and ipratropium [AACE, 2013].

NOTE: Adrenaline is also known as epinephrine, particularly in American texts.

1.4.1 Auto-injectors

Patients who are known to have anaphylactic reactions may have been provided with their own adrenaline auto-injector. Common systems in the UK include Jext® and Epipen® and are typically available as 300 microgram adult and 150 microgram child doses. Depending on your service, you may be authorised to administer these, but even if you are not, it is important that you are aware of the procedure and can ensure that patients administer their own adrenaline properly.

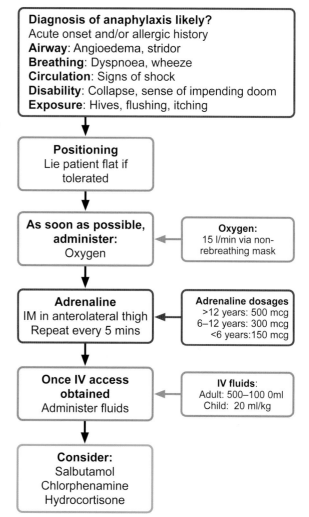

Figure 1.1 Emergency management of anaphylaxis

Procedure for Jext autoinjector [ALK-Abello, 2013]

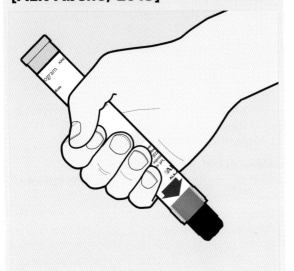

1. Grasp the Jext injector in your dominant hand (the one you use to write with) with your thumb closest to the yellow cap

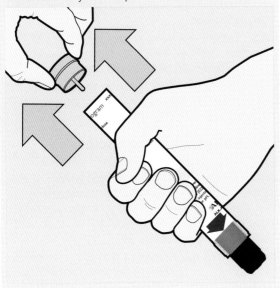

2. Pull off the yellow cap with your other hand

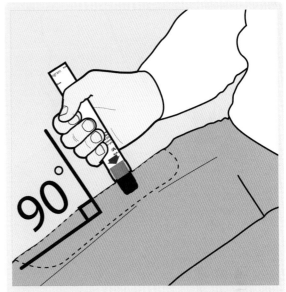

3. Place the black injector tip against your outer thigh, holding the injector at a right angle (approx 90°) to the thigh

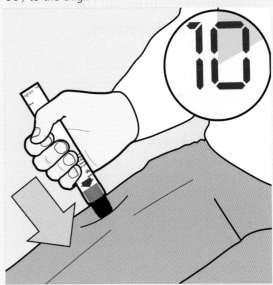

4. Push the black tip firmly into your outer thigh until you hear a 'click' confirming the injection has started, then keep it pushed in. Hold the injector firmly in place against the thigh for 10 seconds (a slow count to 10) then remove. The black tip will extend automatically and hide the needle

Procedure continued →

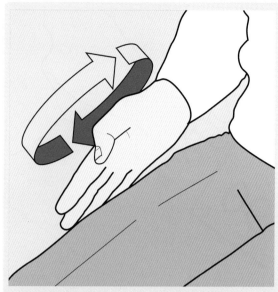

5. Massage the injection area for 10 seconds

2 Diabetes

2.1 Learning objectives

By the end of this lesson you will be able to:

- Describe the types and causes of diabetes
- Describe two diabetic emergencies
- Explain how to record a blood sugar measurement.

2.2 Introduction

Diabetes mellitus is a common metabolic disorder typified by chronic high blood sugar (hyperglycaemia). It is a major cause of morbidity and premature death due to long-term complications such as heart attacks, stroke, kidney failure and blindness [Holt, 2010]. There are around 3.2 million people in the United Kingdom known to have diabetes, 6% of the population [Diabetes UK, 2014].

2.3 Types and causes of diabetes

Types of diabetes

There are two types of diabetes [WHO, 1999]:

- Type 1: Previously referred to as insulin-dependent diabetes (IDDM). Patients with type 1 diabetes are unable to produce any insulin, usually due to autoimmune disease which destroys the insulin-producing beta cells in the pancreas [Holt, 2010]. Insulin is a hormone that

increases transport of glucose across cell membranes and is released by the beta cells. It targets the muscle, fat and liver cells to promote the creation of glucose [Tortora, 2008].

- Type 2: Previously referred to as non-insulin dependent diabetes (NIDDM). Patients with type 2 diabetes have a relative insulin deficiency due to varying degrees of insulin resistance. This is by far the most common type of diabetes, accounting for around 90% of all people with diabetes in the UK.

Causes/risk of diabetes

Underlying causes of diabetes generally fall into four categories [Holt, 2010]:

- Genetic: A family history of type 1 diabetes or other autoimmune disease is linked to a higher risk of developing type 1 diabetes in the family. Likewise, type 2 diabetes also has a familial component, although this connection is rather more complicated

- Obesity: This increases the risk of developing type 2 diabetes, particularly in people with a body mass index over 25 kg/m^2 or large waist circumference

- Age: People are living longer and beta cell function declines with age, leading to a chance of developing diabetes in old age

- Ethnicity: Some ethnic groups are at higher risk of developing diabetes, particularly those of South Asian and Afro-Caribbean origin.

2.4 Diabetic emergencies

Blood sugar is typically maintained within a narrow range of 3.0 to 5.6 mmol/l [AACE, 2013]. Diabetic patients are generally encouraged to keep their blood sugar at 4.0 or higher, with a target range of 4.0–8.0 mmol/l for children and 4.0–7.0 mmol/l for adults [NICE, 2004].

There are two main types of diabetic emergency that you will encounter on an ambulance:

- Hypoglycaemia
- Severe hyperglycaemia.

2.4.1 Hypoglycaemia

Although diabetic patients are generally encouraged to keep their blood sugar at 4.0 or higher, some will experience symptoms of hypoglycaemia at blood sugar levels higher than this, making recognition important. Some signs and symptoms of hypoglycaemia include [Deary, 1993]:

- Sweating
- Palpitations
- Shaking
- Hunger
- Confusion
- Drowsiness
- Odd/aggressive behaviour
- Speech problems
- Headache
- Nausea.

Management

If the patient is still conscious and able to take oral glucose, then administer 10–20g of glucose. You can find 10g of glucose in [BNF, 2014; AACE, 2013]:

- 55 ml Lucozade Energy Original
- 100 ml Coca-Cola
- 18 ml Ribena Blackcurrant (diluted to taste)
- NB: none should be diet/sugar-free varieties!
- 2 teaspoons of sugar
- 3 sugar lumps.

In addition, commercial preparations of glucose are available including Glucogel, Dextrogel and Hypo-Fit. Administration of oral glucose can be repeated after 10–15 minutes, if required.

If the patient is unable to take oral glucose due to impaired consciousness, is uncooperative or there is a risk of aspiration, then either IM glucagon or IV glucose should be administered. This decision will be a judgement call by the senior clinician and will depend on whether IV access can be obtained.

2.4.2 Severe hyperglycaemia

Hyperglycaemia, or high blood sugar levels, is a classic symptom of diabetes. However, chronically high levels of blood glucose can lead to potentially life-threatening complications such as diabetic ketoacidosis and hyperosmolar hyperglycaemic syndrome. You don't need to know what these are, but you should appreciate that patients with these conditions can still appear reasonably well [Holt, 2010].

Signs and symptoms of severe hyperglycaemia include [AACE, 2013]:

- High blood sugar reading (compare to patient's normal value)
- Excessive urination (polyuria)
- Excessive thirst (polydipsia)
- Increased appetite
- Lethargy, confusion and ultimately, loss of consciousness
- Dehydration, dry mouth and, in severe cases, hypovolaemic shock
- Hyperventilation.

Management

These patients should be managed in hospital. The senior clinician may elect to administer intravenous fluids if the patient is showing signs of shock, but generally this will be undertaken while en route to hospital. Oxygen is also administered if the patient is suffering from hypoxaemia [AACE, 2013].

2.5 Blood sugar measurement

Procedure - Accu-Chek® Aviva blood glucose meter

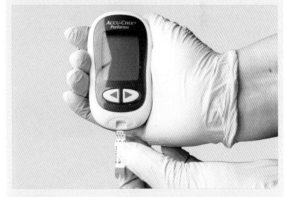

1. Wash and dry your hands or use alcohol gel and put on gloves. Select an appropriate site, which is typically the side of a finger in an adult or older child and the heel of the foot in a younger child or infant. Clean the area with water or a water-soaked gauze. Insert the test strip into the meter and check that the meter turns on automatically

Procedure continued →

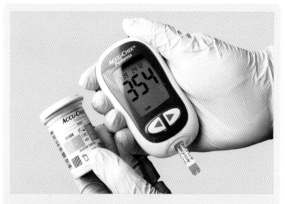

2. Ensure that the code number of the display matches the code number on the test strip container

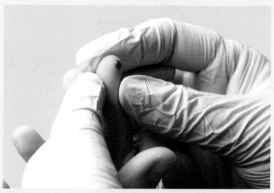

5. With the patient's hand facing downwards, gently squeeze their finger to assist the flow of blood

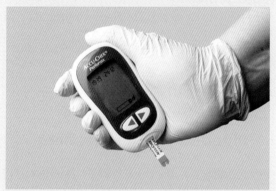

3. On the screen, an icon showing the test strip and a flashing blood drop will appear. Ask the patient to dangle their arm down at their side to encourage blood flow to their fingertips

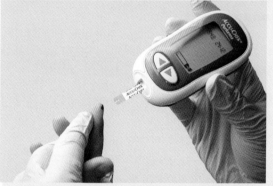

6. Touch the blood drop to the front edge of the yellow window of the test strip. When you have enough blood, you will see an egg timer icon flash

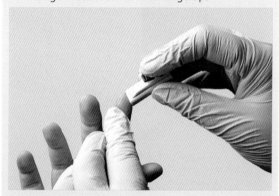

4. Prick the target area with a lancet, disposing of it in a sharps bin after use

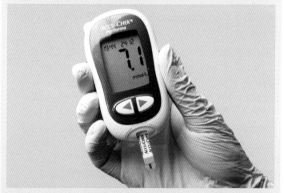

7. The blood sugar result will appear on the display. Note this value on the patient report form

3 Sepsis

3.1 Learning objectives

By the end of this lesson you will be able to:

- Explain what sepsis and septic shock are and how they occur
- State how you would recognise a patient with sepsis or septic shock
- Describe the out-of-hospital management of sepsis.

3.2 Introduction

Sepsis is a life-threatening condition that arises when the bodys response to an infection injures its own tissues and organs. It leads to shock, multiple organ failure and death if not recognised early and treated promptly [Czura, 2011]. Sepsis is estimated to cause 36,00064,000 deaths a year and is responsible for more deaths than lung, bowel and breast cancer [Daniels, 2011a]. Around 90% of patients with sepsis arrive by ambulance, most commonly presenting with a respiratory tract infection [Gray, 2013; Daniels, 2011b] and 3540% of these patients will die in hospital [Daniels, 2011a; Vincent, 2006; Levy, 2010]. Septic shock is a subset of sepsis which has a higher risk of mortality than with sepsis alone [Singer, 2016]. Septic shock causes particularly profound circulatory, cellular, and metabolic abnormalities. Since determining the presence of septic shock can be difficult out-of-hospital, a pragmatic alternative is to treat any patient who is hypotensive despite fluid resuscitation as if they have septic shock. These patients are high risk, as are others with any of the red flag signs/ symptoms shown in Figure 15.2. To ensure that these patients receive urgent attention, it is important the term Red flag sepsis is used when communicating with other healthcare professionals [UKST, 2016].

3.3 Recognition and management

To simplify the identification of sepsis (particularly red flag sepsis), a screening tool has been developed for pre-hospital use (Figure 15.2) [UKST, 2016]. Since use of the National Early Warning Score (NEWS) is widespread, this has been included in the screening tool. However, it is perfectly acceptable for you to use the tool if the patient looks sick. Next, you should consider whether there is an infection present; it is not necessary for you to identify the exact source of the infection. Finally, the presence of any red flag signs/symptoms should be sought out to determine the presence of red flag sepsis. Patients who do not meet the criteria for red flag sepsis but have sepsis still require further assessment and appropriate management to prevent their clinical condition deteriorating. Identifying sepsis before arrival at the ED and, even more importantly, ambulance crews stating that they suspect the patient has sepsis reduces patients time to receive antibiotics and the sepsis care bundle in the ED [Studnek, 2012; Band, 2011].

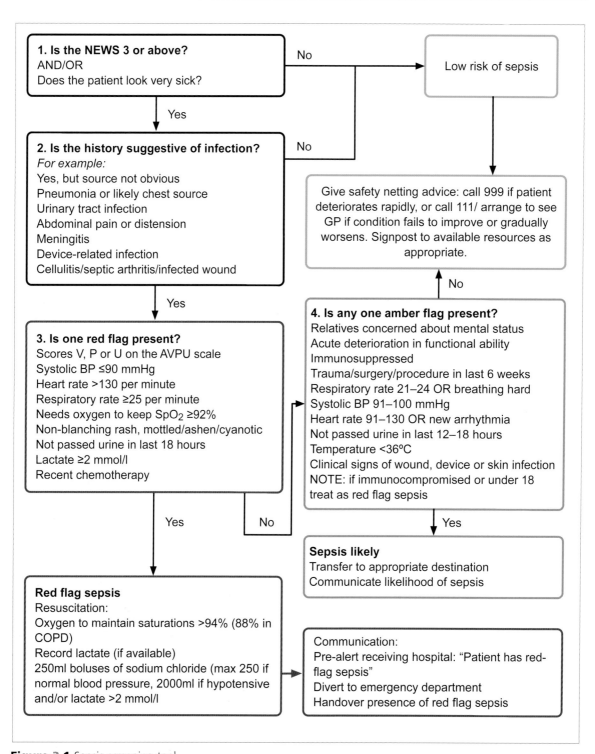

Figure 3.1 Sepsis screening tool

Chapter 15: **Trauma**

1 **Mechanism of injury**

1.1 **Learning objectives**
By the end of this chapter you will be able to:
- Define trauma
- Define mechanism of injury and outline the different types
- Explain the kinetics associated with trauma
- Describe the mechanisms that can cause injury to the head, spine, chest, abdomen and pelvis.

1.2 **Introduction**
Trauma is the acute physiological and structural change (injury) that occurs in a patient's body when an external source of energy transfers to the body faster than the body's ability to sustain and dissipate it. The mechanism of injury (MOI) is defined as the physical forces that act on the body to cause damage [Pilbery, 2013]. Since human tissue, organs and systems can only withstand a limited range of physical, environmental and physiological stress, when the energy delivery to the body exceeds these limits, injury occurs. This tolerance to external energy delivery is dependent on which type of tissue(s) have been targeted, the age and physical health of the patient, and the type, magnitude and duration of the energy that has been transferred [Greaves, 2008].

Types of trauma
Trauma is generally divided into two types [NAEMT, 2014]:
- Blunt: Injuries that do not cause penetration of the skin by an external object. Typical mechanisms of blunt trauma include road traffic collisions (RTC) involving vehicles, pedestrians, motorcyclists etc., fall from height, serious sports injuries and blast injuries (although this mechanism often also causes penetrating trauma, the other type)
- Penetrating: Injuries caused by projectiles penetrating the skin. Examples include stab and gunshot wounds and blast injuries involving shrapnel and secondary projectiles.

1.3 **Kinetics**
Kinetics is the study of the relationship between motion and its forces.

In a road traffic collision there are three collisions. The first occurs when the vehicle a person is travelling in collides with another object. Newton's first law of motion states that a physical body will remain at steady speed and direction (i.e. velocity) or at rest until an external force acts upon it. In the case of a person driving their car, this force may be due to a collision with another car, vehicle or other object, such as a tree. During a head-on collision with a tree, for example, the vehicle stops abruptly, but the occupant inside will still be moving at the same velocity as they were prior to the collision until they come into contact with the vehicle (the second collision). The third collision occurs when the person's internal organs and tissues make contact with the body's hard surfaces, such as the skull or chest wall [NAEMT, 2014].

Newton's second law states that the force an object exerts is equal to its mass multiplied by its acceleration, or in the case of a collision, mass multiplied by the deceleration. Thus rapid decelerations, such as a car hitting an immovable object, or striking another vehicle travelling in the opposite direction at speed, for example, lead to large forces being exerted.

Newton's third law states that for every force, there is an equal and opposite force, meaning that the force applied to the tree in our head-on collision example is exerted on the vehicle too, leading to damage to the vehicle and, potentially, the occupants [Pilbery, 2013].

1.4 **Energy**
Energy is a measure of an object's ability to do work, or transfer energy to another object. The law of conservation states that energy cannot be destroyed, only transformed.

Energy comes in at least five forms [Greaves, 2008]:
- Kinetic: Related to motion, and the most common type of injury-causing energy

- Thermal: Kinetic energy of molecular motion, measured as temperature. The cause of burns
- Electrical: The flow of electrical charge. This type of energy mainly causes damage through conversion to thermal energy
- Chemical: Energy created or consumed during the alteration of electrical charge in chemical reactions. Explosions are often due to chemical reactions
- Nuclear: Energy released as a result of nuclear fission (the splitting of an atom into smaller parts, with associated energy release).

In trauma, it is usually kinetic energy that is of interest and this can be represented by the formula [NAEMT, 2014]:

$$\text{kinetic energy} = 1/2mv^2$$

where m is the mass of the object and v its velocity. From this, it is clear that it is the velocity of the object that makes the greatest difference to the amount of kinetic energy available to be transformed. Human tolerance to kinetic energy is influenced by the magnitude of the energy (the force applied) and the duration of the exposure, specifically the change in velocity. This is typically deceleration, for example a person's feet hitting the floor after a fall from height, or when a car strikes a large tree at speed. However, excessive acceleration can also cause injury, for example when a pilot is ejected from a jet aircraft [Greaves, 2008].

1.4.1 **Energy transfer**

The energy exchanged during trauma is the same, whether it is blunt or penetrating. Cavitation, the formation of a cavity or hollow, occurs during trauma as tissues in the body move away from the point of impact and their usual position. If this energy is dispersed over a wide area then penetration of the skin may not occur. Thanks to the elastic properties of tissues, body shape of the torso in particular often returns to its usual position, i.e. the cavitation is temporary. However, this may hide serious internal injury to organs and tissues that have had the kinetic energy of the impact transferred to them. Other denser tissues, such as bone, may remain deformed, giving clues to the presence of injury [Greaves, 2008].

In penetrating trauma, temporary cavitation also occurs, but there is also a permanent cavity

which remains once the temporary cavity has collapsed due to the elasticity of the tissues. In low-energy penetrating trauma, such as a stab wound, temporary cavitation may be minimal, but with higher energies, such as those in a gunshot, the temporary cavity can become significant in terms of injury to surrounding tissues and by generating a sub-atmospheric pressure within, causing external debris and dirt to be 'sucked in' to the wound [Greaves, 2008].

The mechanical damage that remains after trauma does not necessarily correlate to the severity of injury either. For example, a screwdriver plunged through the chest that damages the heart may leave only a small external injury, but is likely to be more serious than a gunshot wound to the patient's knee (Figure 1.1).

Penetrating projectiles do not always follow a straight path and can ricochet off internal organs and bone as the projectile decelerates. Although entrance and exit wounds are sometimes visible, determining which is which is not clinically important. Note that the absence of an exit wound means that much of the projectile's kinetic energy has been transferred to the body [NAEMT, 2014].

1.5 **Mechanisms that cause injury**

There are many mechanisms that can result in a host of isolated and multiple injuries to the human body. Some of the more common mechanisms and the injuries they cause to the

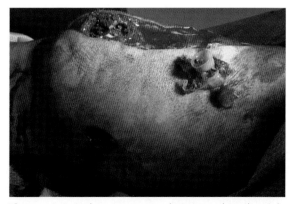

Figure 1.1 A close-range gunshot wound to the right knee, with a shotgun. Note the smaller entrance wound towards the bottom of the picture and the much larger exit wound.

head, spine, thorax, abdomen and pelvis are covered in this section.

1.5.1 Head

If the head is travelling ahead of the body, such as during a headfirst fall, it is the first structure to receive the force of the impact and energy transference. The continued movement of the rest of the body results in compression, which can damage the scalp and skull. If the skull fractures, bony fractures can end up damaging the brain. The same damage can also be caused by the application of an external force, such as occurs as a result of a blow to the head during an assault [NAEMT, 2014].

The brain is soft and compressible and can move following the application of external forces. This can lead to shearing of brain tissue as well as rupture of the blood vessels surrounding the brain, leading to intracranial haemorrhage.

If a projectile penetrates the skull, the damage can be very severe as the kinetic energy is distributed within the confines of the skull. Small calibre bullets, for example, may not have enough energy to exit the skull, but instead contour around it, leading to extensive damage [NAEMT, 2014].

1.5.2 Spine

The main mechanisms that cause spinal injury can be divided into abnormal flexion, extension, rotation and compression. Extension or flexion with rotation are the main causes of injury to the cervical spine [Greaves, 2008; Pilbery, 2013; NAEMT, 2014].

Flexion

Hyperflexion injuries are typically caused by RTCs where lap-belts (rather than three-point belts) are used, direct blows to the occiput and rapid deceleration in flexed positions such as diving and contact sports like rugby. Hyperflexion on its own is uncommon in the cervical spine, since the chin abutting the chest limits flexion.

Flexion with rotation

The design of the first two cervical vertebrae allows for significant rotation. Injuries due to this mechanism are considered unstable as there is little in the way of bony or soft-tissue support. Not surprisingly, this mechanism is much more likely to produce significant cervical injury and is

often caused by lateral impact RTCs or direct trauma. Note that rotation rarely occurs in isolation.

Extension

These injuries are generally only found in cervical and lumbar regions and can be caused by hanging, striking the chin on a steering wheel during a collision or a rear impact collision where the headrest is improperly positioned [NAEMT, 2014].

Compression

Wedge fractures are the most common type of fracture of the lumbar and thoracic spine, but if a weight falls on the head or if the patient lands on their head after a fall, then the cervical vertebrae can be fractured and/or ligaments ruptured. Most fractures caused by compression are stable, but spinal cord injury can occur if the vertebral body is shattered and fragments of bone become embedded in the cord [Pilbery, 2013].

1.5.3 Thorax

Severe blunt thoracic trauma most commonly occurs as a result of RTCs (about 70–80%) where high speeds are involved, leading to rapid deceleration. This causes shearing forces that can rupture large blood vessels, tear the bronchial airways and damage the lungs, causing pneumothoraces, for example. Even with lower velocity mechanisms, such as direct blows to the chest, fractures of the rib cage and sternum as well as bruising to the underlying structures including the heart and lungs can occur [NAEMT, 2014].

In penetrating trauma, the most serious consequences arise as a result of rupture of the major blood vessels, which can lead to serious haemorrhage. Projectiles penetrating the chest wall can also cause open pneumothoraces [Greaves, 2008].

1.5.4 Abdomen

Abdominal injury is most commonly caused by blunt trauma, usually due to RTCs, and often as part of a multi-system pattern of injuries. If the abdomen comes into contact with the steering wheel during rapid deceleration, crush injuries can occur. Compression of the abdominal organs increases the intra-abdominal pressure, which in turn can rupture the hollow organs and/or the diaphragm. Penetrating trauma is less common, and in the UK is more likely to be as a result of a stab wound than gunshot. Fortunately, less than half of all stab wounds actually penetrate the peritoneum (the lining of the abdominal cavity) [Greaves, 2008].

1.5.5 **Pelvis**

As with any trauma patient, you should consider the MOI to provide an indication as to possible underlying injuries. Pelvic ring fractures usually require high forces, so it is no surprise that the most common cause is RTCs. Front-seat passengers in head-on collisions, and those on the side of impact in T-bone type collisions in cars, are most common. These are closely followed by motorcyclists, pedestrians and falls from heights [Gabbe, 2011; Papadopoulos, 2006]. However, a significant sub-group are the elderly, who will typically fall from standing and may have osteoporosis [Garlapati, 2012].

Figure 1.2 shows three main types of pelvic ring fracture (there is an additional type, which is just a combination of the other three) and the direction of forces required to cause them [Burgess, 1990]:

- Lateral compression (LC) fractures: These are the most common type of pelvic ring fracture and are caused by internal rotation of the pelvic ring due to a direct force applied to the iliac crests, or indirectly via the femoral head [Garlapati, 2012]. These forces typically result in pubic rami fractures on one or both sides anteriorly, which places severe strain on the sacroiliac joints. If these become displaced, the pelvis will be unstable. The typical mechanism of injury is a side-impact RTC or fall from height.
- Anterior–posterior compression (APC) fractures: These are most commonly caused by a frontal collision between a pedestrian and a vehicle, front-seat passengers in a frontal RTC and crush injury [NAEMT, 2014]. With these mechanisms, either the pubic rami are fractured or the symphysis pubis is disrupted, resulting in the pelvic bones springing apart and externally rotating. This is often called an 'open book' injury. Posteriorly, the sacroiliac ligaments can be torn and/or the posterior

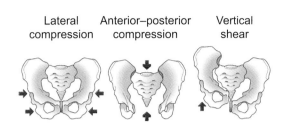

Figure 1.2 Types of pelvic fracture. The red arrows indicate the direction of the forces

aspect of the pelvic bones fractured [McCormack, 2010].

- Vertical shear (VS) fractures: These are the least common type of injury, but are the most likely to kill your patient [NAEMT, 2014]. These fractures occur when one of the pelvic bones is displaced vertically, leading to a fracture of the pubic rami and disruption of the sacroiliac joint on the same side. These are typically caused by falls from height, with the patient landing on one leg first. Because of this, blood vessels are often torn, leading to severe retroperitoneal haemorrhage (which can easily accommodate the body's entire blood volume [Luke, 2010]) and severe damage to soft tissues.
- Combined mechanical (CM) fractures: These are a combination of other types of fractures, typically caused by a multitude of forces applied in different directions, for example during a rollover RTC.

1.5.6 **Blast injury**

Blasts (or explosions) cause complex multi-system injury due to the significant transfer of kinetic,

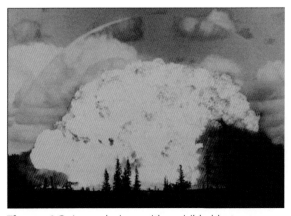

Figure 1.3 An explosion, with a visible blast wave

heat and other energies. Injuries are generally classified into the five types shown in Table 1.1 [NAEMT, 2014; AACE, 2013].

2 Integumentary system anatomy and physiology

2.1 Learning objectives

By the end of this lesson you will be able to:
• Describe the anatomy and physiology of the integumentary system.

2.2 Introduction

The integumentary system (or skin) is the largest organ in the human body, in terms of both surface area and weight. In adults, skin has a surface area of 2 m² and weighs 5 kg [Tortora, 2008]. It is composed of two main layers, the epidermis and dermis. Under the skin is a supportive subcutaneous layer, known as the hypodermis or superficial fascia (Figure 2.1) [Dykes, 2002].

2.3 Epidermis

This is the outermost layer and consists of five sublayers. Most of the cells (90%) are

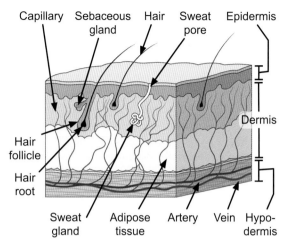

Figure 2.1 Cross-section of the skin

keratinocytes, which produce a tough, fibrous protein (keratin). This helps protect the skin and tissues from heat and microbes. Keratinocytes also produce lamellar granules which decrease water entry and loss, and prevent entry of foreign material. Around 8% of the cells are melanocytes, which produce melanin. This is taken up by keratinocytes, protecting the cell's

Table 1.1: Blast injury categories

Category	Cause	Possible injuries
Primary	Injuries caused by patient contact with blast shock wave (Figure 1.3)	Gas-containing organs may be damaged, including lungs, gastrointestinal tract
Secondary	Injuries due to flying fragments and debris striking the patient	Entire body can be affected, leading to lacerations and fractures Penetrating injuries
Tertiary	Blast wave propels patient against objects Crush injuries secondary to structural damage and building collapse	Blunt and crush injuries
Quaternary	Other explosion-related injuries and illnesses	Burns Toxic gas and exposure to other chemicals
Quinary	Injuries resulting from additives, for example bacteria and radiation ('dirty bombs')	

nucleus from the harmful effects of ultraviolet (UV) light. Keratin is either a yellow-red or brown-black pigment and contributes to skin colour. The remaining cells consist of Langerhans cells, which help in the body's immune response, and Merkel cells, which are involved in touch perception [Tortora, 2008].

It takes around 2–3 weeks for a cell starting at the lowest layer of the epidermis to become a keratinocyte and migrate up to the top layer (stratum corneum) and slough off [AAOS, 2011].

2.4 Dermis

This deeper layer of skin mostly consists of connective tissue, elastin and an extracellular matrix, which provides strength and pliability. However, it also contains blood and lymphatic vessels, nerve fibres, hair follicles and sebaceous and sweat glands. The dermis is divided into two regions, the papillary and the reticular. The papillary region consists of connective tissue that anchors the epidermis and a dense network of capillaries and small blood vessels, in nipple-like projections called dermal papillae. These play an important part in temperature regulation. In addition, the dermal papillae also contain free nerve endings, which act as pain and fine touch receptors (Meissner corpuscles) [Tortora, 2008].

The reticular region makes up 80% of the dermis and consists of dense, irregular connective tissue. Interlocking collagen fibres run in various planes, forming 'lines of cleavage'. Surgeons try to make incisions parallel to these lines, since the skin does not gape as much, resulting in less scarring [Thompson, 2008].

2.5 Hypodermis

Also known as the superficial fascia, this layer contains subcutaneous fat, connective tissue, sweat glands, muscle and bone. It helps to insulate the body, absorbs shocks to the skeletal system and enables the skin to move easily over underlying structures [AAOS, 2011].

2.6 Physiology

The skin provides a range of functions, which any damage can impair [Tortora, 2008; Thompson, 2008]:

- Protection against infection by forming a physical barrier to microbes and foreign material

- Sensory perception of pain, pressure, heat and cold
- Thermoregulation using nerves, blood vessels and sweat glands to control body temperature
- Excretion of trace amounts of water and body waste, while helping to prevent dehydration
- Maintainance of mineralisation of bones and teeth and synthesis of vitamin D
- Absorption of lipid-soluble substances such as fat-soluble vitamins and drugs through the skin.

3 Wounds and bleeding

3.1 Learning objectives

By the end of this lesson you will be able to:
- Describe the types of bleeding
- Explain how to appropriately assess and manage bleeding
- Explain how to detect concealed bleeding
- Describe various types of wounds and how to manage them
- Discuss the implications of foreign objects in wounds
- Explain complications associated with bleeding and wounds.

3.2 Introduction

Wounds and bleeding are a common reason for an ambulance to be requested. Even in the emergency ambulance service, these calls will vary in their severity, from wounds and bleeding that require basic first aid only, through to life-threatening wounds and bleeding that require prompt and more advanced intervention in order to prevent death.

3.3 Bleeding

Bleeding is the loss of blood from a damaged blood vessel. You will often hear the term 'haemorrhage' used, which is bleeding, but in medical circles is usually reserved for severe bleeding. Bleeding is often classified by the type of vessel involved (i.e. artery, vein or capillary) or whether it is external or internal [SJA, SAA, BRC, 2014].

3.3.1 Assessment
Sources of bleeding
Bleeding can be defined by whether it is visible on the outside of the body and/or which type of vessel is responsible [Gregory, 2010a; SJA, SAA, BRC, 2014]:

- Internal: This bleeding is concealed within the body and can be hard to detect [Greaves, 2008]. The thorax, abdomen, pelvis and long bones provide good hiding places for significant volumes of blood. The mechanism of injury and the presence of shock without signs of external haemorrhage can help with diagnosis. These patients need to be in hospital to stop the bleeding
- External: This bleeding is visible and should be detected during your primary and/or secondary survey. This bleeding can usually be controlled
- Arterial: Blood inside the arteries is under relatively high pressure and so bleeding can lead to significant blood loss. It is characterised by bright red (oxygenated) spurting, in time with the heart beat
- Venous: Since veins carry blood back to the heart, they typically carry deoxygenated blood and so bleeding is a darker red. Since the pressure is lower, blood does not spurt but flows freely. However, blood loss can still be severe, particularly from veins in the neck and legs
- Capillary: These are the smallest blood vessels in the body and carry a mixture of oxygenated and deoxygenated blood, so the colour of bleeding will vary. Blood loss tends to be small as blood oozes from wounds.

Estimating blood loss
Estimating blood loss accurately is very difficult and ambulance staff (and doctors/nurses/midwives) generally do not do this well [Frank, 2010; Bose, 2006; Tall, 2003; Moscati, 1999]. Table 3.1 provides examples of what various volumes of blood loss look like (this was originally designed for estimating obstetric blood loss) [Bose, 2006]. Fractures can cause significant blood loss, depending on the bone(s) affected and whether the fracture is open or closed (Table 3.2) [NAEMT, 2014]. Remember to check for signs and symptoms of shock (this was covered in the COMMON CARDIOVASCULAR CONDITIONS lesson in chapter 11, CIRCULATION).

3.3.2 Management
The mnemonic ABC has been in use for many years, identifying the patient management priorities in the primary survey. However, in the military, there has been a change of priorities, to include early control of catastrophic haemorrhage (<C>) before the airway, when both cannot be managed simultaneously [Hodgetts, 2006].

Once the scene assessment has been completed, you need to check for, and manage, any actual or potential catastrophic haemorrhage. Only once this has been completed can you return to the normal AcBC (i.e. airway with consideration of the cervical spine, breathing and circulation) approach.

During the assessment of circulation (the second C), any interventions to manage catastrophic haemorrhage must be reassessed to ensure that bleeding is being controlled appropriately. Don't forget the bleeding you cannot see. 'Blood on the floor plus four more' is a good way to remember the areas where significant blood loss can accumulate, i.e. the thorax, abdomen, pelvis and long bones [Greaves, 2010].

Most external haemorrhage can be controlled with simple first aid measures such as direct pressure and elevation of the bleeding extremity. In some cases, additional interventions are required, but these should be introduced in an incremental fashion, as shown in the haemostasis escalator (Figure 3.1) [Lee, 2007b; Moorhouse, 2007].

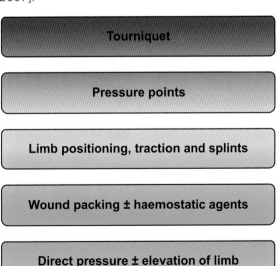

Figure 3.1 The haemostasis escalator

Table 3.1: Visual guide to estimating blood loss

Blood loss (ml)	
30	
60	
100	
250	
500	
1000	

1500	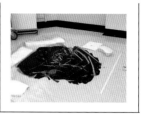

Table 3.2: Approximate internal blood loss due to fractures

Fracture	Blood loss (ml)
Rib	125
Radius or ulna	250–500
Humerus	500–750
Tibia	500–1000
Femur	1000–2000
Pelvis	1000–5000

If direct pressure and elevation fails to stem the bleeding, then wound packing should be undertaken and may be supplemented with haemostatic agents. This is achieved by inserting a sufficient quantity of gauze into the wound, to create mechanical pressure on the injured vessel and provide a structure for coagulation.

If this fails, assess limb positioning and consider whether the use of splinting may help reduce bleeding. Careful handling and the splinting of fractures will help in controlling haemorrhage. If this is still not sufficient, consider using pressure points to indirectly reduce distal blood flow. This involves compressing a proximal artery against a bone. Compression of the artery in this way may help reduce blood flow to the bleeding point, but still allow some degree of circulation to reach the distal tissues.

If indirect pressure fails to stem the haemorrhage, then a tourniquet should be applied.

3.3.3 Tourniquets

The use of tourniquets (Figure 3.2) has caused controversy, but they do have a place in civilian ambulance services for use in specific circumstances [Lee, 2007b]:

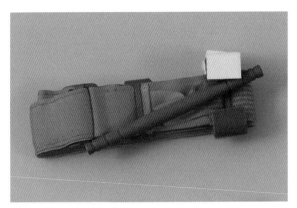

Figure 3.2 A tourniquet

- Extreme life-threatening limb haemorrhage, or limb amputation/mangled limb with multiple bleeding points, to allow immediate management of airway and breathing problems. Following treatment of any airway or breathing problems, the need for a tourniquet can be reassessed in the circulatory assessment and may be converted to a simple method of haemorrhage control
- Life-threatening limb haemorrhage not controlled by simple methods
- Point of significant haemorrhage from limb is not peripherally accessible due to entrapment (and therefore it is not possible to initiate simple methods of haemorrhage control such as direct pressure)
- Major incident or multiple casualties with extremity haemorrhage and lack of resources to maintain simple methods of haemorrhage control.

However, incorrectly applied tourniquets can actually increase blood loss if venous, but not arterial, vessels are occluded. This is a risk for tourniquets sited below the knee and elbow joints, which may not be successful in controlling haemorrhage, as the arteries can run or slip between the tibia/fibula and radius/ulna and thus not be compressed by the tourniquet. Even correctly applied tourniquets, if used when not clinically indicated, can cause local tissue injury from direct contact with the tourniquet, and, when left in place for more than 2 hours, can

lead to muscle and skin damage [Walters, 2005]. In addition, tourniquets cause severe pain and patients must receive adequate analgesia.

Procedure

The following steps are a suggested method for applying a tourniquet. As yet, there is no consensus on the most appropriate location to place a tourniquet, so follow local guidance [SWAST, 2]:

1. Identify the need for a tourniquet during the primary survey, assessing for catastrophic haemorrhage
2. Apply the tourniquet as close to the injury as possible, leaving a gap of at least 5 cm between the injury and the tourniquet, except when injuries are close to the knee and elbow joints. In this case, apply the tourniquet above the joint
3. Tighten the tourniquet until the bleeding stops
4. Record the time of tourniquet application
5. Reassess during the assessment of circulation. If bleeding continues, apply a second tourniquet proximal to the first and over a single bone (i.e. humerus or femur)
6. Frequently reassess and tighten tourniquet as required. Provide analgesia.

3.3.4 **Haemostatic agents**

Where direct pressure and wound packing are ineffective, and in areas such as the groin, neck and axilla, where tourniquet application is not possible, haemostatic agents can be used to control haemorrhage [Greaves, 2008; Cox, 2009; Rossaint, 2010]. Haemostatic agents usually come in the form of granules and may additionally be impregnated into a dressing. They work by either concentrating clotting factors or acting as a precursor to coagulation, or are mucoadhesive [Granville-Chapman, 2011]. In pre-hospital medicine, the most common agents in use are QuikClot® and Celox® (Figure 3.3).

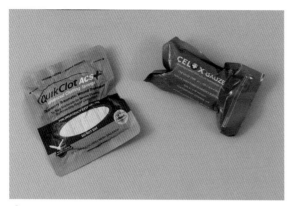

Figure 3.3 Haemostatic dressings

Celox® is extensively used within UK military practice and is a complex polysaccharide made from shellfish. The active element is chitosan, which acts as a mucoadhesive around bleeding vessels. It has been suggested that this haemostatic agent is preferable in severe trauma, as it does not rely on clotting factors to work. In severe haemorrhage, clotting factors may be in short supply due to direct blood loss and haemodilution following fluid therapy [Granville-Chapman, 2011].

Haemostatic agents are placed into the wound, as close to the bleeding point as possible. Direct pressure must then be applied to the wound site for at least 3 minutes to ensure adhesion and stable clot formation. Ideally, constant pressure should be maintained after this time with a suitable elastic bandage.

3.4 **Wounds**

A wound is an injury to living tissue, breaking its continuity. There are seven basic categories [Dougherty, 2011; Gregory, 2010b; Pilbery, 2013]:

- Contusion (bruises): Caused by bleeding from damaged blood vessels under the skin. They cause a bluish/purple discolouration beneath the skin and are typically caused by blunt trauma
- Abrasion (grazes): Injuries caused by friction shearing the skin away. These usually involve the superficial layers of the skin, but can go much deeper. They can be very painful and are often dirty, with embedded grit and mud

- Laceration (tear): Tearing or splitting of the skin due to blunt trauma. These cause a ragged wound, which can extend through the skin surface to the underlying structures
- Incision (cut): A break in the continuity of the skin by a sharp implement, such as broken glass or a knife. These are usually clean wounds (unless the implement is dirty) with neat edges
- Puncture (stab): A penetrating wound caused by an object that is pointed and narrow, such as a nail or knife. Although these wounds are typically small, they can be deep, causing serious damage to vessels and other body structures below the skin
- Burn: An injury caused by energy transfer to the body's tissues, causing necrosis and an associated inflammatory reaction (covered in the BURNS lesson later in this chapter)
- Gunshot: A complicated wound caused by a projectile moving at speed. The wound consists of an entry point, with varying amounts of tissue destruction and cavitation underneath the skin, and, if there is sufficient energy left, an exit wound

There are a range of external and internal factors that can lead to wound formation [Thompson, 2008]:

- External: Mechanical (friction), chemical, electrical, temperature extremes, radiation and microorganisms
- Internal: Circulatory system failure, endocrine (e.g. diabetes), neuropathy, haematological, malignancy (cancer).

3.4.1 **Management**

Wound management will be determined by the size and nature of the wound and the presence of complicating factors. The main initial problems are bleeding, pain and the risk of infection [Purcell, 2010]. Always enquire about tetanus immunisation in any patient who has a wound with a higher risk of infection, such as a dirty wound, or a wound caused by a bite (human or animal) or involving a puncture by a dirty object [SJA, SAA, BRC, 2014].

If the wound is small and bleeding easily controlled, clean the wound, if dirty, before placing a sterile, non-adherent dressing over the site. If the wound is suitable for treatment at home, or at a minor injuries unit, the clinician may advise that a wet dressing be applied over the wound, although this is typically reserved for wounds where treatment will commence promptly (for example within 30–90 minutes) [Pilbery, 2013].

If there is a foreign object in the wound, it may be possible to remove it, if it's small (e.g. grit), by irrigating the wound with water, or using tweezers. However, larger objects or those which appear firmly embedded should not be removed but left in place, and a sterile, non-adherent dressing applied. These objects do need to be removed as they may lead to infection, so follow local guidance and your clinician as to the next step in the patient's management [Purcell, 2010].

4 Assessment and management of the trauma patient

4.1 Learning objectives

By the end of this lesson you will be able to:
- Explain the assessment and management of patients with a range of traumatic injuries
- Describe the complications associated with a range of traumatic injuries.

4.2 Introduction

The approach to the trauma patient is similar to that of all patients, with an initial scene assessment, followed by a primary and secondary survey. However, there are some aspects of this process that are specific to trauma and they are going to be covered in this lesson. In addition, there are a range of complications that can arise as a result of traumatic injury to specific regions and a number of these are going to be covered in this lesson, specifically injuries to the head, spine, thorax, abdomen and pelvis.

4.3 Scene assessment

The SCENE mnemonic that was reviewed in the SCENE ASSESSMENT AND SAFETY lesson (chapter 7) can be used to ensure that you cover all aspects of an initial trauma scene assessment [AACE, 2013]:

- **S**: Safety. A dynamic risk assessment should highlight current as well as potential dangers. If you are not equipped in terms of kit and expertise to deal with the scene, withdraw and request specialist help, for example from the hazardous area response team (HART). Remember to continually reassess safety as the situation can change quickly. Make sure you are wearing appropriate personal protective equipment (PPE)

- **C**: Cause, including mechanism of injury (MOI). Finding out what happened is important in order to appreciate likely injuries and energy transfer. However, ensure that the scene matches the story you are being told, as you may have come across a crime scene or case of abuse

- **E**: Environment. Consider whether there are any environmental factors that need to be taken into account. These may complicate your extrication by affecting access to and from the scene and/or increase the risk of harm to the patient, due to increased risk of hypothermia, for example

- **N**: Number of patients. Determine the number of patients early on in your assessment to help you determine whether you can manage the scene on your own. It may also help to identify patients who have either wandered off from scene or who have been ejected from a vehicle, for example, and are currently hidden from view

- **E**: Extra resources needed. Depending on the number of patients, the severity of their injuries and the nature of the incident, you may need additional help from other emergency services, such as the police to keep a scene safe, or additional ambulances, including the air ambulance, for patient transport.

4.4 Primary survey

The aim of the primary survey is to identify threats to life promptly and intervene as soon as they are found. The steps of the primary survey should be undertaken sequentially, unless there are enough personnel to allow for simultaneous assessment and treatment [Greaves, 2008].

Procedure

Take the following steps to undertake a primary survey in the trauma patient:

1. **General impression**: As you approach the patient, perform a global assessment. Are they sitting up and watching you approach, with well-perfused skin, or are they lying unresponsive, pale and clammy with an expanding pool of blood leaking from a wound?

2. **Catastrophic haemorrhage**: This is bleeding that is likely to cause death within minutes, so cannot wait until airway and breathing have been addressed. Typically, bleeding can be controlled with direct pressure and elevation of the bleeding site, but may require the use of haemostatic dressings or tourniquets (see the lesson on WOUNDS AND BLEEDING above)

3. **Airway with cervical spine consideration**: If a patient has suffered significant blunt trauma or the MOI suggests that the cervical spine may have been damaged, provide prompt manual in-line stabilisation. Assess the airway by looking for obvious obstruction, listening for noisy airflow (snoring or gurgling) and feeling for air movement.

4. Manage the airway using appropriate airway manoeuvres, such as:
   - Jaw thrust–chin lift
   - Suction
   - Naso- and oropharyngeal airways.

5. **Breathing**: Administer high-flow oxygen to patients to obtain a target saturation of 94–98%, even if they have COPD.

6. Examine the neck for:
   - **T**racheal deviation
   - **W**ounds and swellings
   - **E**mphysema (surgical/subcutaneous)
   - **L**aryngeal crepitus
   - **V**eins.

7. If you have enough personnel, a cervical collar can be applied, if appropriate, once this has been completed

8. Look for obvious chest injuries, wounds, bruising or flail segments. Assess the rate, depth and quality of respiration:
   - Ventilate with a BVM if respirations absent or less than 10 breaths/min
   - If respirations are greater than 30 breaths/min it may also be clinically appropriate to ventilate the patient. Follow the advice of the clinician

   - If respirations 10–30 breaths/min monitor closely.

9. Listen (auscultate) over both axilla for air entry. If bilateral air entry is not heard, the clinician may use percussion to indicate the underlying problem

10. Feel for equality of chest movement and note any instability

11. **Note:** This assessment should include examination of the back of the chest, although it may not be appropriate to log roll the patient to do this. If the patient is supine, feel as much of the back as you can without excessively moving the patient

12. Manage breathing problems as you find them. This may include:
    - Applying non-occlusive dressings to sucking chest wounds
    - Insertion of a cannula into the chest by a clinician to decompress a tension pneumothorax
    - Positioning to support a patient with a flail segment (not possible if the patient has a suspected spinal injury).

13. **Circulation**: If a catastrophic haemorrhage was encountered at the start of the primary survey, reassess this now.

14. Assess both central and distal pulses (carotid and radial, typically), noting rate, rhythm and volume. Note the skin colour, temperature and the presence of clamminess. If additional personnel are available, the blood pressure can also be measured

15. Assess for signs of blood loss, remembering the phrase 'blood on the floor plus four more':
    - Externally: Don't forget to consider bleeding into clothing, splints and dressings
    - Chest: Completed during assessment of breathing
    - Abdomen: Look for bruising or external marks and feel for rigidity and to elicit tenderness
    - Pelvis: This should not be manipulated or 'sprung' to assess for instability. The MOI is sufficient to immobilise the pelvis
    - Long bones: Assess long bones, particularly the femurs, but do not be distracted by fractures at this stage

16. Manage bleeding appropriately (see lesson on WOUNDS AND BLEEDING above). Ideally splint pelvic fractures prior to moving the patient. Limb fractures can wait until you are en route if the patient is critically injured.

Procedure continued →

17. The clinician may wish to gain intravenous access now if fluids and/or tranexamic acid are required

18. To minimise clot disruption, patient movement should be kept to a minimum. Use an orthopaedic (scoop) stretcher where possible.

19. **Disability**: Calculate the Glasgow Coma Scale (GCS) score for the pre-hospital major trauma triage tool. Assess pupil size, equality and reaction to light. Don't forget to check the blood glucose.

20. **Exposure/environment**: To identify all injuries, it is necessary to remove the patient's clothing. In cases of severe injury or suspected spinal injury, clothes should be cut off the patient to minimise movement. Take care to prevent hypothermia as this can dramatically increase their chances of dying (up to 3 times higher if core body temperature drops below 35°C [Ireland, 2011]). It may be more appropriate to remove patients to a heated ambulance before completing this step.

4.5 Secondary survey

The secondary survey should only commence once all life-threatening injuries identified in the primary survey have been addressed and, in the case of severely injured patients, once they are on the way to hospital [NAEMT, 2014; AACE, 2013; Greaves, 2008].

Procedure

Take the following steps to perform a secondary survey in the trauma patient:

1. **Vital signs and history**: Obtain a full set of observations, a history of the injury-inducing event and a brief medical history (e.g. SAMPLE)

2. **Head**
   - Reassess the airway to ensure patency and check the mouth for bleeding, lacerations and loose teeth
   - Look at and feel the entire head and face to identify lacerations, bruising, fractures and burns
   - Re-check the pupils and GCS
   - Inspect the nose and ears for the presence of blood and cerebrospinal fluid (CSF) leakage as this may suggest a basal skull fracture. Other signs, such as bilateral bruising around the eyes or behind the ears, can take 12–36 hours to appear

3. **Neck**: To examine the neck properly, it is necessary to remove a cervical collar. Manual in-line stabilisation will need to be maintained while this occurs. The clinician may examine the spinous processes of the cervical spine and, depending on the result, elect to discontinue cervical spine immobilisation

4. Reassess for signs of life-threatening injury, indicated by:
   - **T**racheal deviation
   - **W**ounds and swellings
   - **E**mphysema (surgical/subcutaneous)
   - **L**aryngeal crepitus
   - **V**eins

5. **Chest**: Repeat the assessment carried out in the primary survey. Look for obvious chest injuries, wounds, bruising or flail segments. Note the presence of seat-belt marks

6. Assess the rate, depth and quality of respiration:
   - Ventilate with a BVM if respirations absent or less than 10 breaths/min
   - If respirations greater than 30 breaths/min it may also be clinically appropriate to ventilate the patient. Follow the advice of the clinician
   - If respirations 10–30 breaths/min monitor closely

7. Listen (auscultate) over as much of the chest (front and back) as possible. If bilateral air entry is not heard, the clinician may use percussion to indicate the underlying problem

8. Feel for equality of chest movement and note any instability

9. **Abdomen**
   - Look for open wounds, bruising and seat-belt marks. Try to view as much of the front and back as possible
   - Feel the whole abdomen for tenderness, guarding and rigidity

10. **Pelvis**
    - Check for blood loss from the urethra or vagina
    - Note the presence of bruising around the perineum and scrotum (in males)
    - Discourage urination

11. **Extremities**: Thoroughly examine the lower and then upper limbs. Look for wounds and fractures. Check motor, sensory and circulatory (MSC) function in all four limbs:
    - Motor: Ask the patient to move the limb
    - Sensory: Apply light touch to evaluate sensation
    - Circulation: Assess a distal pulse and skin temperature.

4.6 **Head injuries**

Common causes of traumatic brain injury (TBI) include road traffic collisions, direct blows to the head, falls from heights and sports-related injuries. The worst outcomes are associated with [Moppett, 2007]:

- Penetrating injuries
- Non-accidental injury in children aged under 5 years
- Pedestrians and pedal cyclists
- Ejection from a vehicle.

Other clues at scene include a 'bulls-eye' pattern on a vehicle windscreen and significant damage to protective helmets, if a patient was wearing one at the time of the injury [AACE, 2013].

Once a primary brain injury has occurred, it cannot be undone. Fortunately, good pre-hospital management can help minimise the impact of secondary brain injury. It can be broken down into 3 areas:

- Recognise the injury that will indicate that a traumatic brain injury may be present
- Understand the pathophysiology relating to traumatic brain injury
- Manage the patient appropriately.

4.6.1 **Recognition**

Suggestive signs and symptoms of TBI include [Pante, 2010]:

- Lacerations, contusions or haematomas to the scalp
- Boggy areas when palpating the scalp
- Visible fractures or deformity of the skull
- Battle's sign or 'panda eyes' (not apparent for several hours)
- Cerebrospinal fluid and/or blood leaking from the nose or ears
- Cushing's Triad: Rising blood pressure, reducing heart rate and irregular respirations
- Dizziness
- Nausea and vomiting
- Abnormal pupils and/or pupil reaction
- Visual disturbances (double or blurred vision, seeing 'stars')
- Severe headache
- Altered level of consciousness

- Perseveration (repeatedly asking the same questions)
- Amnesia
- Paraesthesia/paralysis of the extremities
- Convulsions
- Posturing
- Abnormal respirations.

4.6.2 **Pathophysiology**

In the traumatically injured brain, autoregulation starts to fail and affected areas of the brain become pressure passive, relying on higher than normal mean arterial pressures to maintain cerebral blood flow.

If cerebral oedema or haematoma develops, CSF is displaced and the level of venous blood in the cranium is reduced. In the early stages of rising intracranial pressure (ICP), blood pressure will be fairly stable. However, in the later stages when the cardiovascular centre in the medulla becomes ischaemic, the Cushing reflex is triggered, resulting in peripheral vasoconstriction and a rise in blood pressure. This in turn leads to a reflex bradycardia. Respiration is also affected, leading to irregular respirations [Moppett, 2007].

4.6.3 **Management**

The mainstay of management for patients with TBI is preventing hypoxia, treating hypotension and transporting patients quickly to definitive care. There is a link between head injury and injury of the cervical spine, so an assumption of spinal injury should be made, unless your clinician is confident at clearing the patient's cervical spine on scene [NICE, 2014]. Cervical collars can raise ICP, but little can be done to reduce this in the pre-hospital environment [Hammell, 2009].

Airway compromise is common after severe TBI and needs to be managed. Watch for any vagal stimulation such as suction and laryngoscopy as they will increase intracranial pressure. A single drop in the patient's oxygen saturations under 90% doubles their chance of dying. Provide 100% oxygen via a non-rebreathe mask and aim for oxygen saturations of 94–98% [AACE, 2013]. Continuous monitoring of oxygen saturations is important. Assess adequacy of ventilation and provide assistance if required. If you are able to monitor $EtCO_2$, aim for normocapnia, as both hypocapnia and hypercapnia have been shown to increase mortality [Hammell, 2009].

As with oxygen saturations, a single drop of systolic blood pressure to less than 90 mmHg doubles the patient's risk of death [Moppett, 2007]. Make sure you keep your clinician informed if you notice the blood pressure close to this value.

4.7 Spinal injuries

Spinal injuries, or more specifically spinal cord injuries (SCI), are rare, with around 1000 new cases per year [Harrison, 2007]. In adult major trauma, approximately 10% of patients will sustain a spinal fracture/dislocation, but less than 2% will sustain an SCI. The most common cause is a fall (46%), although, significantly, a third of these are falls of LESS than 2m in height. Falls are closely followed by road traffic collisions (RTC, 40%) and the other, much rarer, causes, such as sports injuries (under 3%), stabbings (1%) and shootings (0.6%). SCIs most commonly occur at the cervical level (45%), followed by thoracic (29%), lumbar (24%) and multi-level injuries (2%) [Hasler, 2011].

Risk factors for SCI include [Hasler, 2011:

- Male sex
- Under 45 years of age
- Reduced Glasgow Coma Scale score
- Accompanying chest injury
- Dangerous mechanism (falls greater than 2 m, sports injury, RTC, shooting).

4.7.1 Recognition

The signs and symptoms also depend on the completeness of the SCI. The classic picture in complete SCI is vasodilation, flaccidity of muscles and loss of sensation below the injury, as well as loss of temperature regulation mechanisms such as vasodilation and sweating. This can lead to a poikilothermic state, where the body adopts the temperature of the surrounding environment (whether hot or cold). Depending on how high the SCI injury is the blood pressure can dramatically fall, for example to 80 mmHg systolic in high cervical injuries, but there is no compensatory tachycardia, since the sympathetic signals are blocked. In fact, parasympathetic division dominance leads to bradycardia, further reducing cardiac output. In an incomplete SCI,

there is a mixed picture of paralysis and paraesthesia, but not profound hypotension or bradycardia, making the absence of these signs unreliable in excluding SCI in unconscious patients [Harrison, 2007].

4.7.2 Pathophysiology

Key to the maintenance of homeostasis within the autonomic nervous system (ANS) are the cerebral cortex and hypothalamus, which provide appropriate excitatory and inhibitory inputs to various areas in the medulla, which plays a crucial role in cardiovascular control. This relies on feedback from afferent sensory impulses from central and peripheral baroreceptors. Thus, it is not difficult to see that SCI, depending on the level and completeness of the injury and cord interruption, can dramatically affect the body's ability to keep control of the ANS [Krassioukov, 2012].

Despite the common use of words like 'transection', 'cutting' and 'severing' of the spinal cord after a traumatic injury, in reality a spinal cord lesion (abnormality or damage) is primarily caused by ischaemic necrosis. Traumatic injury mechanisms include displacement of one or more vertebral bodies, causing compression and/or stretching of the cord, which may result in no visible injury, but leads to oedema and vascular disruption. However, not all SCI is due to trauma. Other causes include spinal tumours, transverse myelitis, vascular thrombosis or haemorrhage, and infection and abscesses caused by tuberculosis or meningitis [Gupta, 2009].

It's very cosy within the vertebral canal and an oedematous spinal cord is soon compressed. This disrupts blood and oxygen flow, resulting in ischaemic tissue and, ultimately, necrosis. The rapid cessation of signal transmission that this process causes leads to a range of signs and symptoms, which are termed 'spinal shock' [Harrison, 2007].

Nerves originating from T1 to T5 are responsible for most heart and vascular control, and injuries below this level typically do not have such a dramatic effect on the ANS. However, an injury at T6 or above can lead to interruption of sympathetic division control from the brain. Parasympathetic innervation of the heart arises from the brain and so is typically unaffected, making the parasympathetic division dominant.

4.7.3 **Management**

All patients who are suspected of having a spinal injury should be immobilised as soon as possible. Remember that the whole spine must be immobilised. The techniques and equipment involved in order to perform this safely are described in the SKELETAL IMMOBILISATION lesson below [AACE, 2013].

Remember that spinal immobilisation is not a risk-free procedure. Potential complications of spinal immobilisation include [AACE, 2013]:

* Airway problems (including increased risk of aspiration)
* Increased intracranial pressure
* Restricted respiration
* Dysphagia
* Skin ulceration/pressure sores
* Pain.

Patients with isolated penetrating trauma to the head or limbs do not require immobilisation, but if, in torso or neck trauma, it is possible that the projectile could have passed near or through the spinal cord and there are signs of spinal cord injury, then immobilisation is appropriate.

In blunt trauma, there are guidelines that allow clinicians to discontinue immobilisation, so you may on occasion be asked to stop immobilising a patient once a thorough assessment has been completed [AACE, 2013].

4.8 **Thoracic injuries**

Thoracic trauma accounts for 25–50% of all trauma and is a contributing factor to around half the deaths through injury. Major causes are road traffic collisions, industrial accidents and domestic and sporting injuries [Greaves, 2008]. The most common problem associated with severe thoracic injury is hypoxia [AACE, 2013]. This can occur due to respiratory and/or cardiovascular causes, which are summarised in Table 4.1 [Greaves, 2008].

4.8.1 **Pneumothorax**

The lungs are surrounded by a pleural membrane. The outer layer (parietal pleura) lines the chest wall, and the inner layer (visceral pleura) covers the lungs. Between them is the pleural space, which is lubricated to ensure that the surfaces glide smoothly over one another as well as creating a surface tension that results in the surfaces 'sticking together'.

Pneumothorax, or air in the pleural space, is generally classified as being spontaneous, if there is no obvious causal factor, or traumatic, if there is an external cause [Noppen, 2010]. In the event that air within the alveoli can escape into the pleural space, or there is an external breach of the thoracic cavity allowing atmospheric air to enter the pleural space, the normal physiology of ventilation is disrupted and the lung collapses [Ryland, 2014].

Traumatic pneumothoraces are caused by penetrating trauma, such as stab and gunshot wounds or impalements; blunt trauma that leads to rib fractures and increased intrathoracic pressure; and bronchial rupture and barotrauma, where changes in pressure of the air delivered to the lungs leads to expansion. This phenomenon has been reported in air crew and SCUBA divers [Sharma, 2008].

Open pneumothorax

In an open pneumothorax, air enters the pleural space thanks to a communication between atmospheric air and the pleural space, for example as a result of penetrating trauma. As the chest expands during inspiration, air enters the pleural space. If the wound is large enough, there may be free movement of air into and out of the affected lung during respiration. If the wound is similar in size to the glottic opening to the lower airway, then atmospheric air preferentially enters via the wound, leading to ineffective ventilation of the alveoli. The sound heard as air moves into and out of the wound has led to these types of injury being referred to as 'sucking chest wounds' [NAEMT, 2014; Greaves, 2008].

Table 4.1: Causes of hypoxia from thoracic injury

Respiratory	Cardiovascular
Tension pneumothorax	Tension pneumothorax
Open pneumothorax	Large haemorrhage
Massive haemothorax	Pericardial tamponade
Ventilatory failure (e.g. flail chest)	Rupture of major blood vessels
Pulmonary contusion	Myocardial contusion

Tension pneumothorax

Tension pneumothorax is an uncommon, but life-threatening, condition which can prove rapidly fatal to patients, particularly those who are being ventilated with positive-pressure. It most often occurs in [MacDuff, 2010]:

- Ventilated patients in intensive care
- Trauma
- Cardiac arrest
- Acute exacerbations of asthma and COPD
- Blocked or clamped chest drains
- Non-invasive ventilation.

As with other types of pneumothorax, air enters the pleural space on inspiration, but cannot escape during expiration due to the presence of a one-way valve formed by a pleural defect. This leads to increasing intra-pleural pressure on the affected side of the chest, worsening the lung collapse and causing diaphragmatic depression. In severe cases, and dependent on mediastinal distensibility, this can compress the contralateral lung.

It's worth noting that tension pneumothoraces typically develop far more slowly in spontaneously breathing awake patients, compared to ventilated and sedated patients, who can experience hypotension and a rapid decline in oxygen saturations in just a few minutes, hastened by the administration of positive-pressure ventilation [Leigh-Smith, 2005; MacDuff, 2010].

Assessment

Arguably, the most important type of pneumothorax to recognise is one under tension. However, the clinical course of a tension pneumothorax is not the same for all patients, with the progression of clinical deterioration for an awake, spontaneously breathing patient likely to be considerably longer than for those who are being ventilated with positive-pressure ventilation [Leigh-Smith, 2005].

Signs and symptoms of a tension pneumothorax in awake patients include:

- Pleuritic chest pain (sharp pain, worse on breathing in and out)
- Air hunger
- Respiratory distress
- Tachypnoea (rapid breathing rate)
- Tachycardia (rapid heart rate)

- Falling oxygen saturations (SpO$_2$)
- Agitation
- On the same side as the injury:
  - Hyper-expansion
  - Hypo-mobility
  - Decreased breath sounds
- Pre-terminal (near death):
  - Decreasing respiratory rate
  - Hypotension
  - Decreasing level of consciousness.

Do not rely on tracheal deviation or distended neck veins as these can be difficult to determine [Spiteri, 1988].

In ventilated patients, the clinical deterioration is likely to be far more alarming. In addition, ventilated patients are more likely to suffer a cardiac arrest, whereas awake patients tend to suffer from respiratory arrest initially [Leigh-Smith, 2005].

Management

Patients with a simple pneumothorax with no signs of cardiovascular compromise, suggesting tension, can be managed conservatively out-of-hospital, but should be closely monitored en route to hospital [Lee, 2007a]. All patients with a pneumothorax should receive oxygen at the appropriate target range (usually 94–98%, except for patients at risk of carbon dioxide retention, who should be managed at either 88–92% or their usual range [AACE, 2013]). If there is an open pneumothorax, then the wound should be covered with a commercial chest seal or an occlusive dressing, taped on three sides to act as a one-way valve [Lee, 2007a]. However, these can block, so closely monitor the patient and remove the dressing if the patient shows signs of tension pneumothorax. Patients with signs of a tension pneumothorax require prompt decompression by needle thoracentesis, which involves inserting a large-bore cannula (typically a 14 gauge needle) into the patient's chest, which should be performed by clinicians only.

4.8.2 Haemothorax

Haemothorax, or blood in the thoracic cavity, usually occurs due to penetrating trauma. Life-threatening haemorrhage can occur in cases of severe lacerations of the lung, large vessels in the mediastinum and the heart. Each hemithorax (literally, half of the chest) can easily accommodate half of the patient's circulating blood volume before the physical signs are obvious [Greaves, 2008].

However, this amount of bleeding will lead to the signs and symptoms of shock, and since blood occupies space usually reserved for the lung, lung collapse occurs, leading to absent or decreased lung sounds and reduced chest wall expansion on the injured side [Greaves, 2008].

There are few treatment options available outside of hospital; usually, expedient transport to the nearest major trauma centre is indicated.

4.8.3 Flail chest

Blunt chest trauma can lead to multiple rib and sternal fractures. In the event that two or more ribs are broken in two or more places, the chest wall will lose the rigid structure that usually supports the chest. A flail segment will start to move paradoxically, that is, it will move inwards during inspiration and outwards on expiration. If this area is large enough, it results in compromised ventilation. However, it is usually bruising of the underlying lung that leads to hypoxia and there can also be significant blood loss, with each rib fracture causing around 100 ml of blood loss [Greaves, 2008].

The flail segment is not always obvious as muscular spasm can support the segment until the muscles are exhausted. However, these injuries are painful and your clinician is likely to want to provide intravenous analgesia [AACE, 2013]. Do not attempt to splint the flail segment as this is likely to further impair ventilation [NAEMT, 2014].

4.9 Abdominal injuries

The abdominal cavity extends from the diaphragm to the pelvic bones and from the vertebral column to the muscles of the abdomen and flanks (Figure 4.1). Organs are classed as peritoneal if they are covered by a lining called the peritoneum. These include the spleen, liver, stomach, gallbladder, parts of the large intestine and most of the small intestine, and the female reproductive organs [NAEMT, 2014]. The retroperitoneal space is the area behind the peritoneum. This area contains the kidneys, ureters, pancreas, parts of the small and large

intestine and the aorta and vena cava [AACE, 2013].

In blunt trauma, the spleen, liver and structures that are firmly fixed, such as the retroperitoneal organs, are most commonly injured due to shearing forces associated with rapid deceleration. Penetrating trauma can also cause serious damage and severe bleeding. Depending on the angle at which the penetrating object enters, thoracic injury is also possible, particularly in upper abdominal stab injuries [NAEMT, 2014].

Patients suffering from abdominal trauma may not exhibit many symptoms initially, although you should suspect internal injury in any shocked patient with a suggestive mechanism of injury. Look at the abdomen for signs of injury, such as bruising, abrasions and seat-belt marks. Gently feel the abdomen for signs of tenderness, but don't be reassured by a normal examination [AACE, 2013].

There is no specific management of blunt abdominal trauma, but in penetrating trauma, if the injury has caused the bowel to protrude out of the abdomen, you should not push it back in.

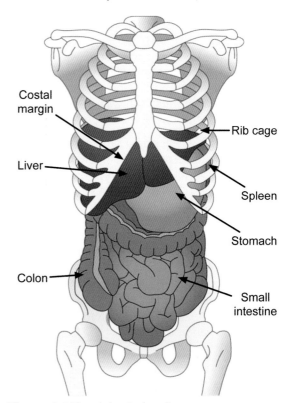

Figure 4.1 The abdominal cavity

Instead, cover it with a dressing soaked in warm saline [NAEMT, 2014].

If the penetrating object is still in place in the patient's abdomen, do not attempt to remove it. Instead, secure it appropriately, although if it is pulsating, allow some movement of the object, but not its removal [AACE, 2013].

4.10 Pelvic injuries

All pelvic fractures cause some bleeding, although the source can vary. Bleeding from cancellous bone that has been fractured is common, but bleeding can also occur from lacerations to retroperitoneal veins and the internal iliac arteries. Arterial bleeding accounts for up to 25% of haemodynamically unstable pelvic ring fractures [McCormack, 2010], but most bleeding is actually low-pressure bleeding (i.e. not arterial) and usually responds well to appropriate stabilisation (such as with a pelvic binder or external fixator) and tamponade [Abrassart, 2013]. Reducing the pelvic volume is an important step in controlling bleeding, as just a 3 cm gap at the symphysis pubis can lead to an increase in pelvic volume of 1.5 litres [Mears, 1986].

Associated abdominal injuries

As well as the potential vascular damage that pelvic ring fractures can cause, the soft tissues are also vulnerable, and injuries to the anorectum, vagina, urethra and nerves can occur. The most common is bladder injury, typically caused by compression or tearing of the bladder wall. Urethral and anorectal injuries are more common with straddle injuries, for example when a motorcyclist straddles the fuel tank during an RTC, resulting in the separation of the two pelvic bones and severe tearing of the pelvic floor [Luke, 2010].

Pelvic binders

If your clinician elects to apply a pelvic binder, make sure it is positioned correctly. Generally, the binder should be placed over the greater trochanters, but it is commonly placed too high [Bonner, 2011], such as over the iliac crests, which can actually compound pelvic fractures. Where possible, pelvic binders should be placed directly against the patient's skin. The correct application of pelvic binders is reviewed in more detail in the SKELETAL IMMOBILISATION lesson.

5 Skeletal immobilisation

5.1 Learning objectives

By the end of this lesson you will be able to:

• Describe how to perform a range of skeletal immobilisation techniques.

5.2 Introduction

Skeletal immobilisation is an important skill to learn and has the following benefits when performed correctly [NAEMT, 2014; Greaves, 2008]:

• Reduces pain
• Reduces risk of further damage to soft tissues, nerves and blood vessels
• Helps to control bleeding
• Reduces risk of fat embolism.

In this lesson you will learn how to perform the following techniques and/or use the equipment listed:

• First-aid techniques
  • Triangular bandages
• Spinal immobilisation
  • Manual methods
  • Cervical collar application
  • Crash helmet removal
  • Spinal board
  • Orthopaedic (scoop) stretcher
  • Vest-type extrication devices
• Using splints:
  • Box splint
  • Pelvic splint
  • Traction splint.

5.3 First-aid techniques

Effective splinting does not have to require expensive equipment, which may or may not be available. Sometimes, it is preferable to use basic first-aid methods, such as triangular bandaging for the management of upper limb injuries.

5.3.1 **Triangular bandages**

Triangular bandages have three main uses:

- Folded as a broad- or narrow-fold bandage to immobilise and support a limb or to secure a splint or bulky dressing

- Opened to form a sling

- Folded into a pad and used as a dressing.

In the ambulance service, it is probably most commonly used to make a sling to hold an injured limb close to the body and take some of the weight of that limb to prevent pain. Usually, the arm sling is used for injuries at the elbow or below and the elevated sling for injuries above the elbow. However, there is little evidence to support the benefit of either technique over the other and it is acceptable to adopt the technique that is most comfortable for the patient [Gregory, 2010b].

Procedure – Arm sling

Take the following steps to apply an arm sling [SJA, SAA, BRC, 2014; Gregory, 2010b]:

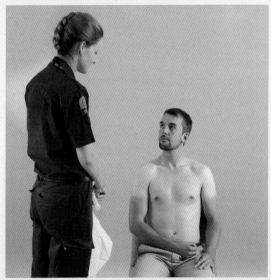

1. Explain the procedure to the patient and obtain informed consent. Provide analgesia as required to enable the sling to be applied. Prepare the triangular bandage

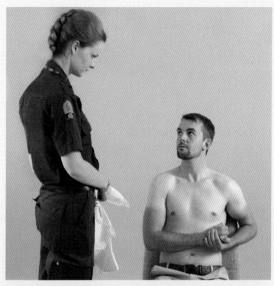

2. With the patient supporting their injured arm with the uninjured arm, ask them to flex the elbow to 90° if possible

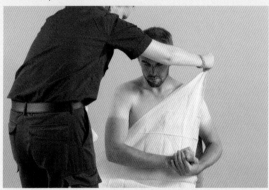

3. Slide the triangular bandage under the patient's arms so that the point is under the injured arm and the base (the long edge) is on the side of the uninjured arm

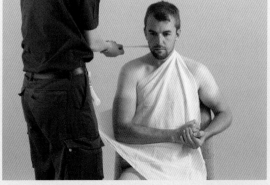

4. Slide the upper end of the triangular bandage around the neck towards the injured shoulder

Procedure continued →

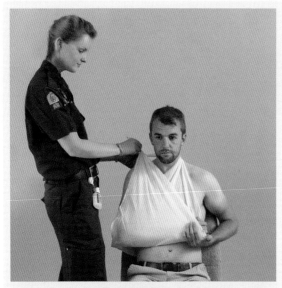

5. Fold the lower end of the bandage up over the forearm and bring it to meet the other end of the bandage at the shoulder

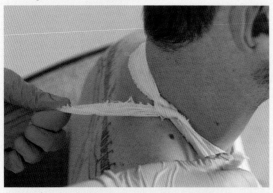

6. Tie the ends together using a reef knot. Consider applying a pad under the knot, if required

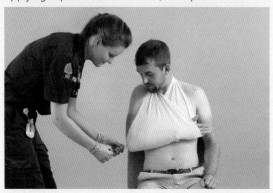

7. Holding the point of the bandage beyond the elbow, twist the point of the bandage until it fits the elbow snugly, then tuck it into the bandage. An alternative is to use tape or a safety pin

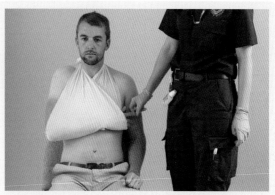

8. Re-check and record motor/sensory/circulation (MSC) function

Procedure – Elevated sling

Take the following steps to apply an elevated arm sling [SJA, SAA, BRC, 2014; Gregory, 2010b]:

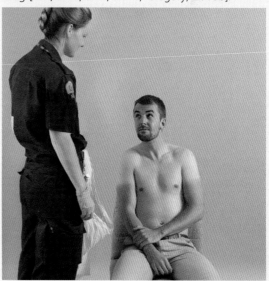

1. Explain the procedure to the patient and obtain informed consent. Provide analgesia as required to enable the sling to be applied. Prepare the triangular bandage

Procedure continued →

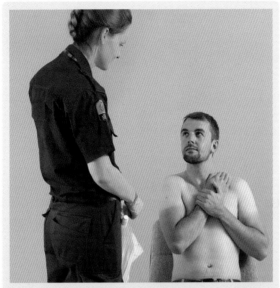

2. Ask the patient to support their injured arm across their chest, with the fingers of the injured arm resting on the opposite shoulder

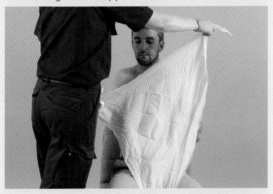

3. Place the sling over the injured arm so that the point of the bandage lies just beyond the elbow

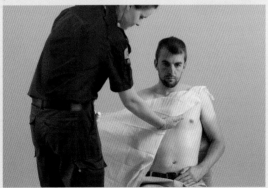

4. Ask the patient to let go of their injured arm. Tuck the base of the bandage under their lower arm

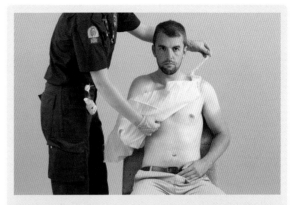

5. Bring the lower end of the bandage up diagonally across the patient's back to meet the other end at the shoulder

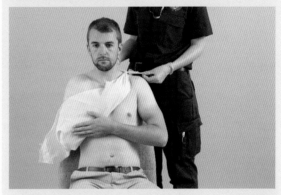

6. Tie the ends together using a reef knot. Consider applying a pad under the knot, if required

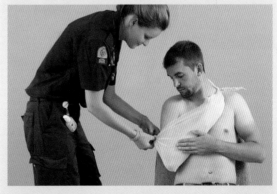

7. Holding the point of the bandage beyond the elbow, twist the bandage until it fits the elbow snugly, then tuck it into the bandage. An alternative is to use tape or a safety pin

Procedure continued →

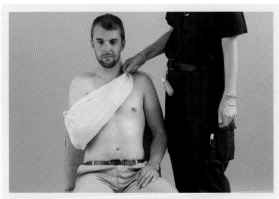

8. Re-check and record motor/sensory/circulation (MSC) function

5.4 Spinal immobilisation

Spinal immobilisation should be considered for any trauma patient with [EEAST, 2014]:

- A mechanism of injury consistent with spinal injury (mechanism may be minimal in the elderly or those with fragility conditions e.g. osteoporosis)
- Glasgow Coma Scale score of less than 15
- Complaints of neck or back pain
- Signs or symptoms of spinal cord injury
- Drug/alcohol intoxication.

5.4.1 Manual in-line stabilisation

Manual in-line stabilisation (MILS) with adequate back support is one of two acceptable methods of immobilisation. The other requires the use of several items of equipment [AACE, 2013]. Therefore, MILS will almost always be the first form of spinal immobilisation to be applied to a patient with a suspected spinal injury.

Procedure

Take the following steps to apply manual in-line stabilisation [NAEMT, 2014; Pilbery, 2013]:

1. Use appropriate PPE as required. Advise the patient not to move their head, explain that you are about to hold their head, and gain their consent if possible.
2. If the patient is supine (lying on their back) either kneel or lie on the ground behind the patient's head. If seated, move behind the patient. Hold the head firmly with both hands. Support the lower jaw with your fingers and support the head with your palms. Try to rest your lower arms on a surface (such as the ground or the back of a seat) as maintaining MILS can be tiring.

3. If the patient's head is not facing forwards and the patient is conscious, ask them to slowly move their head into a neutral, in-line position (eyes looking straight ahead and nose in line with umbilicus). If the patient is unconscious, gently move the head into a neutral position. If there is any pain or resistance to this manoeuvre, stop immediately.
4. Do not let go until instructed to do so by a clinician.

5.4.2 Cervical collars

The most important thing to know about cervical (semi-rigid) collars is that they do not fully immobilise the cervical spine [NAEMT, 2014; James, 2004]. Until head blocks and a back support are in place, manual in-line stabilisation must be used.

Procedure in the SITTING position – Ambu Perfit adjustable collar for extrication (ACE)

Take the following steps to apply a cervical collar when the patient is in a sitting position [Ambu, 2011]:

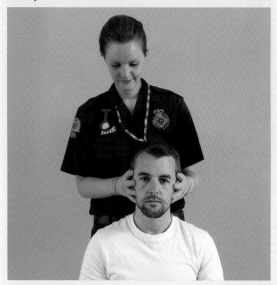

1. Use appropriate PPE as required. Inform the patient and obtain consent, if possible. One crew member should maintain manual in-line stabilisation while the other prepares the collar

Procedure continued →

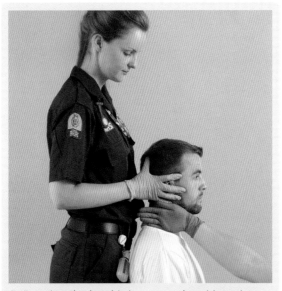

2. Ensuring the head is in a neutral position, size the collar by measuring the distance with your fingers between an imaginary line drawn horizontally and immediately below the patient's chin, and another immediately on top of the patient's shoulder

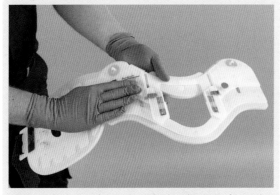

3. Compare this distance with the distance from the collar sizing line to the lower aspect of the plastic collar (NOT the foam)

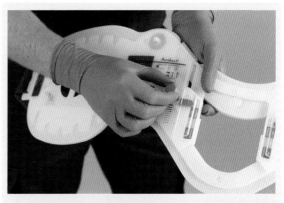

4. The Perfit ACE collar is preset to neckless size 3. If a larger size collar is needed, disengage the safety locks by pulling UP on the buttons

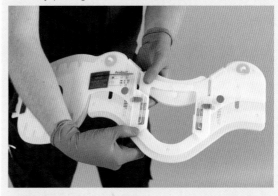

5. Adjust the collar to the correct size. There are 16 ratchet settings: simply pull the collar apart until the distance between the sizing line and the plastic collar body is the same as your finger measurement in step 2

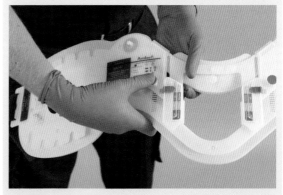

6. Engage the safety locks by pushing DOWN on the safety buttons

Procedure continued →

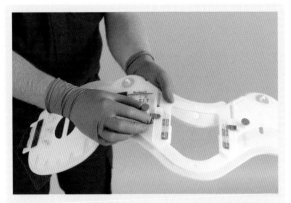

7. If the collar requires resizing, disengage the safety locks and pull OUT on the ratchet latches. Once resized, push the arrows IN and the safety locks DOWN

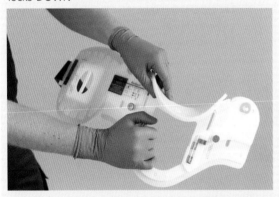

8. Assemble the collar by holding it near the tracheal opening and flip over the chin piece from the back of the collar to the front

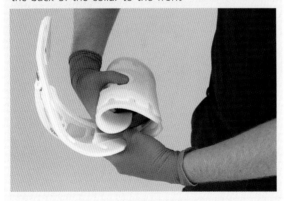

9. Preform the collar

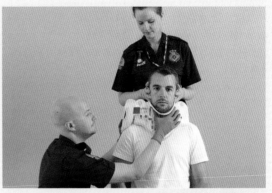

10. Slide the front of the collar along the patient's chest and position the chin piece so that the chin is supported. The collar body should rest on top of the patient's shoulder and against the sternum without gaps. The patient should remain in neutral alignment

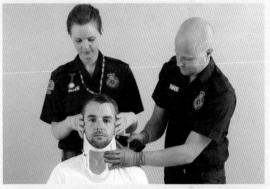

11. While holding the front of the collar in place, wrap the back of the collar around the back of the patient's head and neck and secure to the front of the collar with the Velcro tab. Maintain MILS

Procedure in the SUPINE position – Ambu Perfit adjustable collar for extrication (ACE)

Take the following steps to apply a cervical collar when the patient is in a supine position [Ambu, 2011]:

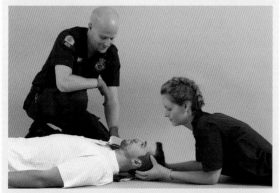

1. Follow steps 1 to 9 above. Slide the back portion of the collar directly behind the patient's neck until the velcro can be seen on the opposite side of the patient's neck

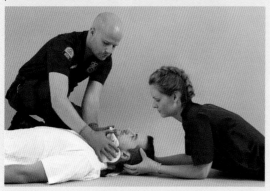

2. Position the chin piece under the chin

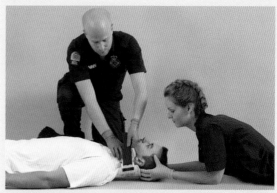

3. While maintaining proper positioning of the front of the collar with one hand, attach the Velcro with your other hand, to form a snug fit. Maintain MILS

5.4.3 Orthopaedic (scoop) stretcher

Orthopaedic stretchers (Figure 5.1) are the preferred tool to immobilise and transport patients who require spinal immobilisation [AACE, 2013]. This results in less movement of the spine while placing the patient onto the device, compared to the spinal board, and is also more comfortable [Krell, 2006].

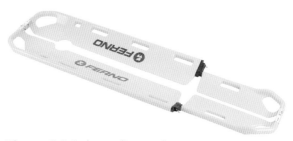

Figure 5.1 Orthopaedic stretcher

Procedure

Take the following steps to apply the orthopaedic stretcher [Pilbery, 2013; Ferno, 2006]:

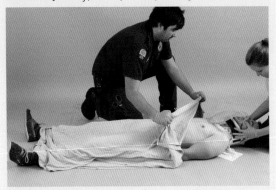

1. Explain the procedure and obtain the patient's informed consent, if possible. In major trauma, you should remove the patient's clothes ('skin to scoop') and maintain in-line stabilisation (MILS). Assess distal motor, sensation and circulatory (MSC) function in each extremity. Apply a cervical collar

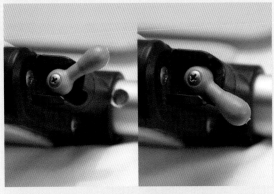

2. Adjust the length of the stretcher before uncoupling the halves. This ensures equal adjustment to both halves:

- Move the lock-pin lever on each side of the frame to the unlocked position.
- Pull the foot section outward to the desired length, stopping near one of the locking positions located at the holes along the foot-section frame
- Return both lock-pin levers to the locked position
- Push or pull the foot section a little until it locks into place
- Make sure both sides are securely locked

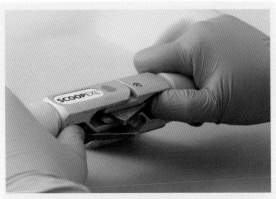

3. To separate the stretcher halves, unlock the Twin Safety Lock® coupling by pressing both levers of the Twin Safety Lock® and pull the coupling halves away from each other. Place one half on either side of the patient

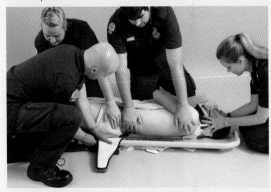

4. Gently insert each side of the orthopaedic stretcher under the patient. This may require a 10° tilt. If applying a pelvic binder to the patient, do this at the same time (Note: the tilt has been exaggerated in the photo and is in excess of 10°)

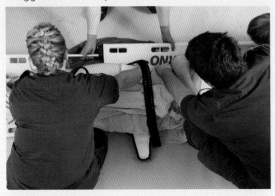

5. Return the patient to the supine position and repeat step 4 with the other half of the orthopaedic stretcher

Procedure continued →

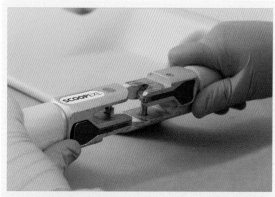

6. To rejoin the stretcher halves, align the right and left halves of the head and foot couplings and push them together until the Twin Safety Locks® engage

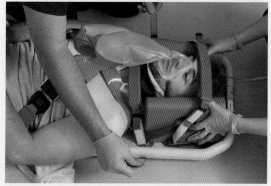

7. Insert appropriate head padding. Secure the patient to the stretcher by applying straps in the following order: chest, pelvis, thighs, ankles (tie the straps in a figure-of-eight), head blocks and straps. Reassess MSC function

5.4.4 Spinal board

Long extrication/spinal boards should only be used as an extrication device. Supine patients should be placed on an orthopaedic stretcher, if available, unless the transfer time is very short (total time on the spinal board less than 30 minutes) [Connor, 2013].

Procedure – Extrication in a time-critical situation

Take the following steps to extricate a sitting patient in a time-critical situation [EEAST, 2014; Gregory, 2010b]:

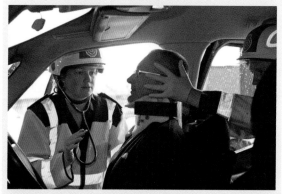

1. Explain the procedure and obtain the patient's informed consent, if possible. Maintain in-line stabilisation (MILS) and apply a cervical collar. Ensure that the spinal board has a head pad in place

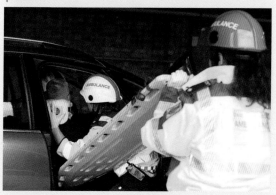

2. Place the foot end of the spinal board next to the patient's buttocks at right angles to their torso. Place the ambulance trolley under the spinal board. With the rescuer who is applying MILS giving the commands, turn the patient so that they are in line with the spinal board and slowly lower them onto it

Procedure continued →

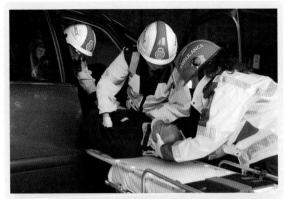

3. Slide the patient up the spinal board until they are centrally positioned. Remove the patient from the spinal board using an orthopaedic stretcher and secure the patient by applying straps in the following order: chest, pelvis, thighs, ankles (tie the straps in a figure-of-eight), head blocks and straps. Reassess MSC

5.4.5 Vest-type extrication devices

Vest-type extrication devices are the preferred option for the seated trauma patient (such as a driver involved in an RTC who is still in their vehicle) who does NOT have life-threatening/time-critical injuries [NAEMT, 2014].

Procedure – Kendrick Extrication Device® (KED)

Note: For clarity, the images below were not taken inside a vehicle. Application of vest-type extrication devices in the confined environment of a car interior is likely to be more challenging.

Take the following steps to extricate a patient using a KED [NAEMT, 2014; Ferno 2001]:

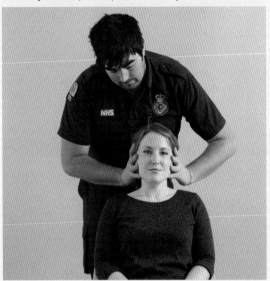

1. Explain the procedure and obtain the patient's informed consent, if possible. Maintain in-line stabilisation (MILS) from behind the patient. Assess distal motor, sensation and circulatory (MSC) function in each extremity. Apply a cervical collar and prepare the KED for use

Procedure continued →

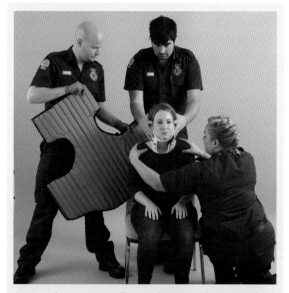

2. In order to optimally use the KED, three people are required. One rescuer should apply MILS. The second should grasp the KED at the top of the head flap and the top corner of the torso flap closest to the patient. Then, they can tilt the KED at about a 45° angle and slide it behind the patient, while a third rescuer on the other side of the patient moves the patient a hand's width forward to reduce friction, enabling the KED to slide in more easily

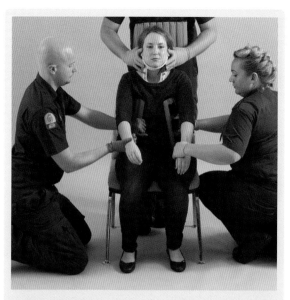

4. Wrap both torso flaps around the patient's torso, lifting the patient's arms only as much as needed to slide the flaps beneath them. The top of the flaps should be just below the patient's armpits

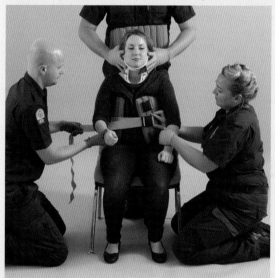

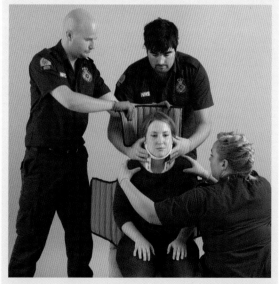

3. The second rescuer moves the KED to the vertical position. Note that this may require the rescuer applying MILS to lift their elbow slightly, providing clearance for the KED while taking care not to move the patient's head

5. Before beginning to fasten the torso straps, make sure the patient is sitting back against the KED as fully as his/her body structure and condition allow. Fasten the middle (yellow) strap and then the bottom (red) strap

Procedure continued →

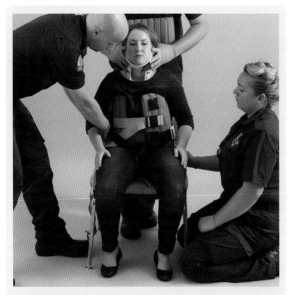

6. Fasten the leg straps. Pass the leg straps between the leg and car seat (make use of a gap if there is one). Using both hands, 'see-saw' one strap into position under the patient's leg and buttock. Reach behind the patient and make sure the strap lies straight downward from its anchor point on the KED, as close as possible to the body midline. Either clip the strap into the buckle on the same side, or cross over to the other side of the KED and use the opposite buckle

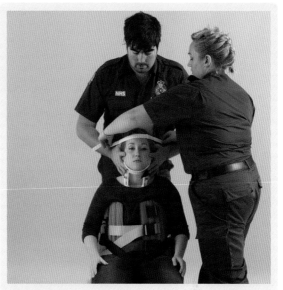

8. Secure the patient's head. Grasp a head strap with both hands and turn the centre pad fully inside-out so the rubber will be against the patient's forehead. Position the strap at the patient's eyebrows and secure the strap to the head flap fastening strips at a downward angle. Place the second strap under or on the chin area of the cervical collar and position the strap ends as horizontally as possible. Secure the strap ends to the fastening strips on the head flaps and ensure the patient can still open their mouth

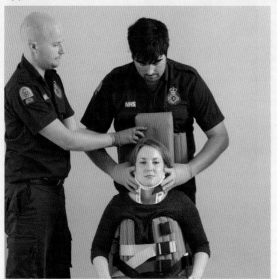

7. If there is a gap between the KED and the patient's head, the cervical collar, or the patient's shoulders, fill the gap with the pad provided with the KED, or rolled towels

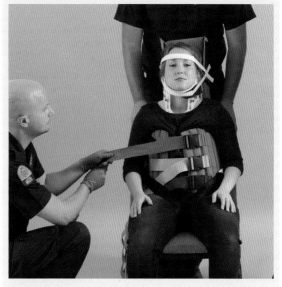

9. Apply the top (green) strap and tighten all the other straps

Procedure continued →

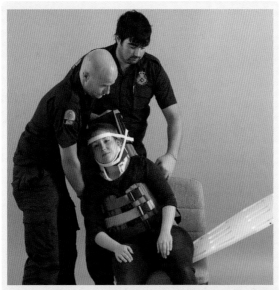

10. If attempting a vehicle extrication, bring the ambulance trolley with spinal board to the opening of the vehicle door. Slide the spinal board under the patient's buttocks. Rotate the patient so that their back faces out of the vehicle and lower them onto the waiting spinal board. Slide the patient into the correct position and loosen the leg and top (green) strap. Fully immobilise the KED and patient onto the spinal board

5.4.6 **Crash helmet removal**

Patients who are wearing crash helmets need to have them removed in order to assess and manage their airway and ventilation. In addition, hidden bleeding at the back of the head can be identified and the head moved into a position of neutral alignment. Note that some degree of spinal motion will occur, even in optimal circumstances [NAEMT, 2010].

Procedure

NOTE: Unless immediate airway intervention is required, a single rescuer should not attempt helmet removal [Pilbery, 2013].
Take the following steps to remove a crash helmet:

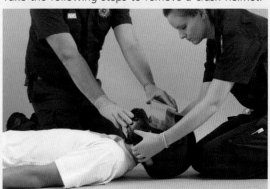

1. Explain the procedure and obtain the patient's informed consent, if possible. Rescuer one should position themselves above the patient's head. Their palms should be pressed on the sides of the helmet and fingertips curled underneath. The helmet, head and neck should be maintained in as near to an in-line neutral position as possible. Rescuer two should remove the face shield, glasses (if worn) and chin strap

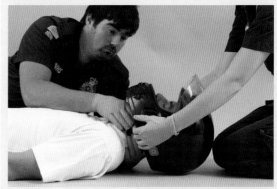

2. Rescuer two should move their thumb and first two fingers up to support the mandible. Their other hand should be placed behind the head at the back of the helmet

Procedure continued →

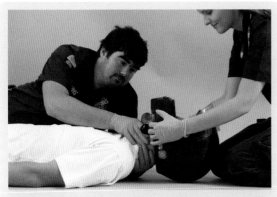

3. Rescuer one pulls the side of the helmet slightly apart and gently tilts the helmet up and down while applying traction to remove the helmet. This should be slow and deliberate. Take care as the helmet clears the patient's nose

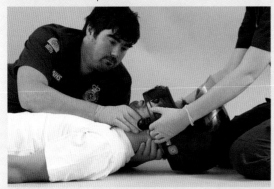

4. Once the helmet has reached the halfway point, rescuer one should stop moving the helmet, while rescuer two repositions their hands from the back of the helmet to the occiput. Take care, the head is heavy!

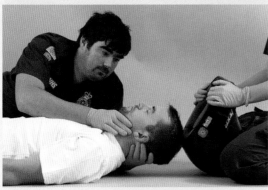

5. Once rescuer two has repositioned their hands and has control of the patient's head, rescuer one should continue to remove the helmet

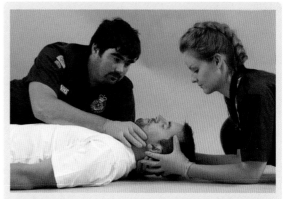

6. Once the helmet has been removed, rescuer one takes back control of the head and gently moves it into an in-line neutral position

5.5 Splints

Splinting forms an important part of fracture management, particularly in the lower limbs.The benefits of splintage include reducing [Greaves, 2008]:

- Pain
- Blood loss
- Pressure on skin
- Pressure on adjacent neurovascular structures
- Risk of fat embolism
- Risk of further damage.

Basic principles of immobilisation should consist of assessment and reassessment of the neurovascular status before and after any manipulation or handling of the fracture, and immobilisation of the joints above and below the fracture.

Note: It is not possible to show the application of every type of splinting device in this text. Instead, a selection of commonly used devices are explained. This is not a substitute for hands-on training with your service's splints.

5.5.1 Box splints

Box splints are simple devices that are most commonly used for lower leg fractures (Figure 5.2). They are only suitable for the immobilisation of straight limbs as they will not conform to the shape of deformed limbs [Gregory, 2010b].

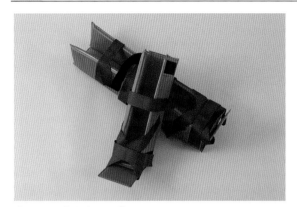

Figure 5.2 A box splint

Procedure

Take the following steps to apply a box splint [EEAST, 2014; Gregory, 2010b]:

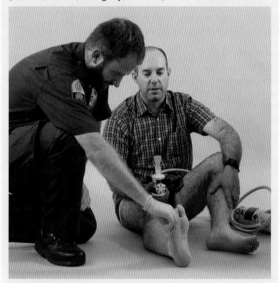

1. Gain the patient's informed consent. Provide analgesia if required prior to the procedure. Ensure the splint is clean and undamaged. Check motor/sensory/circulation (MSC) function

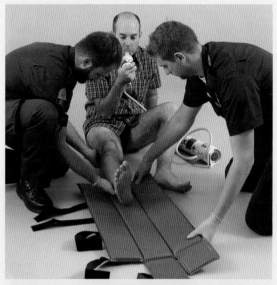

2. Expose the injured limb and remove footwear where possible. Support the limb manually and raise it carefully while the splint is passed under it

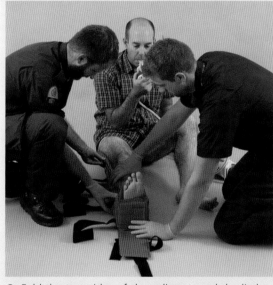

3. Fold the two sides of the splint around the limb to form a box to support the limb

Procedure continued →

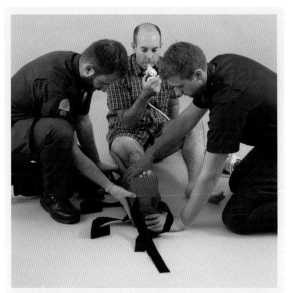

4. Ensure the foot piece is placed against the sole of the foot at 90° or in a position comfortable for the patient

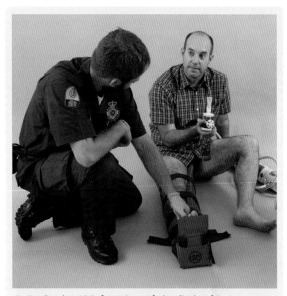

6. Recheck MSC function of the limb after application of the box splint

5.5.2 Pelvic splints

Commercial pelvic splints (commonly called pelvic binders) have been shown to reduce stable, open book and rotational and vertically unstable fractures adequately (Figure 5.3), with no important displacement of fractures, irrespective of device [Knops, 2011]. Concerns have been expressed with their use in lateral compression fractures, but there is no good evidence that their use is detrimental to the patient with these fractures [Toth, 2012]. That said, there is no conclusive evidence that the use of pelvic binders reduces morbidity or mortality from serious trauma either [Stewart, 2013].

In the absence of a commercial device, sheets (and binding the legs together at the knee and ankles) [Simpson, 2002] or an inverted Kendrick Extrication Device® (KED) can be used, although these make access to the pelvis and abdomen difficult [McCormack, 2010].

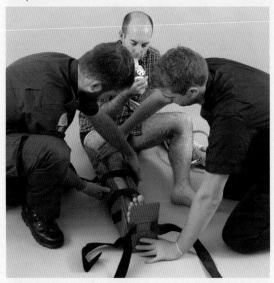

5. The Velcro straps should be carefully placed over the limb, avoiding the area of injury. The footstrap should be passed over the top of the foot

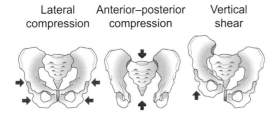

Lateral compression   Anterior–posterior compression   Vertical shear

Figure 5.3 Types of pelvic fracture. The red arrows indicate the direction of the forces

Procedure – SAM pelvic sling II

Take the following steps to apply the SAM pelvic sling II [EEAST, 2014]:

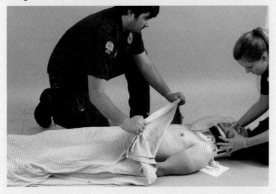

1. Use appropriate PPE as required. Inform the patient and obtain consent, if possible. Prepare the SAM splint. Fully expose the patient as the splint needs to be placed directly on the patient's skin. Cover the patient to preserve their dignity and prevent heat loss

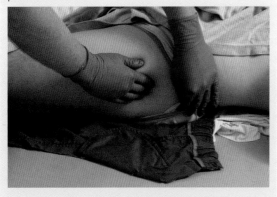

2. Identify the level of the greater trochanters

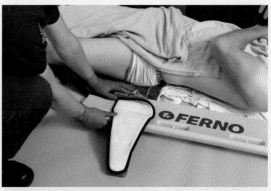

3. Place the buckle side of the device level with the greater trochanter and facing away from the direction of the first roll. Fold the tail end of the splint 90° so that the tail strap points down towards the patient's feet, forming an L-shape. Slide one half of the orthopaedic stretcher under the splint, so both can be inserted under the patient during the log roll

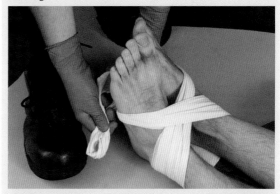

4. As long as there are no lower limb fractures, tie the patient's feet together prior to securing the splint

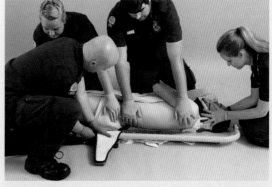

5. Log roll the patient 10°, place the SAM splint on the orthopaedic stretcher and insert both items under the patient (Note that the degree of tilt has been exaggerated in this photo)

Procedure continued →

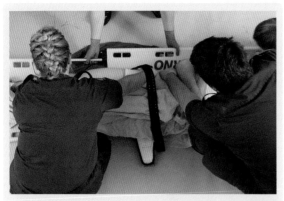

6. Roll the patient onto their back and then roll 10° in the other direction. Pull the tail of the SAM splint through and ensure it is at the correct level. Insert the remaining half of the orthopaedic stretcher and connect both together

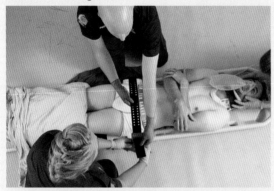

7. Log roll the patient onto their back. Place the black strap through the buckle and pull completely through

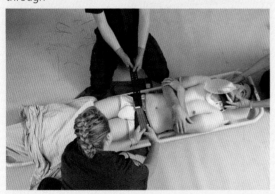

8. Hold the orange strap and pull the black strap in the opposite direction until you hear and feel the buckle click. Maintain tension and immediately press the black strap onto the surface of the SAM splint to secure. You may hear a second click as the sling secures

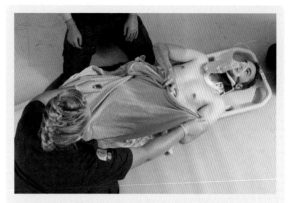

9. Re-cover the patient to maintain dignity and minimise heat loss

5.5.3 Traction splints

Traction splints apply longitudinal force to long bones (normally the femur). Correctly splinting the femur using this method helps to reduce [AACE, 2013]:

- Pain

- Haemorrhage and damage to blood vessels and nerves

- Movement of bone fragments and the risk of a closed fracture becoming an open fracture

- The risk of a fat embolus

- Muscle spasm.

Indication

- Suspected fracture of the femoral shaft.

Contraindications [NAEMT, 2014]

- Suspected pelvic fractures (except the Kendrick traction device)

- Suspected femoral neck fracture

- Avulsion or amputation of ankle and foot

- Fractures close to, or below, the knee

- Dislocated knee (not just patella).

Procedure – Kendrick traction device (KTD)

Take the following steps to apply the KTD [EEAST, 2014]:

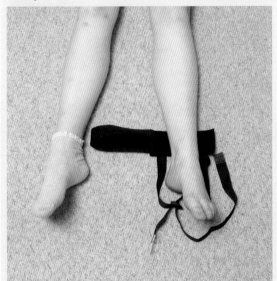

1. Use appropriate PPE as required. Inform the patient and obtain consent, if possible. Remove the patient's shoes and clothing to expose the injured leg. Check motor, sensation and circulation (MSC) below the injury. Prepare the KTD

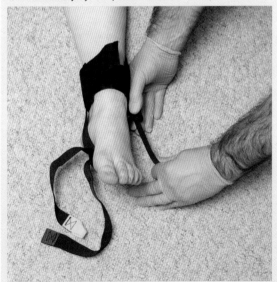

2. Apply the ankle hitch around the injured leg, just above the anklebone, and tighten the stirrup by pulling the GREEN tabbed strip until snug under the heel

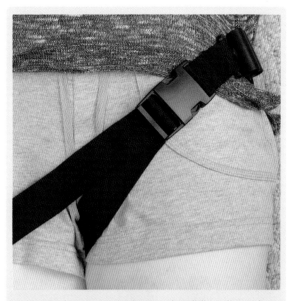

3. Apply the upper thigh strap by sliding the male buckle under the knee, seesaw the strap upwards until it rests in the crotch area and click the ends together. Tighten the strap until the traction pole receptacle is positioned at the level of the pelvic crease. Make sure male genitals are clear of the strap

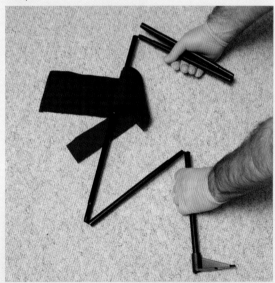

4. Snap out the traction pole, ensuring each joint is securely seated

Procedure continued →

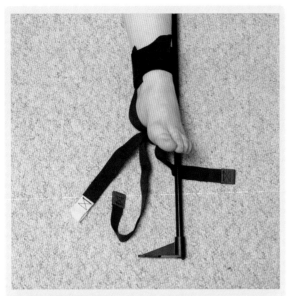

5. Place the traction pole alongside the leg so that one section extends below the foot

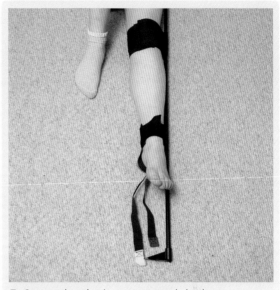

7. Secure the elastic strap around the knee

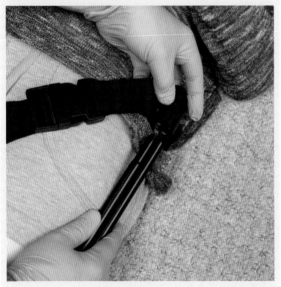

6. Adjust the length of the pole and place the ends into the traction pole receptacle

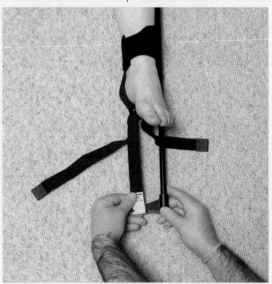

8. Place the YELLOW tab over the dart end

Procedure continued →

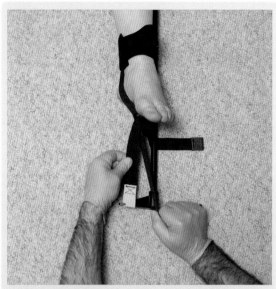

9. Apply traction by pulling on the RED tab. As a guide, apply around 10% of body weight (up to 7kg) tension. Use patient comfort as the main objective. Traction can be applied smoothly by grasping the strap either side of the buckle and simultaneously feeding and pulling with equal pressure

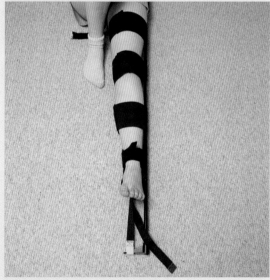

10. Finish packaging by applying upper and lower straps. Re-check and record MSC

6 Burns

6.1 Learning objectives

By the end of this lesson you will be able to:

- Explain what is meant by the term 'burn'
- Describe the types of burn and their causes
- Explain the safety considerations when dealing with burns
- State the rules associated with estimating the size of burns
- Explain time-critical factors that affect the management of burns
- Explain the complications associated with burns
- Explain the treatment of burns
- Explain why burns patients are transported to definitive care.

6.2 Introduction

A burn is an injury caused by energy transfer to the body's tissues, causing necrosis and an associated inflammatory reaction [Greaves, 2008].

It is estimated that there are 250,000 burn injuries a year in the United Kingdom, resulting in 175,000 visits to an emergency department [NBCRC, 2001]. In England and Wales, serious burn injury (defined as requiring at least a 72-hour stay in hospital) is responsible for 5.4% of all serious trauma [Kalson, 2012].

Burn injury most commonly occurs in the home (over 30%) with the kitchen being the favoured location. The most common sources of injury are [NBCG, 2008]:

- Cup of tea in children
- Petrol ignition in adults
- Bathing, kettle spills and central heating radiators in elderly people.

Burns are commonly split into a number of types [AACE, 2013]:

- Chemical
- Cold
- Electrical
- Friction
- Radiation
- Thermal.

Note: Cold injury was discussed in the EXTREMES OF TEMPERATURE lesson (chapter 13).

6.3 Assessment of burns

History

It is important to identify the mechanism, including the cause of the burn, how it came into contact with the patient and any first aid undertaken. Note when the injury occurred, how long the patient was exposed to the source and the duration of any cooling. Don't forget to be alert for signs of non-accidental injury.

Assessment

Pre-hospital estimation of total body surface area (TBSA) of burn injury is poor, with the 'rule of nines' (Figure 6.1) underestimating burns of less than 20% and overestimating burns over 40%; also, it is not suitable for children under 14 years of age [Hettiaratchy, 2004; AACE, 2013].

The whole hand (palm and fingers) represents about 0.82% TBSA in adults and 0.77% in children, making accurate calculations tricky. However, the palm alone is 0.5% TBSA [Muehlberger, 2010] and is suitable for estimating burns less than 15% or greater than 85% TBSA. Note that these methods will generally underestimate %TBSA in obese patients [Berry, 2001].

Lund and Browder charts are more accurate, but these are cumbersome to complete in the back

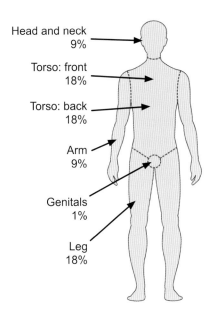

Figure 6.1 The 'rule of nines'

Head and neck
9%

Torso: front
18%

Torso: back
18%

Arm
9%

Genitals
1%

Leg
18%

of an ambulance. An alternative that has been advocated is serial halving [Allison, 2004]. This involves determining whether greater than or less than 50%, 25% and finally 12.5% of the TBSA is burnt. This approximation is sufficient to determine whether the patient requires referral to a burns unit (if direct access is an option) and the need for intravenous fluids. Erythema (reddening) should not be included when calculating TBSA of burn injury [Enoch, 2009].

6.3.1 Classification

Although important for subsequent burns management, the depth of a burn does not affect pre-hospital treatment, but may provide some indication as to the cause (Table 6.1) [NZGG, 2007].

6.3.2 Burns requiring transport to hospital

The National Network for Burn Care (NNBC) has set out a suggested minimum threshold for patients who may require specialised burn care services. These patients will usually require transport to hospital, but check with your own ambulance service's local arrangements [NNBC, 2012]:

- All burns ≥2% TBSA in children or ≥3% in adults
- All full thickness burns
- All circumferential burns
- Any burn not healed in 2 weeks
- Any burn with suspicion of non-accidental injury
- All burns to hands, feet, face, perineum or genitalia
- Any chemical, electrical* or friction burn
- Any cold injury
- Any unwell/febrile child with a burn.

*May not apply to low (domestic) voltage injury

6.4 Thermal burns

Pathophysiology

The most common type of thermal burns are flame, scald and contact. Flame burns are more common in adults and are often associated with smoke inhalation and other traumatic injuries. These are more likely to result in deep dermal or full-thickness burns.

Table 6.1: Burns classification

Classification	Other names	Example causes	Appearance	Sensation
Epidermal	Superficial, 1st degree	Ultraviolet light	Dry and red, blanches with pressure, no blisters	May be painful
Superficial dermal	Superficial, partial thickness, 2nd degree	Scald (spill or splash)	Pale pink, fine blisters, blanches with pressure	Very painful
Mid-dermal	Superficial, partial thickness, 2nd degree	Scald (spill), flame	Dark pink with large blisters, delayed capillary refill	May be painful
Deep dermal	Deep partial thickness, 2nd degree	Scald (spill), flame	Blotchy red, may blister, no capillary refill	No sensation
Full thickness	3rd degree	Scald (immersion), flame, steam, high-voltage electricity	White, waxy or charred. No blisters or capillary refill Children: dark lobster red with mottling	No sensation

Scalds are the most common cause of burn in children, usually due to spillages of hot drinks or immersion in hot bath water. They generally cause epidermal or superficial dermal burn injury [Hettiaratchy, 2004].

Direct contact burns are caused by brief contact with a very hot object, or (more commonly) prolonged contact with a cooler object. Typical patient groups include epileptics and those who misuse alcohol or drugs.

Irreversible damage to the epidermis can be caused by exposure to 44°C heat for six hours, or 65°C for one second [Moritz, 1947]. Burns injuries are characterised by a local response and, if the total body surface area (TBSA) burned is greater than 20%, a systemic response [Greaves, 2008].

Local response

At skin level, burns form three zones of injury [Hettiaratchy, 2004]:

- Zone of coagulation: The point of maximal injury, with irreversible damage to tissue due to protein coagulation

- Zone of stasis: Surrounding the zone of coagulation and characterised by reduced tissue perfusion. Potentially salvageable with adequate resuscitation
- Zone of hyperaemia: Surrounds the zone of stasis and is characterised by increased tissue perfusion. Usually recovers.

The zones spread out from the point of injury in three dimensions, including deeper into dermal tissue.

Systemic response

The level of inflammatory response is related to the %TBSA that is burned. Once the burn covers more than 20% TBSA, the inflammatory response can exert systemic effects. Capillary permeability increases, leading to loss of intravascular proteins and fluid into interstitial space. Peripheral and splanchnic vasoconstriction occur and myocardial contractility decreases. Combined with fluid loss from the burn, this results in hypotension and end-organ hypoperfusion. In the lungs, there can be bronchoconstriction and the development of acute respiratory distress syndrome in any severe burns. Initially, there is a reduction in metabolic rate ('ebb phase'), but this can double in the days following burn injury ('flow phase') [Sheridan, 2012].

Acute smoke inhalation injury

Smoke inhalation is a killer. Between 80% and 90% of fire-related fatalities are attributed to smoke inhalation, and it has a greater contribution to overall mortality and morbidity of burn injuries than either %TBSA or age [Kimmel, 1999]. Naso-oropharyngeal and mucosal burns are common [Toon, 2010], but thermal injury below the vocal cords is rare since heat is effectively exchanged in upper airway passages [Prien, 1988]. When air, steam and/or smoke are at sufficiently high temperatures to cause thermal injury to the lower airways, rapid oedema of the glottis develops, resulting in fatal airway obstruction.

Systemic toxins are the products of incomplete combustion and include carbon monoxide (CO) and hydrogen cyanide. CO is an odourless, colourless gas that binds to haemoglobin with 250 times the affinity of oxygen. This results in a decrease in the oxygen-carrying capacity of the blood. Cyanide adversely affects internal respiration by preventing aerobic production of adenosine triphosphate (ATP, the energy source for cells) [Toon, 2010].

Particulates and irritants have the greatest effect on the pathophysiological processes that occur due to smoke inhalation. Soot impregnated with toxins can reach the alveoli suspended in air. The types of chemicals vary, depending on what has been burning, but they trigger a cascade of events, resulting in pulmonary oedema and other respiratory problems [Murakami, 2003]. Water-soluble gases such as ammonia and hydrogen chloride react with the mucous membranes, producing strong alkalis and acids, leading to intense and prolonged inflammatory reactions. Lipid- (fat) soluble irritants act more slowly as they dissolve into cellular membranes.

Friction burns

Although friction burns are strictly speaking a thermal burn, they are the result of heat production caused by friction between the skin and another object. This can result in not just a burn, but abrasions too (see the lesson on WOUNDS AND BLEEDING above) [Gregory, 2010b].

6.4.1 Management

Safety first! The patient needs to be removed from the source of the burn if it is safe to do so, but don't get burnt yourself. Clothing should be removed unless it is sticking to the patient, as should jewellery, which may become constrictive as tissues swell.

Follow the <C>ABC approach for burns as you would any traumatic injury. However, inhalation injury is a particular concern and occurs in around 22% of all burns, 60% if facial burns are present [Toon, 2010].

Signs of inhalation injury include [Singer, 2010]:

- Full thickness or deep dermal burns to face, neck or upper torso
- Singed nasal hair
- Soot in sputum or oropharynx
- Dyspnoea, hoarseness, cough or stridor
- Cyanosis
- Altered level of consciousness.

Administer high-flow oxygen via a non-rebreathe mask. CO poisoning may make pulse oximetry readings unreliable [AACE, 2013].

Cooling

Thermal burns should be cooled for 20 minutes [Bartlett, 2008], preferably with running water (between 8°C and 15°C) [NZGG, 2007]. There is little evidence that ice causes damage to underlying tissues, but it runs the risk of making the patient hypothermic so is not recommended [Cuttle, 2008, 2009]. Cooling should commence immediately after the burn has occurred, but there is limited evidence to suggest that cooling up to an hour after the burn has occurred is still beneficial [Cuttle, 2010]. If running water is not available or practicable, then gel-based body blankets can be used without causing hypothermia [NZGG, 2007; Singer, 2006; Martineau, 2006].

Covering/dressing

Patients with burns lose heat from non-epithelialised areas of skin due to evaporation. With the thermoregulatory function of the skin disrupted, patients are at risk of hypothermia, even on a warm day [AAOS, 2011]. Hypothermia is part of the lethal triad in trauma, and for each 1°C reduction in body temperature the mortality rate increases significantly [Lonnecker, 2001], although there is no evidence currently to suggest that pre-hospital cooling causes hypothermia [Lonnecker, 2001; Singer, 2010]. Once cooling has been completed, cover the burn with a clean sheet or Clingfilm, but take care not to apply it circumferentially as it can become constrictive as oedema develops [NZGG, 2007].

Time-critical features

A blue light transfer to the most appropriate location is required for any of the following conditions [AACE, 2013]:

- Any major ABCD problems
- Airway burns
- History of hot air or gas inhalation
- Respiratory distress
- Evidence of circumferential (completely circling the neck, torso or limb) burns
- Significant facial burns
- Burns more than 15% TBSA in adults or 10% TBSA in children
- Presence of other major injuries.

Note that transfer may not be to your nearest hospital, but to a major trauma or specialised burns centre. Check local guidance.

6.5 Chemical burns

Chemical burns generally result from exposure to acids, alkalies and other corrosive materials. Alkali burns are generally more serious as they penetrate more deeply than other chemicals [ATLS, 2008]. Their severity depends on the concentration of the chemical, the duration of exposure and the speed in applying first-aid measures [Greaves, 2008].

6.5.1 Management

Safety first! It is important that you do not become exposed to the chemical. If in doubt, do not approach the scene but wait for the Hazardous Area Response Team (HART) or the fire and rescue service to attend.

Speed is of the essence when treating chemical burns so flush the exposed area with copious quantities of water as soon as possible. However, brush off any chemical powder from the patient first. In industrial settings, decontamination showers may be available, but at home, the shower or a hosepipe is an alternative. While flushing, contaminated clothing should be removed, although do not pass anything over the patient's head; cut it off [Pilbery, 2013].

Chemical burns should be irrigated for at least 15 minutes, and ideally for up to an hour (although alkali burns may require much longer periods of irrigation), but watch for hypothermia [NZGG, 2007].

6.6 Radiation burns

Radiation burns are most commonly caused by ultraviolet radiation from the sun or sunlamps (sunburn). However, in rare cases, it can be caused by exposure to radioactive materials [Gregory, 2010b].

Approximately 80% of skin cancer is preventable, and avoiding sunburn is key [Simon, 2010]:

- Take care not to burn
- Cover up with loose cool clothing, a hat and sun glasses
- Seek shade during the hottest part of the day
- Apply high-factor sunscreen (at least sun protection factor 15) to sun-exposed body parts
- Take extra care to protect children in the sun.

6.6.1 Management

Safety first! If the burns are due to exposure to radioactivity, do not approach but wait for the Hazardous Area Response Team (HART).

Sunburn

Basic first-aid measures are usually sufficient [SJA, SAA, BRC, 2014]:

- Cover the patient's skin with light clothing or a towel. Move them out of the sun, preferably indoors
- Encourage them to drink frequent sips of cold water while cooling the affected area with cold water. If the area of sunburn is large, it may be more practical for the patient to soak the area in a cold bath for 10 minutes
- If burns are mild, calamine or an after-sun lotion may help. Patients should be advised to stay inside or in the shade.

Most sunburn will manifest as reddening of the skin (erythema), but blistering is evidence of a partial thickness burn and transport to hospital should be considered if it meets the criteria for review by specialised burns care services [NNBC, 2012].

6.7 Electrical injuries

Electrical injuries are thankfully uncommon, but they cause significant damage and even death when they occur. The majority of electrical injuries in adults occur in the workplace and involve high voltages, whereas in children most injuries occur in the home with domestic voltage. Electrocution from lightning strikes is very rare, leading to around 1000 deaths each year worldwide [Nolan, 2010].

Electrical burns arise when a source of electrical power makes contact with the patient's body. They are frequently more serious than they appear, since rapid heat loss from the surface of the skin may leave it relatively undamaged, whereas the underlying tissues may have sustained serious injury, particularly between the entry and exit points (don't forget to look for both!) [ATLS, 2008].

6.7.1 Management

Safety first! Do not approach the patient until you are certain that the source of electricity has been cut off.

When dealing with electrical injuries, the thermal burns sustained may not be your highest priority. The patient may be in cardiac arrest, have airway or facial burns, have cardiac arrhythmias (also perform electrocardiogram monitoring) and be traumatically injured (fractures, serious internal injuries) that will need addressing first. Associated thermal burns can be managed as previously described.

6.8 The problem with burns

Without appropriate intervention and management, patients with serious burns can die due to [Sheridan, 2012]:
- Burn shock due to excessive fluid loss in the first 24 hours
- Respiratory failure in the subsequent 3–5 days
- Burn wound sepsis in the following few weeks.

Thankfully, because of prompt transfer by ambulance staff to burn centres and the subsequent specialised management that patients receive, this is less common. However, it does underline the importance of transporting patients to definitive care.

There are four general phases of burn care, with the ambulance service only playing a small part in the initial management stage [Sheridan, 2012]:
- Initial evaluation and resuscitation (0–72 hours)
- Initial surgery and temporary closure of wounds created by removal of full-thickness burns (days 1–7)
- Definitive wound closure (weeks 1–6)
- Rehabilitation and reconstruction (up to 2 years).

Chapter 16: Assisting the Paramedic

1 Assisting the paramedic: Airway

1.1 Learning objectives

By the end of this lesson you will be able to:

- Explain your role in assisting the paramedic with advanced airway procedures
- Explain the function of equipment associated with advanced airway procedures
- Describe the safety checks relating to advanced airway adjuncts
- Explain your role in infection prevention and control.

1.2 Introduction

Having completed the AIRWAY chapter, you already know about airway anatomy and have knowledge of a range of manual airway manoeuvres and adjuncts. This lesson will cover three other airway procedures in which you may be required to assist a paramedic:

- Nasopharyngeal airway (NPA) insertion
- Supraglottic airway insertion
- Endotracheal intubation.

1.3 Nasopharyngeal airway (NPA)

When to do it (indications)

- An unresponsive patient, or a patient with a reduced level of consciousness who has an intact gag reflex.

When not to do it (contra-indications)

- Patients who do not tolerate the procedure.

Cautions

- Patients who have a basal skull fracture
- Patients with nasal polyps.

Advantages

- Can be suctioned through
- Can be tolerated by patients who are not unconscious
- Does not require the mouth to open.

Disadvantages

- Poor technique can cause bleeding
- Does not protect against aspiration.

1.3.1 Inserting an NPA

Procedure

The following steps demonstrate the correct insertion technique of a nasopharyngeal airway (NPA) [Nolan, 2012; Pilbery, 2013; Gregory, 2010b]:

1. Adopt standard precautions
2. Prepare equipment. You will need the following:
   - An appropriately sized NPA, which is generally considered to be a 7.0 for an average adult male and 6.0 for an average adult female
   - Water-soluble gel
   - Suction
3. If the NPA you are using comes with a safety pin, insert it through the non-bevelled end to avoid accidentally inserting the NPA too far
4. Lubricate the NPA ensuring that the gel does not go over the open ends of the airway
5. The NPA will be inserted with the bevel facing the nasal septum. This means that the right nostril is usually used, although if the left is clearly larger, then this can be used. In this instance, the NPA will be initially inserted 'upside down' and then rotated through 180° once it enters the nasopharynx (Figure 1.1)
6. Confirm position by listening for breath sounds and ensuring the chest rises and falls
7. Check for blanching of the patient's nostrils. If this occurs, the NPA should be removed and a smaller diameter NPA inserted instead
8. Correct technique will minimise the risk of bleeding, but if this occurs, have suction ready.

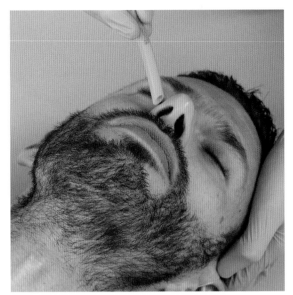

Figure 1.1 Insertion of the NPA in the right nostril.

1.4 Supraglottic airway devices

Supraglottic airway devices (SADs) have been used by anaesthetists in operating theatres for over 20 years and have proven to be safe and reliable. SADs generally lead to better ventilation and less air entering the stomach than bag-valve-mask (BVM) ventilation, particularly in the hands of the inexperienced [Nolan, 2012].

When to do it (indications)

- When BVM ventilation is not effective, is unable to be performed by an experienced person and/or prolonged ventilation is required
- When intubation fails and BVM ventilation is not possible (can't intubate, can't ventilate).

When not to do it (contra-indications)

- Any patient who has a gag reflex
- Any patient who is not deeply unconscious.

Advantages

- Better oxygenation than BVM with an oropharyngeal airway (OPA) [Cook, 2006; Dixon, 2009]
- No need to maintain continuous manual airway seal
- Easier than endotracheal intubation and does not require laryngoscopy
- Provides protection from airway secretions.

Disadvantages

- Does not protect against vomiting
- May leak when high ventilatory pressures are required, such as in obese, asthmatic and chronic obstructive pulmonary disease (COPD) patients.

A common SAD in use in ambulance services is the i-gel and the technique for insertion is described here. However, there are others in use and you should be familiarised with the devices relevant to your service.

1.4.1 i-gel insertion technique

When to do it (indications)

- An unresponsive patient with an absent gag reflex in whom more basic airway manoeuvres are inadequate
- Airway of choice in cardiac arrest as easy to insert.

When not to do it (contra-indications)

- Trismus
- Patients with limited mouth opening.

Advantages

- Easy to place
- Straightforward insertion without needing to interrupt chest compressions
- Small suction catheter can be placed down side-port to drain oesophageal secretions.

Disadvantages

- May leak, particularly if high inflation pressures are required
- Does not protect against vomiting.

Equipment

Figure 1.2 shows the equipment you will require in order to insert an i-gel.

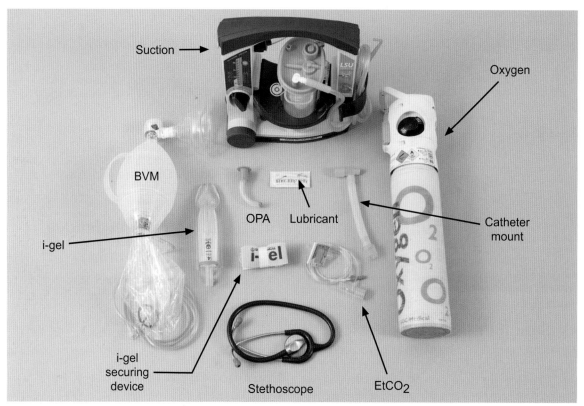

Figure 1.2 Equipment for i-gel insertion

Procedure

Take the following steps to insert an i-gel [EEAST, 2014]:

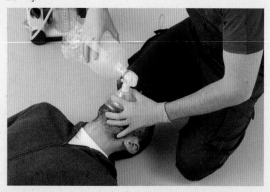

1. Pre-oxygenate the patient while preparing your equipment

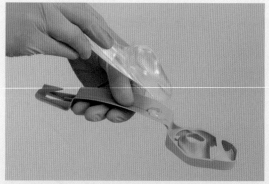

2. Choose the correct size i-gel: 3 for small adults, 4 for medium adults and 5 for large adults. Weight ranges are provided on the i-gel. Open the packaging and remove the device. Place a small amount of water-based lubricant onto the inner and outer rim of the device

Procedure continued →

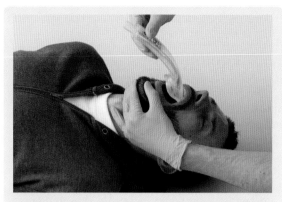

3. With the patient in the 'sniffing the morning air' position, hold the i-gel by the integrated bite block and introduce the green tip into the patient's mouth, directed at the hard palate

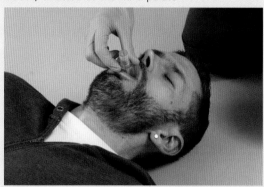

4. Glide the device downwards and backwards along the hard palate with a continuous but gentle push until a definitive resistance is felt. As a rough guide, the bite block should end up at the level of the incisors

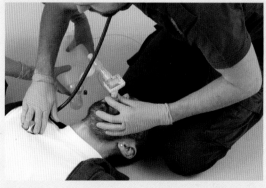

5. Connect the i-gel to your capnography detector, catheter mount and bag-valve-mask. Check for end-tidal carbon dioxide and bilateral chest air entry and movement on ventilating the patient

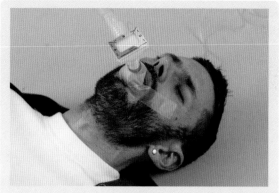

6. Secure the device appropriately

1.5 Endotracheal intubation

Endotracheal intubation involves the insertion of a cuff-sealed tube into the trachea. This provides protection against aspiration of solid or liquid material, but without the assistance of drugs that are not currently in routine use by paramedics, only patients who have a severely depressed level of consciousness (and most likely, in cardiac arrest) can be intubated [Gregory, 2010b]. Evidence of the benefit of performing endotracheal intubation by paramedics is therefore limited [JRCALC, 2008].

When to do it (indications)

- Unconscious patients with no gag reflex, whose airway cannot be managed with more basic airway methods/adjuncts
- Post-return of spontaneous circulation (ROSC) patients who remain unconscious and require transportation.

When not to do it (contra-indications)

- Patients with an intact gag reflex
- In the first few minutes of a cardiac arrest (chest compressions have priority, and usually a basic airway adjunct or a supraglottic airway device will be sufficient).

Advantages

- Provides a secure airway which protects against aspiration.

Disadvantages

- Requires skill and frequent practice to remain competent
- Bypasses physiological functions of the upper airway (filtering, warming and humidifying)

- Unrecognised oesophageal intubation will result in the death of the patient.

1.5.1 Equipment

Preparation is a key competent of (endotracheal) intubation and it cannot be done properly by one clinician. You are vital to the success of this procedure and it starts with assembling the equipment required (Figure 1.3). The airway is not sterile, but the equipment used should be clean, not damaged and in date, in the case of disposable items, such as the endotracheal tube. Care needs to be taken to ensure that equipment that is going to end up inside the patient's airway is kept as clean as possible. Try not to place items directly onto the floor, and where possible keep items in their packaging (although opened) until required for use.

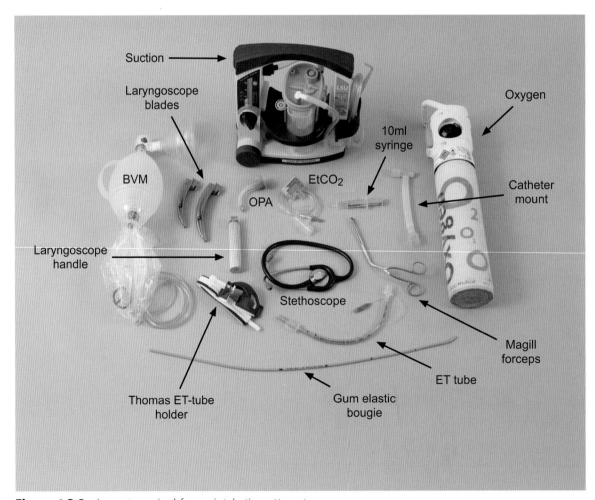

Figure 1.3 Equipment required for an intubation attempt

Endotracheal tube

The endotracheal tube (Figure 1.4) consists of a bevelled end, which is inserted into the patient, and the opposite end with an adaptor that can be connected to a catheter mount and/or ventilation device such as a bag-valve-mask, without the mask.

The inflation port includes a one-way valve into which air can be injected by use of a syringe. The pilot balloon gives an indication as to whether the inflatable cuff is inflated or deflated once it has been inserted into the trachea.

Endotracheal tubes come in a variety of sizes with adults typically requiring a tube size of 7.0–8.0 for an adult female and 8.0–9.0 for an adult male [Pilbery, 2013].

Laryngoscope blades and handle

Blades also come in different sizes and it is helpful to have a selection available. Size 3 and 4 blades are typically required for adults. Blades can be straight or curved, but the curved variety (Macintosh) are most commonly used for adults. The blade usually has a light source, and the handle contains batteries. The handle and blade are designed to connect together, and when the blade is moved into a perpendicular position the light should come on [Pilbery, 2013].

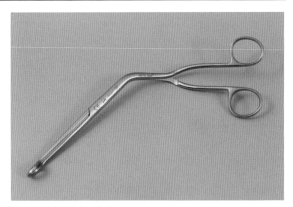

Figure 1.5 Magill forceps

Magill forceps

These are curved forceps that enable the removal of foreign bodies from the airway, or can guide an endotracheal tube under direct vision, without the operator's hands obscuring the view (Figure 1.5) [Gregory, 2010b].

1.5.2 Procedure for endotracheal intubation

Procedure

The following steps are required to perform endotracheal intubation. Note where you are required to assist [Pilbery, 2013; EEAST, 2014]:

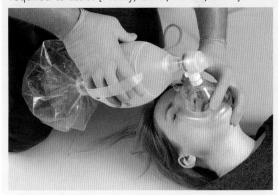

1. Adopt standard precautions (gloves and face shield). The patient will be pre-oxygenated for 2–3 minutes with a bag-valve-mask (BVM) and oxygen

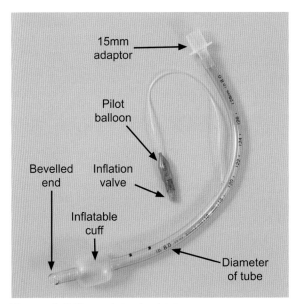

Figure 1.4 The endotracheal tube

15mm adaptor

Pilot balloon

Bevelled end

Inflation valve

Inflatable cuff

Diameter of tube

Procedure continued →

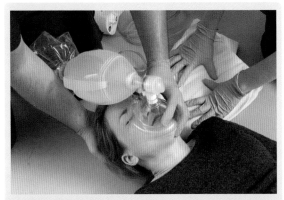

2. The patient's head should be in the 'sniffing the morning air' position to give the best view, if they do not have a cervical spine injury. A towel placed under the head may assist with this

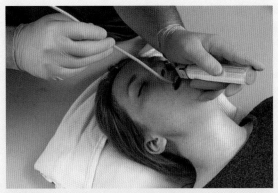

4. By gently lifting the laryngoscope handle, the glottic opening and vocal cords should be visualised. If this is not the case, you may be asked to perform the BURP manoeuvre (see section 1.5.3). Once the glottic opening is visualised, you'll be asked for the bougie, so have it ready. The bougie will have a bent end, which goes into the mouth first, so present it to the paramedic with the bent end closest to the patient's mouth

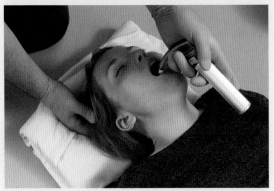

3. The laryngoscope blade will be inserted into the right side of the patient's mouth and then moved to the midline, displacing the tongue to the left

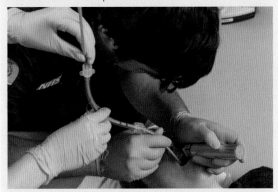

5. With the bougie inserted into the trachea, your next job is to thread the endotracheal tube over the bougie, making sure the bevelled end enters the patient's mouth first. Once the tube is on the bougie, you'll be asked to hold the top of the bougie to prevent it moving while the paramedic inserts the tube into the trachea

Procedure continued →

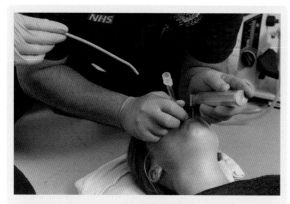

6. Once the paramedic is satisfied that the tube is in the trachea and at the right depth, you'll be asked to remove the bougie

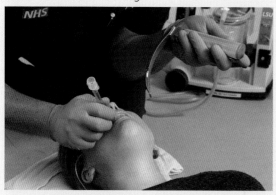

7. The laryngoscope will be removed from the patient's mouth, but the tube will be firmly held at all times to prevent it from becoming displaced. The paramedic may do this, or they might ask you to

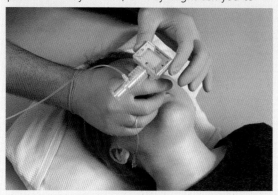

8. The end-tidal carbon dioxide (EtCO$_2$) monitor should be attached to the tube now

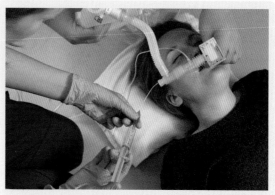

9. A BVM (without the mask) will be attached, either via a catheter mount, or directly to the adaptor on the tube. About 8 ml of air will be injected into the inflation valve with a 10 ml syringe while the patient is ventilated. Depending on the paramedic, you may be asked to squeeze the BVM or inflate the tube cuff

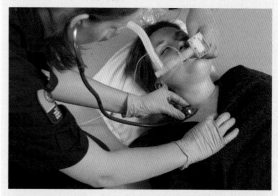

10. In addition to measuring ETCO$_2$, both lung fields should be auscultated to confirm correct tube placement

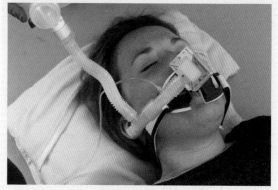

11. Once the paramedic is confident that the tube is correctly placed, it needs to be secured, preferably with a commercial device like the Thomas ET-tube holder, but tape will suffice if this is not available

1.5.3 Additional manoeuvres

The BURP manoeuvre

In the event that the view of the glottic opening is poor, you may be asked to perform the BURP manoeuvre to improve the view. BURP stands for:

- Backwards
- Upwards
- Rightwards
- Pressure.

Place your thumb, index and middle fingers on the patient's thyroid cartilage and push firmly backwards, upwards (towards the head) and then rightwards (Figure 1.6). Alternatively, the paramedic may manipulate the thyroid cartilage themselves while looking for the glottic opening (bimanual laryngoscopy) and ask you to maintain the position of the thyroid cartilage once they have found the position that gives the best view [Walls, 2012].

Sellick's manoeuvre (cricoid pressure)

Paramedics sometimes ask for cricoid pressure (Figure 1.7) when they actually want an improved view of the glottic opening. Sellick's manoeuvre is actually meant to occlude the oesophagus to prevent air going into the stomach during positive pressure ventilation. The technique involves placing your thumb and index finger on the cricoid cartilage and pushing firmly backwards. It actually worsens the laryngeal view and so should not be used for this purpose. Bimanual laryngoscopy or the BURP manoeuvre should be used instead [Gregory, 2010b].

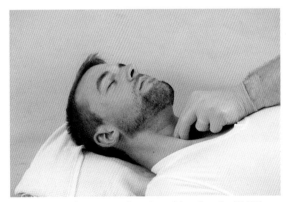

Figure 1.6 The correct hand position for the BURP manoeuvre

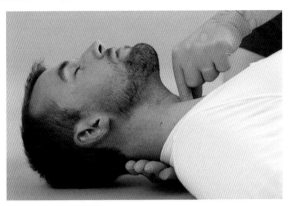

Figure 1.7 Sellick's manoeuvre

Confirming tube placement

Since unrecognised oesophageal intubation will likely result in the death of the patient, it is vital that the correct tube placement is confirmed. This should be done by [Nolan, 2012]:

- Waveform capnography: This is the best way of confirming correct tube placement
- Direct visualisation of the tube passing through the vocal cords
- Observing for bilateral chest movement and auscultating for bilateral air entry in the lungs and absence of air entering the stomach. Note that these are not completely reliable.

2 Assisting the paramedic: Drug administration

2.1 Learning objectives

By the end of this lesson you will be able to:

- Identify relevant legislation and clinical guidelines relating to the administration of medication
- Explain your role in the checking and administration of medication
- Explain your role in assisting the clinician with cannulation and intravenous infusions
- Explain the function of equipment used during cannulation and intravenous infusions
- Describe the safety checks undertaken prior to cannulation and starting intravenous infusions
- Explain your role in infection prevention and control in relation to cannulation and intravenous infusions
- Explain the procedure for administration of oral and nebulised medications.

2.2 **Introduction**

The administration of drugs to patients is a frequent and important part of an ambulance clinician's practice. Although you are limited in terms of the drugs you personally can administer, you have a responsibility to ensure that the necessary checks are carried out prior to drug administration.

In addition, many of the drugs in use by the ambulance service are given directly into a patient's vein. This intravenous method of administration requires the insertion of a cannula directly into the patient's blood stream; if this is not undertaken correctly, it can result in harm to the patient. Your assistance in these procedures can help reduce the risk of this occurring.

2.3 **Legislation and guidelines**

The two key pieces of legislation relating to the administration of medicines in the ambulance service are:

- Medicines Act 1968
- Misuse of Drugs Act 1971.

Both have been amended since their introduction. However, other legislation also relevant when discussing medicines includes the Control of Substances Hazardous to Health 2002 and the Health and Safety at Work etc. Act 1974, but these are not explored further here.

Medicines Act 1968

Under this Act, medicines are classified into three types [Pilbery, 2013]:

- General-sales-list medicines (GSL): These can be sold to the public and do not require a prescription or the supervision of a pharmacist
- Pharmacy medicines (P): These can only be sold under the supervision of a pharmacist
- Prescription-only medicines (POM): These medicines require a prescription from an appropriate practitioner, such as a doctor or non-medical prescriber.

Many of the drugs (medicines) administered by ambulance service crew members fall into the POM category. However, certain drugs can be administered in emergency situations, such as adrenaline, whereas others can be administered by paramedics in specific circumstances, which are typically the indications given in the UK

Ambulance Services Clinical Practice Guidelines [AACE, 2013].

Since you are not (yet) a paramedic, you are not covered by these exemptions, so it is important that you follow your service guidance about which (if any) drugs you can administer without the direction supervision of a clinician. Typically, drugs such as oxygen can be administered by support workers (SW), but you must be familiar with your ambulance service medicines management policy and scope of practice for your role.

Misuse of Drugs Act 1971

This Act covers drugs that are considered to be dangerous or harmful (because of the risk of dependence and/or misuse) and controls their production, supply and possession, which is why the drugs are known as controlled drugs. Drugs are classified into three types:

- Part 1 Class A drugs including cocaine and morphine
- Part 2 Class B drugs including amphetamine and codeine
- Part 3 Class C drugs including diazepam and lorazepam.

The use of these controlled drugs is allowed subject to conditions specified in the Misuse of Drugs Regulations 2001 (and subsequent amendments). These regulations classified controlled drugs into 5 schedules [Pilbery, 2013]:

1. Drugs that cannot be used for medicinal purposes. Their use is typically restricted to research

2. Drugs with high abuse potential, such as morphine and methadone, and stimulants, such as amphetamines.

3. Drugs that are less likely to lead to physical or psychological dependence

4. Drugs such as diazepam and anabolic steroids are in this schedule

5. Drugs in this class are typically preparations of controlled drugs with limited risk of abuse.

Both morphine and diazepam are available for paramedics to administer. It is important that you do NOT prepare or administer any controlled drugs. Only the paramedic is allowed to do this.

2.4 **Routes of administration**

Drugs can be administered to patients via a number of routes. These are typically divided into two types: parenteral and non-parenteral.

Parenteral routes require the skin or mucous membranes to be breached, such as by an intravenous, intramuscular, intraosseous or subcutaneous injection. Non-parenteral routes rely on passive absorption of the drug, such as by inhalation, nebulisation, oral, rectal, sub-lingual, buccal, transdermal or intra-nasal administration [AACE, 2013].

2.5 **Drug administration**

Prior to the administration of any drug, check the following [AACE, 2013; Pilbery, 2013]:

- The patient is not **allergic** to the drug about to be administered
- It is the **correct** drug
- The **dose** of drug required
- The **presentation** of the drug, including its concentration (e.g. 4 mg in 2 ml) and the container it comes in (e.g. ampoule, tablet, prefilled syringe)
- Whether the **packaging** is intact
- If it is a fluid, the **clarity** (except for intravenous diazepam, which comes as a milky-white emulsion)
- The **expiry** date.

Although it is ultimately the responsibility of the clinician for the administration of drugs to the patient, you are part of a team, and spotting and preventing a mistake that can affect patient safety is everyone's responsibility.

2.5.1 **Drawing medication from an ampoule**

You may be asked to draw up some drugs, but this should not generally include drugs that require mixing. However, follow your employer's guidance on this matter. The most common presentation of a drug that requires drawing up in the ambulance service is an ampoule (Figure 2.1). It is important that you can do this efficiently and safely.

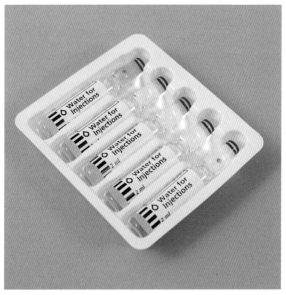

Figure 2.1 Ampoules

Equipment

You will require the following items:

- Appropriately sized syringe
- Either blunt filter needle or 23G needle to prevent glass particle contamination [Zabir, 2008; Preston, 2004]
- Gauze swab or disposable ampoule breaker
- Sharps bin.

Procedure

Take the following steps to draw up drugs from an ampoule [Pilbery, 2013; Gregory, 2010b]:

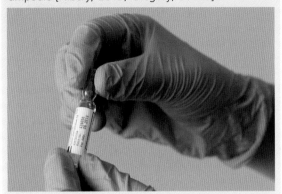

1. Take standard precautions and prepare the equipment. Check the drug:

- Correct drug
- Dose/concentration
- Expiry date
- Integrity of the ampoule

If possible, record the batch number and expiry date of the drug so that the ampoule can be disposed of once the contents have been removed. If any of the drug remains in the top of the ampoule, gently tap the neck

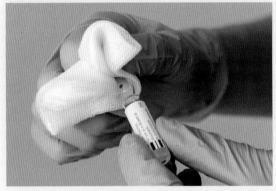

2. Grip the neck of the ampoule using a 10 x 10 cm gauze pad

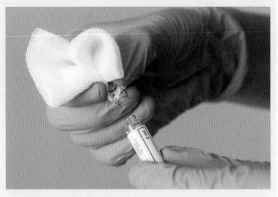

3. With the blue dot (which signifies where the neck of the ampoule has been scored and so is weaker) facing away from you, snap the neck of the ampoule and dispose of the top of the ampoule in the sharps bin

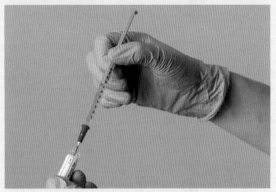

4. Without touching the outer edges of the ampoule, insert the needle into the medication and draw it into the syringe by pulling back on the plunger

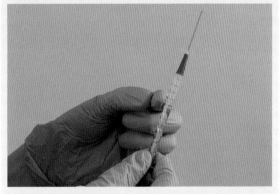

5. Once the ampoule is empty, dispose of it in the sharps bin. Holding the syringe upright, gently tap the barrel to encourage any air bubbles to rise to the top of the syringe

Procedure continued →

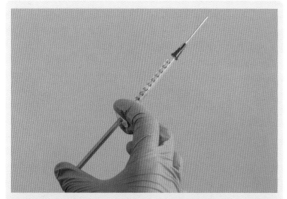

6. Remove the air bubbles by gently pressing on the plunger

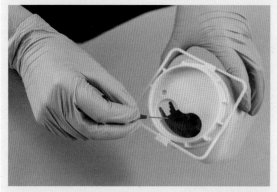

7. Dispose of the needle used to draw up the drug into the sharps bin

2.5.2 Preparing an intravenous infusion

The equipment for an intravenous infusion consists of the administration set (also called a giving set, Figure 2.2) and the fluid to be administered. You may be asked to assemble this while the paramedic is obtaining intravenous access.

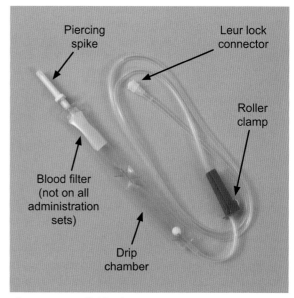

Piercing spike

Leur lock connector

Roller clamp

Blood filter (not on all administration sets)

Drip chamber

Figure 2.2 A fluid administration set

Procedure

Take the following steps to prepare an intravenous infusion [Pilbery, 2013]:

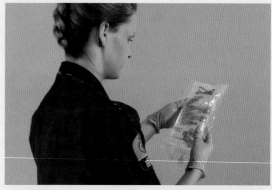

1. Take standard precautions. Confirm with the paramedic that the fluid to be administered is the correct type and concentration, has not expired, has intact packaging, looks clear and is free of contaminants

Procedure continued →

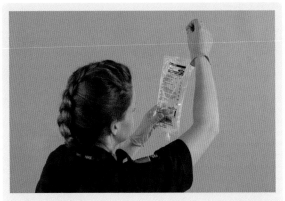

2. Remove the protective packaging and hang up the bag of fluid. This can be achieved using the ceiling mounted hooks or holders in the ambulance, if available, but sometimes bystanders or ingenuity is required. Avoid placing sterile fluid bags on the floor or other contaminated surface

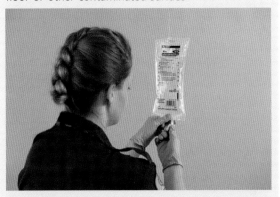

3. Twist and remove the rubber pigtail on the bottom of the bag of fluid. The bag will remain sealed until punctured by the piercing spike

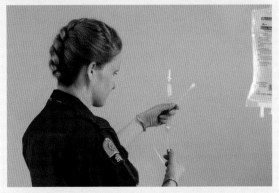

4. Check the administration set for damage and to ensure it has not expired. Open the packaging and close the roller clamp

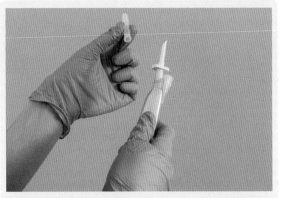

5. Remove the protective cover from the piercing spike. This is sharp and sterile, so don't stab yourself with it or let it come into contact with anything

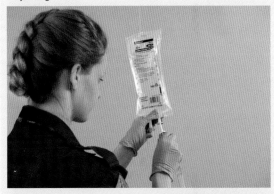

6. Slide the spike into the bag using the port exposed when you removed the rubber pigtail. You will need to hold the bag steady, but keep your fingers clear of the spike. A twisting motion sometimes helps to insert the spike into the bag. You can stop once you see fluid enter the drip chamber

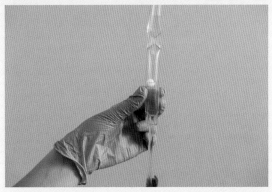

7. Squeeze the drip chamber to fill it halfway

Procedure continued →

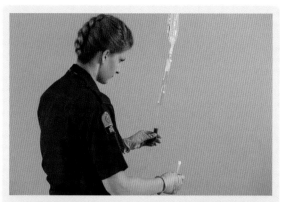

8. Open the roller clamp to allow the fluid to run slowly down the length of the administration set. This will prime the set and remove the air. If air bubbles can still be seen, then remove the protective cover from the Leur lock and run some of the fluid off. This is not ideal, because this end is also sterile and removing the cover increases the risk of infection

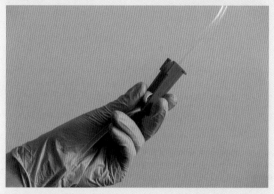

9. Once the tube is primed, stop the flow by closing the roller clamp. Recheck the drip chamber. If it is less than half-full, gently squeeze the chamber to fill it. If it is too full, invert the bag and administration set and squeeze the chamber to return some of the fluid back into the bag

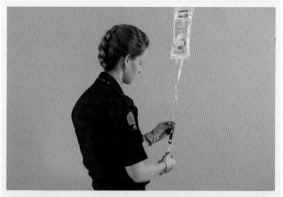

10. Hang up the bag and administration set. Do not let the tubing drop to the floor

2.5.3 Administering oral medication

The majority of your patients' medication at home will be taken orally. They come in a variety of forms including tablets, capsules, lozenges and syrups. If you are asked to assist a patient to administer oral medication, follow the steps below.

Procedure

Take the following steps to administer oral medication [Pilbery, 2013; Gregory, 2010b]:

1. Take standard precautions
2. Ensure consent has been obtained
3. Check the drug:
   - Correct drug
   - Correct dose
   - In date
   - Intact packaging
4. Check that the patient is not allergic to the drug
5. Avoid touching the medication, unless the patient is not capable of self-administering. Ensure you are wearing gloves in this case
6. Present it to the patient with clear instructions:
   - Most oral medication can be swallowed, except aspirin, which should be chewed or dissolved first
   - Sublingual tablets need to be placed under the tongue
   - Buccal tablets should be placed between the gum and cheek
7. Provide water, if indicated and permitted
8. Ensure the administration is documented.

2.5.4 Administering nebulised drugs

Nebulisers enable drugs to be inhaled. In the ambulance service, this will usually be salbutamol and ipratropium for patients suffering from asthma, chronic obstructive pulmonary disease and expiratory wheeze due to allergy, anaphylaxis or smoke inhalation, for example [AACE, 2013].

Procedure

Take the following steps to administer drugs via a nebuliser [Pilbery, 2013; Gregory, 2010b]

1. Adopt standard precautions. Check the medication:
   * Correct drug
   * Correct dose
   * Expiry date
   * Integrity of packaging
2. Add medication into the chamber. This may involve unscrewing the two parts of the nebuliser
3. Connect the nebuliser to the oxygen source and set the flow rate to 6–8 l/min. A fine mist should be generated
4. Place the mask over the patient's face and adjust the elastic to make a good seal
5. Coach the patient's breathing. They should breathe in slowly and deeply and aim to hold their breath for 3–5 seconds before breathing out again
6. Ensure the administration is documented.

Note that the administration of drugs such as salbutamol with the patient's own inhaler is as effective as a nebuliser if they use a spacer (Figure 2.3). This is particularly true of children [BTS, 2012].

2.6 Intravenous cannulation

Intravenous cannulation is the technique of siting a cannula (a plastic tube) into a vein. This is undertaken to administer drugs and/or fluids. This is a technical skill and needs to be as aseptic as possible. Your assistance will be helpful, but if you are not aware of the steps involved, you could inadvertently put you, your colleague and/or the patient at risk from a sharps injury and/or infection.

Equipment

Figure 2.4 shows most of the equipment you will need. However, you will also require a sharps bin for safe disposal of the needle inside the cannula,

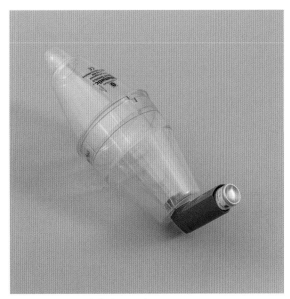

Figure 2.3 An inhaler and spacer

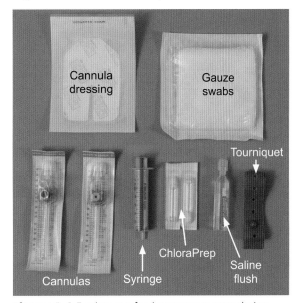

Figure 2.4 Equipment for intravenous cannulation

and you may need to have several cannulas of differing sizes available.

Cannulas

Cannulas come in a range of sizes and types. Many ambulance services use safety cannulas, which will cover the sharp end of the cannula when the needle is withdrawn. However, they offer no protection until the needle is removed, and even afterwards you should treat them as a sharp that can puncture the skin.

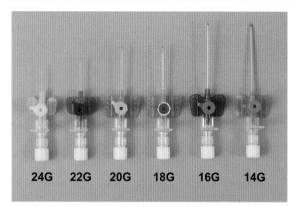

Figure 2.5 Cannulas

Cannulas in common use by the ambulance service are sized from 24gauge (G) to 14G. Somewhat counter-intuitively, a 24G cannula has a smaller diameter than the 14G, which is the largest. Figure 2.5 shows the range of cannulas.

2.6.1 Procedure for intravenous cannulation

The following procedure outlines the steps that the paramedic will take when cannulating a patient and the actions that you may be required to take when assisting [Pilbery, 2013; EEAST, 2014]:

Procedure

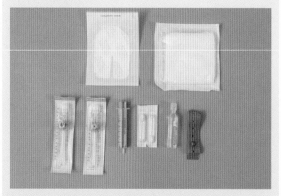

1. The paramedic will explain the procedure and obtain consent (unless the patient is not capable, such as in cases of cardiac arrest). You may be asked to prepare the equipment while the paramedic undertakes the next steps

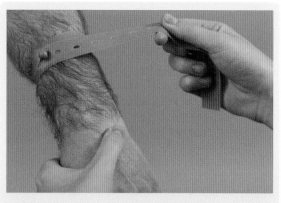

2. A tourniquet will be applied above the cannulation site in order to stop venous flow back to the heart and cause the veins to bulge

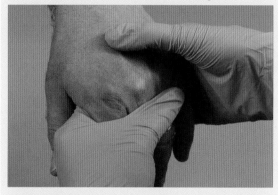

3. The paramedic will wash their hands (or use hand sanitiser) and put on disposable gloves. You should too

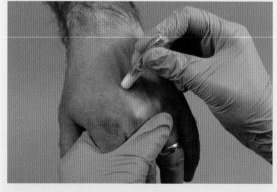

4. The vein will require cleaning with ChloraPrep, so have one ready. Make sure you do not accidentally touch the area cleaned, to avoid contaminating it

Procedure continued →

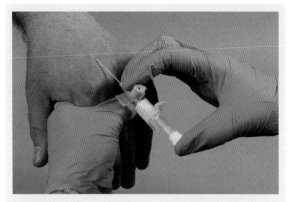

5. You may be asked to open the packaging the cannula comes in. Avoid touching the cannula inside. The paramedic will then insert the cannula

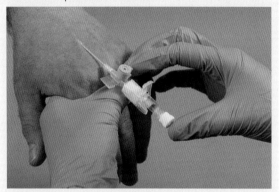

6. A 'flashback' should be observed. This is when blood enters the back chamber of the cannula. If you see a growing lump under the skin where the cannula has been inserted, it is likely that the cannula will need to be removed. Have some gauze ready and remove the tourniquet if asked

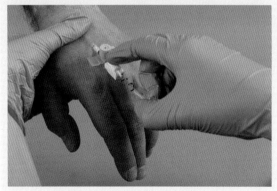

7. The cannula will be advanced over the needle. Make sure the sharps bin is nearby

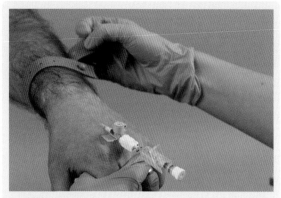

8. Before the needle can be removed, the tourniquet needs removing. You may be asked to do this

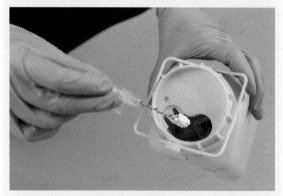

9. The needle will be removed by the paramedic and should go straight into a sharps bin. Try to avoid holding the bin if you can, but if this is unavoidable, ensure your hands are well away from the the top of the bin, so that if the needle misses the hole (because it is dropped for example), you are less likely to get injured

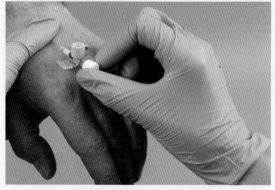

10. A bung needs to be placed on the end of the cannula to prevent blood from running out of the vein. These are sometimes dropped. Do not pick it up. Instead, obtain another one and pass it to the paramedic

Procedure continued →

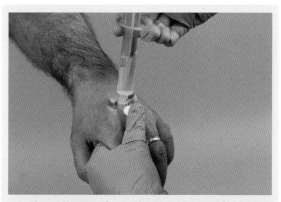

11. The cannula is flushed with 5–10 ml of saline to ensure it is patent. You may be asked to draw this up: the procedure is the same as for drug administration

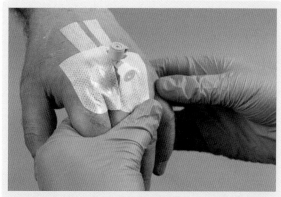

12. Finally, the cannula will then be secured with the cannula dressing

Chapter 17: **Obstetrics**

1 Complications in pregnancy

1.1 Learning objectives
By the end of this lesson you will be able to:
- Briefly explain the following conditions, including how you can assist the clinician:
  - Ectopic pregnancy
  - Ante-partum haemorrhage
  - Miscarriage
  - Pre-eclampsia.

1.2 Ectopic pregnancy
Normal fertilisation and implantation
Once a sperm has penetrated an ovarian egg, the egg is considered fertilised, and makes its way along the fallopian tube to the uterus (womb). Around six days after fertilisation, it loosely attaches itself to the endometrium (the inner lining of the uterus), usually at the fundus of the uterus. As the egg (now called a blastocyst) invades the uterine wall, it divides into two distinct types of cells that form the placenta. One set of cells invades through the endometrial layer of the uterus until they reach the maternal arterioles. The cells constrict the flow through these vessels, digest the vessel wall and form blood-filled cavities called lacunae. Since the lacunae are still connected to the maternal circulation, blood passes through the maternal arterioles and the lacunae before returning via the maternal venules. The second set of cells from the blastocyst form into finger-like projections called chorionic villi. These project into the lacunae and allow diffusion of nutrients and gases to occur between the maternal and fetal circulations [Tortora, 2008].

Maternal blood flow through the placenta is mostly pressure-dependent and so is sensitive to reductions in maternal blood pressure and increases in venous pressure (for example, caval occlusion if a pregnant woman is laid supine).

The placenta affects fetal circulation by altering resistance to blood flow. Increases in placental resistance, due to pre-eclampsia for example, can have a negative impact on umbilical artery blood flow [Vause, 2005].

In an ectopic pregnancy, the egg implants itself somewhere other than the uterus. This occurs in 1–2% of all pregnancies. Risk factors increasing the chance of an ectopic pregnancy include [ALSG, 2010]:
- Pelvic inflammatory disease
- Intrauterine contraceptive device
- Previous ectopic pregnancy
- Sterilisation or reversal of sterilisation
- Endometriosis.

Signs and symptoms of an ectopic pregnancy typically present when the patient is 6–8 weeks pregnant, so the mother will usually have missed only one menstrual period. Signs and symptoms include [AACE, 2013]:
- Acute lower abdominal pain
- Small amounts of bleeding externally or a brownish vaginal discharge
- Signs of blood loss inside the abdomen (signs of shock)
- Unexplained fainting
- Shoulder-tip pain.

1.2.1 Management
The management of a ruptured ectopic pregnancy includes [AACE, 2013; ALSG, 2010]:
- Oxygen administration to maintain an SpO_2 of 94–98%
- Intravenous access and fluids if the mother is hypotensive
- Pain relief
- Reassurance
- Prompt (blue light) transport to an appropriate receiving hospital
- Keep the patient nil by mouth.

You will be able to assist the clinician with many of these, although in time-critical situations, most interventions are likely to be performed en route to the hospital.

1.3 Ante-partum haemorrhage

Maternal physiology

There are a number of maternal changes that occur in pregnancy including [AACE, 2013; ALSG, 2010]:

- Cardiac output at the end of pregnancy increases by 50%
- Average maternal heart rate increases by 10–15 beats per minute
- Systolic and diastolic blood pressures drop by 10–15 mmHg, although by the end of pregnancy, these values usually approach the normal range
- Work of breathing increases, as does respiratory rate, while vital capacity reduces
- Circulating blood volume increases by 50% (although there is a relative anaemia)
- The increase in blood volume results in the pregnant patient tolerating greater blood or plasma loss before showing signs of hypovolaemia. In fact, tachycardia may not develop until blood loss exceeds 1000 ml and blood pressure is usually maintained well beyond this level of loss [Bose, 2006]. However, in order to maintain maternal blood pressure in hypovolaemic states, blood is shunted away from the uterus and placenta, compromising the fetus.

Ante-partum haemorrhage

Ante-partum haemorrhage (APH) is defined as bleeding from the genital tract after the 24th week of pregnancy and is primarily related to three conditions: placental abruption, placenta praevia and uterine rupture [Magill-Cuerden, 2011].

Placental abruption

This occurs when a normally sited placenta separates from the uterine wall, resulting in bleeding from the maternal sinuses (Figure 1.1). The exact cause (aetiology) of abruption is unclear, but there are a number of identified risk factors [Mukherjee, 2008; Walfish, 2009]:

- Trauma to the abdomen
- Multiparity (multiple births previously)
- Substance abuse
- Smoking
- Prior abruption

- Hypertension (high blood pressure)
- Pre-eclampsia
- Preterm pre-labour rupture of membranes.

Placental abruption often causes severe abdominal pain. If the patient is not already in labour then she is likely to start with contractions. The uterus will be tense, feeling hard and woody, and the abdomen, tender. The volume of visible blood loss is not likely to be an accurate indicator of actual blood loss. Any revealed blood loss is typically dark in colour. Suspect concealed haemorrhage if there is a good history and signs of altered mental status or increasing tachycardia, even if the systolic blood pressure is normal [ALSG, 2010].

Placenta praevia

This term refers to a placenta that is partially or completely sited in the lower part of the uterus (Figure 1.2), in some cases over the cervix, making a normal vaginal delivery impossible. There are a number of risk factors including [Walfish, 2009]:

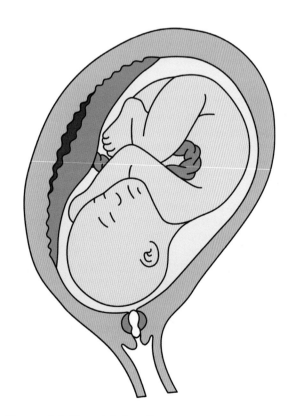

Figure 1.1 Placental abruption

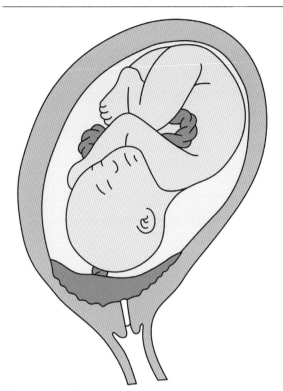

Figure 1.2 Placenta praevia

- Multiparity
- Advanced maternal age
- Previous caesarean section or other uterine surgery
- Previous placenta praevia.

Most blood loss is likely to be revealed and can be significant, particularly if the patient is in labour. Blood loss tends to be bright red. If the patient is not in labour, then the uterus will be relaxed, the abdomen non-tender and the patient may be pain free. However, bleeding can cause uterine irritation, which will result in contractions and associated discomfort. Placenta praevia is usually identified during ante-natal scans and patients deemed at risk booked in for an elective caesarean section. Recurrent bleeding is common.

Uterine rupture

This is a tear in the uterus and most commonly associated with previous caesarean section, but can occur in a first pregnancy (primigravida). It is rare and tends to occur during labour, but is very serious and can result in serious consequences, including death for mother and baby.

Uterine rupture can cause severe localised abdominal pain and rapid onset of maternal hypovolaemic shock. In labour, rupture may present with a sudden cessation of contractions and retraction of any presenting parts [Walfish, 2009].

1.3.1 **Management**

The management of APH includes [AACE, 2013; ALSG, 2010]:

- Oxygen administration to maintain an SpO_2 of 94–98%
- Positioning the mother in a full left-lateral tilt (Figure 1.3)
- Intravenous access and fluids if the mother is hypotensive
- Pain relief
- Reassurance
- Prompt (blue light) transport to an appropriate receiving hospital with obstetric theatres, blood transfusion, intensive care and anaesthetic services immediately available
- Making a pre-alert call to the receiving hospital
- Keep the patient nil by mouth.

You will be able to assist the clinician with many of these, although in time-critical situations most interventions are likely to be performed en route to the hospital.

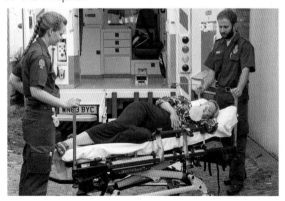

Figure 1.3 A woman who is more than 20 weeks pregnant in the left-lateral position on an ambulance stretcher

1.4 **Miscarriage**

A miscarriage (previously called a spontaneous abortion) is defined as the loss of a pregnancy before 24 weeks' gestation. It is more common, however, in the first 12 weeks [ALSG, 2010].

If products of conception are not completely passed through the cervix, they can become trapped and lead to cervical shock. This is a life-threatening emergency.

Risk factors for miscarriage include [AACE, 2013]:

- Previous miscarriages
- Smoker
- Obesity.

Signs and symptoms

- Bleeding can be light or heavy and there may be clots or jelly-like tissue present
- The patient is likely to have pain, which is typically located in the suprapubic region of the abdomen or the lower back. It may radiate down the back of the patient's legs
- The patient may note that the signs of pregnancy (morning sickness or breast tenderness) have been improving.

1.4.1 Management

The management of a miscarriage includes [AACE, 2013; ALSG, 2010]:

- Oxygen administration to maintain an SpO_2 of 94–98%
- Positioning the mother in a full left-lateral tilt, if over 20 weeks
- Intravenous access and fluids if the mother is hypotensive
- Pain relief
- Reassurance
- Prompt (blue light) transport to an appropriate receiving hospital
- Making a pre-alert call to the receiving hospital
- Keeping the patient nil by mouth.

1.5 Pre-eclampsia

Pre-eclampsia is defined as new hypertension presenting after 20 weeks of pregnancy with significant proteinuria (protein in the urine). It can be classified into mild, moderate and severe based on the mother's blood pressure [NICE, 2011]:

- Mild: Systolic blood pressure 140–149 mmHg and diastolic blood pressure 90–99 mmHg
- Moderate: Systolic blood pressure 150–159 mmHg and diastolic blood pressure 100–109 mmHg
- Severe: Systolic blood pressure 160 mmHg or greater and diastolic blood pressure 110 mmHg or greater.

Pre-eclampsia and eclampsia (generalised convulsions in the pre-eclampsic patient) are the second most common cause of maternal death after sepsis [Cantwell, 2011].

Risk factors for pre-eclampsia include [ALSG, 2010]:

- Primiparity, or first baby with new partner
- Previous severe pre-eclampsia
- Pre-pregnancy hypertension
- Diabetes
- Obesity
- Twins or higher multiple pregnancies
- Kidney disease
- Mother over 40 or under 16 years of age.

Mild and moderate pre-eclampsia is unlikely to require intervention from the ambulance service, but you may be called to a patient with severe pre-eclampsia. In addition to a raised blood pressure, they may also have signs and symptoms of [AACE, 2013]:

- Headache: Severe and frontal
- Visual disturbances
- Epigastric and/or right-sided upper abdominal pain
- Muscle twitches or tremor
- Nausea and vomiting
- Confusion
- Rapidly progressing oedema.

1.5.1 Management

The management of severe pre-eclampsia includes [AACE, 2013; ALSG, 2010]:

- Oxygen administration to maintain an SpO_2 of 94–98%
- Intravenous access, but NO fluids
- Reassurance
- Preparing for eclampsia (convulsions)
- Prompt transport to an appropriate receiving hospital with a consultant-led obstetric unit, although note that strobe lights and loud sirens can lead to eclampsia.

You will be able to assist the clinician with many of these, although in time-critical situations, most interventions are likely to be performed en route to the hospital. Ask specifically about the use of lights and sirens en route to hospital.

2 Normal childbirth

2.1 Learning objectives

By the end of this lesson you will be able to:

- Outline the stages of labour
- Identify the equipment required for delivering a baby
- Outline ways to support the clinician during childbirth
- Describe how to support a woman in labour
- State the components of the APGAR assessment for newborn babies.

2.2 Stages of labour

Normal labour follows a sequence of progressively painful contractions of the uterus that cause the cervix to shorten and dilate, which enables the descent of the fetus through the maternal pelvis, leading to spontaneous vaginal birth of the baby. Afterwards, the placenta and membranes are expelled. Typical time frames are shown in Table 2.1 [Magill-Cuerden, 2011].

First stage

This stage commences with the onset of regular contractions, which cause cervical dilation from 0 to 10 cm. Established labour is signified by regular contractions (about 3–4 in 10 minutes) lasting around 1 minute each. By 8 cm dilated women typically become vocal, requesting epidurals and demanding that the baby is delivered, for example [ALSG, 2010].

Second stage

This stage starts once the cervix is fully dilated and ends with delivery of the baby. Women may have a strong urge to push, which can feel similar to the sensation of wanting to open their bowels … which might also happen, so be prepared!

Third stage

After delivery of the baby, the third stage commences, ending with the delivery of the placenta. If this stage lasts more than 30 minutes, the placenta is classed as being retained. In addition, if the placenta partially separates, life-threatening haemorrhage can ensue (post-partum haemorrhage) [ALSG, 2010].

2.3 Assisting in labour and childbirth

Although the clinician will assume clinical responsibility for the health and well-being of the mother and baby, you have an important part to play supporting them both. You can do this by [AACE, 2013]:

- Providing reassurance: Labour and childbirth can be frightening for women
- Ensuring that pain relief is to hand: Entonox is safe to use in labour (Figure 2.1)
- Supporting the mother to adopt whichever position she finds comfortable, although make sure she does not lie on her back. In this position, a pregnant uterus can compress the inferior vena cava, reducing cardiac output and making the mother's blood pressure drop.
- Cutting the cord: If you are asked to do this, ensure that the cord has stopped pulsating (unless the newborn requires urgent resuscitation), apply two clamps about 3 cm and 15 cm from the umbilicus (where the cord attaches to the baby) and keep the baby's fingers and genitals well away!
- Keeping an eye out for blood loss: Women in late pregnancy typically have a circulating blood volume of around 6–7 litres (compared with the normal 5 litres) to allow for blood loss during delivery. However, while some women can tolerate losses up to 1 litre with no apparent effect on their circulation, others will become symptomatic with much smaller volumes. Alert the clinician to all blood loss you identify [PROMPT, 2012].

Table 2.1: Typical time frame in labour

Stage of labour	First pregnancy	Subsequent pregnancies
First	12–14 hours	6–10 hours
Second	60 minutes	Up to 30 minutes
Third	20–30 minutes	20–30 minutes

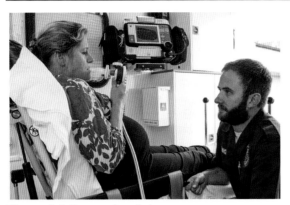

Figure 2.1 Entonox is safe in pregnancy

2.4 Equipment for childbirth

When assisting a clinician with a birth, either in the community or in the back of an ambulance, an important task is preparing the area for delivery and having the correct equipment to hand.

Delivery area

- Drape either the ambulance stretcher or the bed/sofa etc. with incontinence pads as childbirth is messy!
- Open the maternity pack and lay out the contents so they are easily to hand
- Towels: These should be warm and dry. You'll need at least two
- Blankets: To cover the mother to keep her warm and protect her modesty
- Heat: The delivery area should be around 25°C, which is generally uncomfortably hot for you and your colleagues, but is essential to avoid the newborn becoming hypothermic.

Maternity packs

The contents of maternity packs vary so make sure you are familiar with the contents of your service's packs. Typical equipment found in maternity packs as shown in Figure 2.2 consists of:

- Baby wrap: These often have an insert so that it can be placed over the baby's head. If you have plenty of warm towels, you may not need this
- Clinical waste bag
- Umbilical cord clamps: These are used to prevent blood loss from either the baby or the mother via the placenta following birth

- Maternity pad: Multiple uses, but helpful for applying direct pressure during excessive blood loss following childbirth
- Clear polythene bag: Babies who are premature (born at under 28 weeks) should be placed up to their neck in a food-grade clear plastic wrap or bag immediately after birth without drying [Nolan, 2010]
- Scissors: To cut the cord
- Shallow dish: Usually used to catch or place the placenta in. It is important that a midwife checks the placenta to ensure it is complete and no parts have been retained inside the mother
- Suction catheter: Not usually required, but useful for removing excessive secretions from the baby's mouth and nose.

Resuscitation equipment

Most childbirths end with a screaming baby and a happy mother, but ensure you have the following equipment to hand in case there is a need to resuscitate the newborn or support the mother in the event of large blood loss:

- Oxygen
- Paediatric bag-valve-mask
- Suction unit
- Cannulation equipment (adult)
- Intravenous fluids (usually sodium chloride).

2.5 APGAR

Once a baby has been born, he or she requires assessment to identify the need for intervention, up to and including newborn life support. A commonly used tool is the APGAR score, which was devised by Virginia Apgar in 1953 [Apgar,

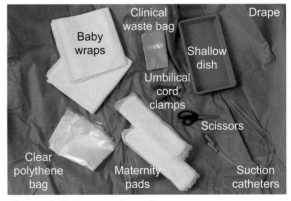

Figure 2.2 A maternity pack

1953]. APGAR is a mnemonic consisting of 5 elements which are helpful in assessing the newborn baby [AACE, 2013]:

- **A**ppearance (skin colour)
- **P**ulse rate
- **G**rimace (response to stimulation)
- **A**ctivity or muscle tone (whether moving spontaneously, or floppy)
- **R**espiratory rate.

APGAR scores are recorded at 1 and 5 minutes following birth and each element awarded a score of 0–2 (Table 2.2) [AAP, 2006; AACE, 2013].

An APGAR score of 8 or more generally means that the newborn baby is in good condition [Magill-Cuerden, 2011].

3 Childbirth complications

3.1 Learning objectives

By the end of this lesson you will be able to:
- Briefly explain the following complications, including how you can assist the clinician:
  - Cord prolapse
  - Shoulder dystocia
  - Breech presentation
  - Post-partum haemorrhage
  - Multiple births
  - Pre-term labour.

3.2 Cord prolapse

If the umbilical cord descends below the presenting part, it is said to be prolapsed. However, the presenting part does not actually

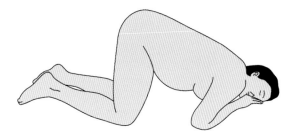

Figure 3.1 Knees to chest position

have to be visible from the entrance to the vagina (introitus). If the cord prolapses, it can become occluded by pressure from the presenting part, resulting in serious fetal morbidity or death. In the absence of a midwife, the only way to know that the cord has prolapsed is if someone checks the introitus, which is why it is vital to perform a visual check to see if the mother's waters have broken (i.e. the membranes have ruptured) [ALSG, 2010].

3.2.1 Management

This is a time-critical emergency. If the woman has been on the phone to a midwife, she may have been advised to adopt a knees to chest position (Figure 3.1), but this is not a practical position to transport the mother in an ambulance.

Assuming delivery is not imminent, get the mother onto the ambulance trolley as quickly as possible. If you can get the trolley alongside, that is great; otherwise walk her to the ambulance. Do not use a carry chair as this can compress the cord.

Table 2.2: APGAR score [AACE, 2013]

Score	0	1	2
Appearance	Blue or pale all over	Blue extremities, body pink	Body and extremities pink
Pulse rate	Absent	<100	≥100
Grimace or response to stimulation	No response to stimulation	Grimace/feeble cry when stimulated	Cry or pulls away when stimulated
Activity or muscle tone	None	Some flexing of arms and legs	Flexed arms and legs that resist extension
Respiration	Absent	Weak, irregular, gasping	Strong cry

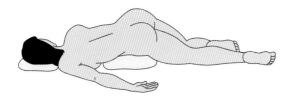

Figure 3.2 Left lateral position with hips raised

Once on the trolley (in or out of the ambulance), place the mother in the left lateral position with hips raised, either with blankets under her hips (Figure 3.2), or by placing the trolley in the Trendelenburg position (i.e. feet end of the trolley raised and head lowered) [ALSG, 2010].

The clinician should make one attempt to replace small loops into the vagina using two fingers. Once this has been completed, cover the vagina with dry pads to prevent further prolapse [AACE, 2013].

The patient should be rapidly conveyed (blue light) to the nearest consultant-led obstetric unit. Make sure a pre-alert call, including notification of a cord prolapse, is made.

3.3 Shoulder dystocia

Shoulder dystocia is a vaginal, head-first delivery that requires additional obstetric manoeuvres after the head has delivered, and a head–body delivery delay of more than 60 seconds [RCOG, 2012]. Shoulder dystocia is difficult to predict prior to birth, with around 50% of cases having no risk factors and in babies of normal birth weight [ALSG, 2010].

In the late second stage of labour, a clue that shoulder dystocia is a possibility is head bobbing, where the fetal head is visible during contractions, but retracts in between. At the time of delivery, you may see the 'turtle neck sign', where the fetal chin retracts tightly onto the mother's perineum and the fetal neck is not visible at all [RCOG, 2012].

3.3.1 Management

The senior clinician will attempt to deliver the anterior shoulder by applying gentle downwards traction. If this is not successful after two contractions, place the mother flat on her back with a pillow under her head and ask her to bring her knees towards her chest (the McRobert's position, Figure 3.3). Due to the size of the mother's uterus, this will cause flexion and

abduction of her hips, increasing the anterior–posterior diameter of the pelvis [RCOG, 2012]. In 60–70% of cases, this position alone will result in successful delivery with gentle downwards and outwards traction while the mother is encouraged to push.

If after another two contractions the baby has still not delivered, you will be asked to apply suprapubic pressure to aid delivery. The procedure is as follows [AACE, 2013]:

- The clinician will identify the fetal back (usually the opposite side to the way the fetus is facing)
- You will be asked to stand on the same side as the fetal back and adopt a CPR-style hand technique with your hands positioned two-finger's breadth above the symphysis pubis, behind the fetal shoulder
- Do not push on the fundus (the superior portion of the uterus) as this could rupture the uterus
- You will be instructed to press down and away to dislodge and rotate the shoulder
- While this is being done, the clinician will apply gentle downward traction on the head.

If the baby has not been delivered after a further two contractions:

- The mother should be encouraged to empty her bladder
- You will be asked to continue applying pressure on the symphysis pubis but, in addition, gently rock backwards and forwards on the symphysis pubis.

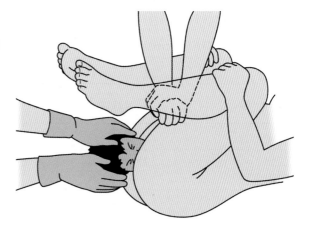

Figure 3.3 The McRobert's position with an assistant applying suprapubic pressure

If the baby has not been delivered after a further two contractions:

- Assist the mother onto all fours (hands and knees). The clinician will apply gentle downward traction to deliver the posterior shoulder (i.e. the shoulder nearer the mother's back).

If the baby has not been delivered after a further two contractions:

- It is time to go!
- The mother should be rapidly transported to the nearest consultant-led obstetric unit. If you cannot get the ambulance stretcher next to the patient, it is acceptable to allow the mother to walk a short distance, but get ready to deliver the baby
- Place the mother in the left lateral position with hips raised
- Provide high-flow supplemental oxygen
- Pre-alert the unit and make sure you tell them it's a shoulder dystocia.

3.4 Breech presentation

In a breech presentation, the fetus enters the birth canal with buttocks or feet first, rather than the more usual head first. The most common presentations are shown in Table 3.1 [Magill-Cuerden, 2011]. Breech presentations are similar to normal labour except that you may see buttocks, feet or the soles of the feet during your assessment of the introitus. In addition, the genitals may look bruised and swollen, and meconium may be present (looking a bit like black toothpaste) [ALSG, 2010].

3.4.1 Management

If delivery is not in progress and the clinician is confident that you can get the mother to hospital, transport the mother to the booked obstetric unit, but continually reassess en route.

If birth is imminent, call for a second ambulance and community midwife and adopt the following principles [AACE, 2013]:

- The golden rule is that breech births should be as hands-off as possible
- Ask the mother to adopt a semi-recumbent position; if she is sitting on a chair or sofa, get her to shift to the edge and support her splayed legs

- The body should deliver spontaneously without intervention, and should rotate so that the baby's back faces the mother. If this does not happen, the clinician should gently rotate the baby, holding onto the pelvis (not the legs or abdomen)
- If asked to clamp or cut the cord, **do not** do this until the head has been delivered
- Once the body has delivered, the clinician will lift the baby by its feet to assist in delivering the head
- Once the baby has been delivered, the childbirth is managed as for a normal childbirth, but breech babies are more likely to be covered in meconium and require newborn life support.

3.5 Post-partum haemorrhage

Primary post-partum haemorrhage (PPH) is defined as a blood loss greater than 500 ml within 24 hours of birth [WHO, 2012]. It affects around 18% of vaginal births, although only 1.3% involve major PPH, which is a blood loss of over 1000 ml [PROMPT, 2012]. Massive PPH is defined as loss of 50% of the mother's circulating blood volume within three hours of delivery [AACE, 2013].

Risk factors

As with many aspects of obstetrics, there is no definitive list as to who will suffer a PPH and who will not, but there are a number of risk factors that make a PPH more likely [ALSG, 2010]:

- Multiparity greater than 5
- Advancing maternal age
- Previous PPH or ante-partum haemorrhage (APH)
- Long labour
- Obesity
- Anything that increases the size of the uterus (multiple pregnancy, large baby, excess amniotic fluid)
- Uterine fibroids
- Partial separation of the placenta.

3.5.1 Management

The management of the PPH depends on the cause of the bleeding, so it is important to determine this early in your assessment. There are four main causes of PPH, known as the four Ts [AAFP, 2012]:

- Tone
- Tissue
- Trauma
- Thrombin.

Tone

Uterine atony (poor tone of the uterus) is the cause of 70–90% of PPHs [AAFP, 2012]. Usually the uterus contracts after birth, occluding the spiral arteries that have provided the blood supply to the placenta during pregnancy.

In order to control the blood loss from an atonic uterus, the upper portion of the uterus (called the fundus) must be massaged to encourage the uterine fibres to contract. If you are asked to perform fundal massage, start at the umbilicus and apply firm pressure backwards towards the aorta and then downwards towards the uterus in a circular cupping motion. This will encourage the contraction of the uterus (Figure 3.4). As this

Table 3.1: Common breech presentation

Presentation	Incidence	Explanation	
Frank	65%	Bottom first with legs flexed at the hip and extended at the knees.	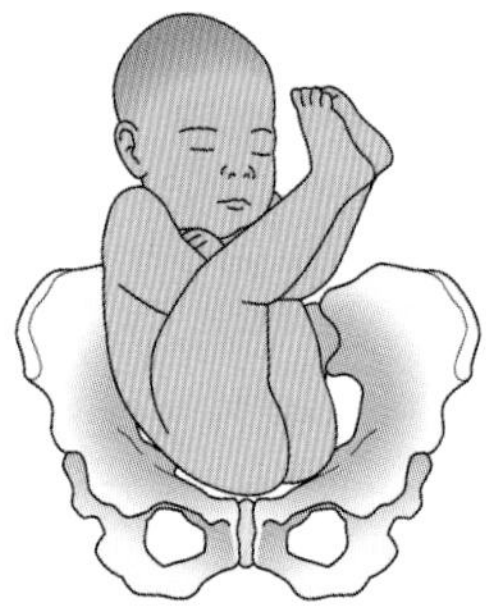
Complete	25%	Hips and knees are flexed resulting in the fetus sitting cross-legged, with feet beside the bottom.	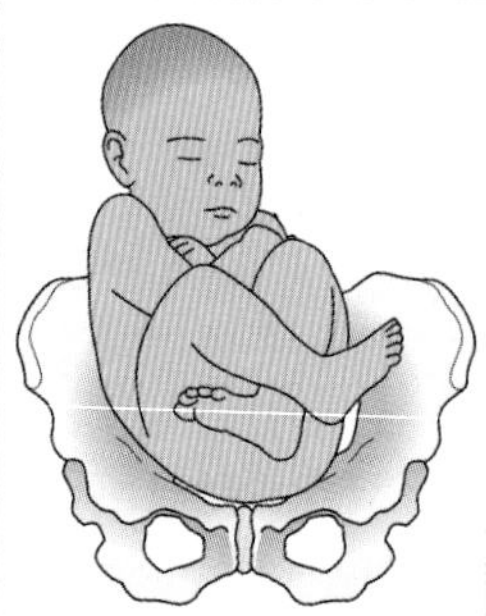
Footling	10%	One or both feet come first, with bottom higher up. Rare presentation at term, but common in premature births	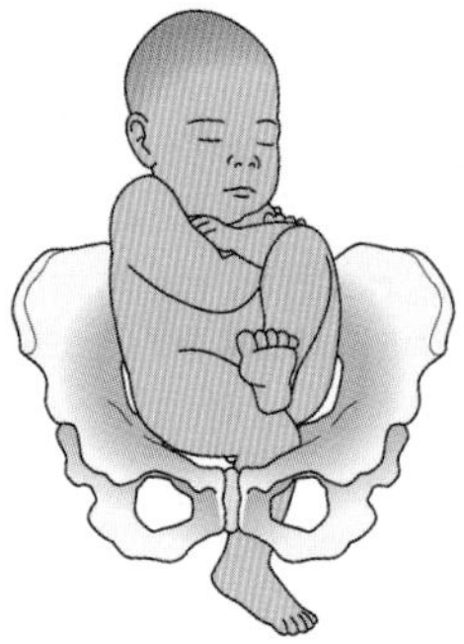

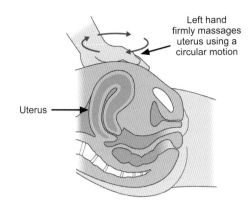

Left hand firmly massages uterus using a circular motion

Uterus

Figure 3.4 Fundal massage

is an uncomfortable procedure, it is important to remember to inform the patient of what you are about to perform and why, gain consent and ensure appropriate analgesia is used. The clinician may elect to use oxytocic drugs such as syntometrine or misoprostol [AACE, 2013].

Tissue

If there are any tissues left behind after the birth, such as the placenta or membranes, the uterus will continue bleeding in order to remove them. This mechanism is responsible for around 10% of PPHs [AAFP, 2012]. These patients should not receive fundal massage as this might cause partial separation of the placenta, causing further bleeding [AACE, 2013]. The completeness of the placenta and membranes is important, so keep the placenta with the mother so that it can be checked to ensure it is complete.

Trauma

Trauma to the genital tract during childbirth occurs in approximately 85% of births [Smith, 2013]. These are wide ranging in terms of severity, from small tears that only involve the skin of the perineum, to deeper tears that affect the muscle layers. Due to an abundant vascular supply, 20% of PPHs are caused by tears [AAFP, 2012]. The bleeding can originate from the tear or from ruptured vessels within the tissue. Definitive management is suturing of the perineum, but direct external pressure with a maternity pad or gauze and the administration of oxytocic drugs such as syntometrine and

misoprostol is the mainstay of pre-hospital treatment.

Thrombin

Clotting problems are rare, being responsible for only 1% of PPHs. These can lead to life-threatening clotting disorders which require urgent hospital management.

3.6 Multiple births

Multiple births (twins or greater) occur in about 1.6% of births in England and Wales each year [ONS, 2013a]. It is uncommon for women with multiple pregnancies to give birth outside of hospital, but premature delivery (before 37 weeks) is more common, increasing the risk of parents being caught out [AACE, 2013].

Complications during a multiple pregnancy are also more likely and include [ALSG, 2010]:

• Pregnancy-induced hypertension, including pre-eclampsia
• Placental abruption
• Placenta praevia
• Post-partum haemorrhage.

Risk factors for multiple pregnancy include [ALSG, 2010]:

• Fertility treatment
• Previous history of twins
• Family history of multiple pregnancies
• Multiparity (having previously given birth twice or more).

3.6.1 Management

If delivery is not imminent, then the mother will be transported rapidly to the nearest consultant-led obstetric unit [AACE, 2013].

If delivery is in progress, however, follow local guidelines to request a community midwife and assist the clinician in delivering the first baby.

Once the first baby has been born, mother and baby need to be transported rapidly to the nearest obstetric-led unit **if** the second baby is not due to be imminently delivered. If the second baby is coming, remain on scene and contact the emergency operations centre (EOC) for an additional ambulance. Remember to make a pre-alert call and ensure the unit knows that it is a multiple pregnancy [AACE, 2013].

3.7 Pre-term labour

Pre-term labour is defined as labour occurring before 37 weeks' gestation. It is a significant cause of neonatal morbidity and death, with babies born before 24 weeks unlikely (although not impossible) to survive [ALSG, 2010].

Risk factors for pre-term labour include [ALSG, 2010]:

- Previous pre-term labour
- Multiple pregnancies (twins or more)
- Maternal smoking
- Lower socioeconomic groups
- Spontaneous rupture of membranes in the current pregnancy.

3.7.1 Management

The destination depends on the gestation (how many weeks pregnant the mother is). If the woman is less than 22 weeks pregnant, then she should be taken to the nearest gynaecology unit. After 22 weeks, the mother should ideally be transported to an obstetrician-led unit [AACE, 2013].

These babies are best born in hospital and the clinician will try to achieve this by asking you to promptly transport the patient. Confirm the destination hospital.

If it is clear that childbirth is imminent, either at scene or en route to hospital, contact the emergency operations centre (EOC) and request a midwife and additional ambulance to your current location.

Once the baby has been born, it should be transported by the second crew immediately. Remember that babies born under 27 weeks should be placed up to their neck in a food-grade clear plastic wrap or bag immediately after birth without drying [Nolan, 2010].

The mother should be transported in your ambulance to the same hospital as the infant.

4 Newborn life support

4.1 Learning objectives

By the end of this lesson you will be able to:

- Demonstrate the resuscitation of the newborn in line with current national guidelines.

4.2 Introduction

The resuscitation of babies at birth is different from that of infants and children, because of the transformation, usually within seconds, from being a fetus with fluid-filled lungs, with all respiratory work undertaken by the mother's placenta, to a baby with air-filled lungs who is capable of ventilating themselves. Childbirth is a hypoxic process for the fetus, but it is resilient and usually will not require intervention. However, if the normal physiological processes fail, then you will need to intervene [Maconochie, 2012].

4.2.1 Management

Normally, your clinician will undertake the following steps, but will still require your assistance as some manoeuvres (such as maintaining a patent airway) are better with two people. In some circumstances (such as post-partum haemorrhage) you may be asked to start resuscitation of a newborn until the mother can be stabilised or further help arrives.

There are 5 stages that the resuscitation moves through systematically (Figure 4.1):

1. Drying and covering the baby
2. Assessing the need for intervention
3. Airway
4. Breathing (aerating the lungs and positive pressure ventilation)
5. Chest compressions.

When a baby is born, unless the clinician feels there is a need for immediate resuscitation, wait until the umbilical cord stops pulsating. Keep the baby warm during this period and then [Maconochie, 2012]:

- Dry the baby quickly. Discard the towel used to dry the baby and wrap it in another, warm and dry towel
- Assess the baby:
  - Respiration: Most babies will spontaneous breathe effectively, such that the heart rate rises above 100 beats/min and leads to 'pinking up' of the torso within 3 minutes of the birth. If the baby is not breathing, or only making occasional gasps, then further intervention is required

Dry the baby
Remove an wet towels and cover
Start the clock or note the time

↓

Assess (tone), breathing and
heart rate

↓

If gasping or not breathing:
Open the airway
Give 5 inflation breaths
Consider SpO₂ monitoring

↕

Reassess
If no increase in heart rate look
for chest movement

↕

If chest not moving:
Recheck head position
Consider two-person airway
control and other airway
manoeuvres
Repeat inflation breaths
Consider SpO₂ monitoring
Look for a response

↓

Reassess
If no increase in heart rate look
for chest movement

↓

When the chest is moving:
If the heart rate is not detectable
or slow (< 60 beats/min)
Start chest compressions
3 compressions to each breath

↓

**Reassess heart rate ever 30
seconds**
If the heart rate is not detectable
or slow (< 60 beats/min) consider
venous access and drugs

Figure 4.1 Newborn life support algorithm
Reproduced with the kind permission of the Resuscitation Council (UK)

- Heart rate: This is best undertaken by auscultating over the cardiac apex (near the baby's left nipple). The exact rate is not necessary, just note whether it is very slow (less than 60 beats/min), slow (60–100 beats/min) or fast (over 100 beats/min). Anything under 100 beats/min is abnormal and will require intervention

- Colour: This is not a reliable sign, but improvements in colour are encouraging

- Muscle tone: Babies should be moving spontaneously and should resist gentle attempts to move their limbs. A floppy baby is not a good sign

- Airway: A newborn baby's head is disproportionately large compared to its body, which leads to flexion of the neck and occlusion of the airway. Worse, overextension of the head can also lead to obstruction. Place the newborn on a folded towel (to about a thickness of 2 cm) to support the shoulders (Figure 4.2). A jaw thrust may be required to open the airway

- Breathing: The first 5 breaths are known as inflation breaths. These are prolonged (2–3 seconds in duration) and are best performed with a 500 ml paediatric bag-valve-mask (BVM) with a blow-off valve set at 30–40 cmH₂0 to prevent excessive airway pressures being generated. Note that the chest may not move for the first to third ventilations as fluid in the lungs has to be displaced. Successful ventilation can be gauged by either a rapidly increasing heart rate after the first 5 breaths, or a heart

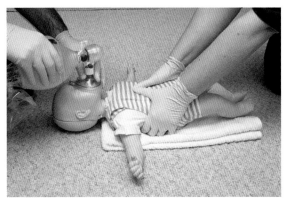

Figure 4.2 Resuscitation of the newborn. Note the use of a towel to help with positioning, the neutral position of the newborn's head, and the use of the encircling technique to provide chest compressions

rate >100 beats/min. Note that you should ventilate with air, NOT oxygen initially

- Chest compressions: If the heart rate remains very slow (<60 beats/min) despite 30 seconds of ventilating the baby and seeing a visible chest rise with each inflation, you will need to start chest compressions. The best way to perform compressions on a neonate is to use the two-thumb encircling technique (Figure 4.2). Compress the chest quickly and firmly by one-third of its depth with a compression-to-ventilation ratio of 3:1. Once the heart rate rises above 60 beats/min, compressions can be discontinued.

Chapter 18: Children and Infants

1 Why paediatric patients are different

1.1 Learning objectives
By the end of this lesson you will be able to:
- Explain how paediatric patients are anatomically, physiologically and developmentally different from adults.

1.2 Introduction
Paediatrics is a speciality of medicine that looks after people from birth to age 18 years. Children are generally divided into 5 main groups [Lissauer, 2007]:
- Infants: From birth to 12 months of age. In the first four weeks after birth, infants may also be called neonates
- Toddler: Approximately 1–2 years of age
- Pre-school: This is a young child aged 2–5 years
- School-age: Generally 5–12 years (or the onset of puberty)
- Teenager: Also called adolescents. Generally from onset of puberty to 18 years, when, in the UK, they become an adult. Some guidance (such as for resuscitation or the administration of some drugs) treats this group the same as adults).

Note that for the purposes of resuscitation, an infant is a patient under 12 months of age and a child is a patient who is 1 year to the onset of puberty (around 12 years) [Maconochie, 2012].

1.3 Anatomy and physiology
As children get older, their bodies change anatomically and physiologically. This is important to remember when undertaking your assessment as you may need to modify your plan for their management.

1.3.1 Airway
Most of the changes in the infant and child airway have been covered in the section on CHOKING IN THE PAEDIATRIC PATIENT (chapter 9).

However, some extra points to consider are provided here.

Face and mouth
Infants' faces are small. This makes sizing of a face mask for resuscitation important if a good seal is to be achieved. It is important that pressure on the eyes is avoided as this can result in damage and a reflex bradycardia. The floor of the mouth is also easy to compress, so care must be taken not to apply pressure to the soft tissues under the mandible during airway opening and positive pressure ventilations (Figure 1.1) [Maconochie, 2012].

Nose and pharynx
In the first 6 months, infants breathe through their nose, meaning that any nasal obstruction can result in increased work of breathing and respiratory compromise [AAP, 2013].

1.3.2 Breathing
Infants and small children have relatively small resting lung volumes, which means they have less oxygen capacity in reserve than adults and have a higher oxygen consumption. In cases of respiratory compromise therefore, the blood oxygen levels in these infants and small children will rapidly decline, making the prompt administration of supplemental oxygen crucial [Maconochie, 2012].

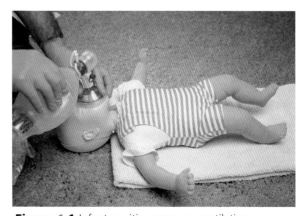

Figure 1.1 Infant positive pressure ventilation

The ribs of infants are cartilaginous and so are very pliable. In addition, they have weak intercostal muscles, which means that the diaphragm is their main muscle of respiration. If the diaphragm is impeded in any way, such as by gastric distension, for example, their ventilation may become ineffective [AAP, 2013].

As children get older, their intercostal muscles become more developed, contributing more to mechanical ventilation. Their ribs ossify, hardening and acting as an anchor for the developing intercostal muscles, making them less likely to collapse during periods of respiratory distress. As a result, intercostal recession in any child over the age of 5 years should be seen as an ominous sign of severe respiratory distress [Maconochie, 2012].

Infants have a relatively high metabolic rate, oxygen consumption and carbon dioxide production, requiring a higher respiratory rate than older children. This can be further increased by pain, fever and anxiety, resulting in changing 'normal' respiratory rates for infants and children (Table 1.1) [Maconochie, 2012].

Table 1.1: Respiratory rate ranges in infants and children

Age (years)	Respiratory rate (breaths/min)
< 1	30–40
1–2	26–34
2–5	24–30
5–12	20–24
> 12	12–20

1.3.3 Circulation

The circulating blood volume in an infant is about 80 ml/kg, which means that in a newborn baby weighing 3 kg, their blood volume is only 240 ml, making small blood losses significant.

Another important point to note is that oxygen delivery to the tissues is dependent on the arterial blood oxygen content multiplied by the cardiac output. In respiratory failure, a reduction in arterial blood oxygen can be compensated by increasing cardiac output. However, in circulatory

failure, it is not possible to increase arterial blood oxygen content so tissue oxygen delivery falls immediately [Fuchs, 2012].

The stroke volume at birth is small, only 1.5 ml/kg, so increasing cardiac output is mainly achieved by increasing heart rate. Thus heart rates in infants and small children are higher than in older children (Table 1.2). In addition, systemic vascular resistance increases as children get older, a change reflected by increased 'normal' blood pressures (Table 1.3) [Maconochie, 2012].

Table 1.2: Paediatric heart rate ranges

Age	Awake (beats/min)	Deep sleep (beats/min)
0–3 months	85–205	80–140
3 months to 2 years	100–180	75–160
2–10 years	60–140	60–90
> 10 years	60–100	50–90

Table 1.3: Paediatric blood pressure ranges

Age	Systolic blood pressure (mmHg)
0–1 month	> 60
1–12 months	80
1–10 years	90 + (2 x age in years)
> 10 years	120

1.4 Cognitive development

Children are also challenging because their brain develops as they age. This means that during your assessment of a child, you will expect different levels of interaction and abilities in a 1-year-old compared to a 12-year-old child [Lissauer, 2007; AAP, 2013; Fuchs, 2012].

1.4.1 Infants

Under 2 months

Infants in this age group will spend the majority of their time feeding and sleeping. They are unable to tell the difference between their parents/carers and others, so do not display stranger anxiety. They will exhibit primitive reflexes such as grasping objects placed in the palm of their hand, or turning their head towards a gentle stimulation of the side of their mouth (rooting).

2–6 months

Infants become more active during this period, making assessment a little easier. They begin to make eye contact, will smile and follow the light of your pen torch or a toy with their eyes. They will also turn their head in response to a loud noise or the voice of their parent/carer. Their motor skills develop and they will start to roll over and reach for objects. They will vocalise with coos and laughs when spoken to.

6–12 months

Infants are much more socially interactive at this age. They may be able to say single words such as "mama" or "dada", but will also develop stranger anxiety in the latter stages (typically after 9 months), so keep the infant with their parent/carer if possible. They will be able to feed themselves, sit unsupported, reach for objects and pass them between hands.

1.4.2 **Toddlers**

There is a rapid change in growth and cognitive development at this age. By 18 months, children will have a vocabulary of around 6–10 words, and will know the name of, and be able to point to, several parts of their body. They should be able to walk steadily and feed themselves with a spoon.

As they reach 2 years of age, children may be able to combine several words together to make a simple phrase. They will start to engage in symbolic play, feeding their teddy for example. Stranger anxiety may be extreme and they are typically illogical thinkers, learning by trial and error, but have no sense of danger. They are self-centred and will be able to label objects as "mine". Toilet training may lead to children being dry during the day.

1.4.3 **Pre-school**

These children are creative and illogical thinkers, often confusing fantasy and reality. They are likely to have misconceptions about illness, injury and bodily functions. In addition, they may fear the dark, being left alone and the presence of monsters under the bed. They have good language skills and can participate in parallel play, taking it in turns with others, but their attention span is short.

1.4.4 **School-age**

Children at this age understand cause and effect and are capable of abstract thought. They can tell you about the progress of their current illness or injury but their ability to understand the seriousness of the situation is limited. They can be involved with their care if explanations are kept simple and clear. Peer-group support becomes important at this age, but they will still have separation anxiety from their parents/carers when ill, and fear pain and loss of control.

1.4.5 **Teenagers**

Teenagers (adolescents) are sometimes compared to toddlers: highly mobile but lacking common sense! However, they are able to rationalise and express themselves and their feelings in words. This is also a period of experimentation and risk-taking. Children at this age will typically transition from relying on their parents/carers for psychological support and development to their friends and peers. This typically leads to feelings of anxiety if they are 'different' from their peers. In addition, they may struggle with anxiety of independence, body image, sexuality and peer pressure.

2 Initial assessment and management of the paediatric patient

2.1 **Learning objectives**

By the end of this lesson you will be able to:

- Conduct an initial assessment of the paediatric patient
- Identify problems with a paediatric patient's airway, breathing, circulation and neurological status
- Describe the principles that underpin the support of a seriously ill paediatric patient
- Demonstrate the procedures to support a clinician to manage a seriously ill paediatric patient.

2.2 Introduction

The assessment of the paediatric patient is much the same as for adults, and you will follow the standard procedure you learnt about in the PATIENT ASSESSMENT PROCESS lesson (chapter 8). As before, the primary survey is a chance to identify and correct life-threatening problems. In infants and children, prompt recognition and intervention when there are signs of respiratory and/or circulatory failure can prevent the majority of paediatric cardiorespiratory arrests [Maconochie, 2012].

2.3 Developmental approach to the paediatric patient

As you found out in the lesson on WHY PAEDIATRIC PATIENTS ARE DIFFERENT, a child's cognitive development changes as they age, which requires modification to your method of assessment. In this section, you will be provided with some suggestions about how to conduct an assessment of the paediatric patient. Don't forget that you will also need to manage and reassure an often anxious and distressed parent/carer.

2.3.1 Infants

Conduct your assessment by taking account of the following principles [AAP, 2013]:

- Keep the environment comfortable, in terms of temperature and security for the infant. Familiar toys and blankets can help
- Use the name of the patient while conducting your assessment
- Where possible, assess an infant in the arms of a parent/carer
- Approach the infant slowly and calmly. Loud voices and fast movements may scare them
- Do not stand over an infant, but sit or kneel at their eye level
- Look, listen and feel, in that order, to minimise infant distress
- Warm your hands, and tools such as stethoscopes
- Be flexible in your assessment. If the infant is calm, count the respiratory rate and listen to the chest first. This is not possible to do accurately when the infant is crying
- Observe the interaction between parent/carer and the infant. Consider if child abuse is a possibility

- Toys can be used to distract the infant
- Older infants may display stranger anxiety, so if you need to expose the infant, ask the parent/carer to do this. Don't let the infant get cold, though
- Save painful procedures (such as blood sugar measurement) until last.

2.3.2 Toddlers

Conduct your assessment taking account of the following principles [AAP, 2013]:

- Use the name of the patient while conducting your assessment
- Approach slowly and don't touch them until they are familiar with you
- Communicate using a firm, but friendly, tone of voice
- Do not stand over a toddler, but sit or kneel at their eye level
- Where possible, place the toddler on the lap of a parent/carer
- Use play and distraction to help you conduct your assessment
- If you need to use equipment, such as a stethoscope, let them hold it and become familiar and comfortable with it
- Communicate directly with the toddler. Admire their clothes or ask about pets. Remember they are self-centred at this age
- Provide limited choices. For example "Do you want me to listen to your belly or chest first?"
- Avoid questions that can be answered with a "NO"
- Examine a toddler from toe-to-head
- Involve the parent/carer. For example, place the pulse oximeter probe on their finger first, and ask them to remove the toddler's clothes or hold an oxygen mask near the toddler
- Do not expect toddlers to sit still and cooperate. Be patient and opportunistic.

2.3.3 Pre-school

Conduct your assessment taking account of the following principles [AAP, 2013]:

- Use the name of the patient while conducting your assessment
- Use simple terms to explain what you are going to do

- Choose your words carefully. Use age-appropriate language and avoid scaring the child
- Teddy or dolls can be helpful to explain what you are going to do
- Set limits on behaviour, if required. For example, "You can cry or scream, but not kick or bite". Praise good behaviour
- Use games and toys to provide distraction. Ambulance bandages can be useful for this
- Focus on one thing at a time and minimise the time between explaining a procedure, especially a painful one, and carrying it out.

2.3.4 School-age

Conduct your assessment taking account of the following principles [AAP, 2013]:
- Use the name of the patient while conducting your assessment
- Privacy becomes important in this age group. Make sure the environment is appropriate, and if you need to expose the child to examine them, cover them up afterwards
- Speak directly to the child first, then include the parent/carer. Ask older children if they would like their parent/carer present
- Involve the child in their care if they want this. Feeling out of control can distress children in this age group. However, do not negotiate unless the child really does have a choice
- Anticipate the fears that the child has and address them straight away. Assure them that becoming ill or injured is not a punishment
- Explain in simple terms what is wrong and what is going to be done
- Explain procedures just prior to undertaking them. Don't lie to the child, for example telling them a procedure won't hurt, when it will
- Praise the child for being cooperative, but do not chastise them if they are not
- Physical assessments in this age group can usually be conducted head-to-toe.

2.3.5 Teenagers

Conduct your assessment taking account of the following principles [AAP, 2013]:
- Use the name of the patient while conducting your assessment

- Speak directly to the teenager and ask them first for information. If they do not know the answer, for example the name of their GP, check with them if it is okay to ask their parent/carer
- Respect their modesty and privacy. Be confidential unless you have a duty to report or pass on their disclosures
- Be honest and non-judgemental. Provide accurate information and allay fears, particularly concerns over body image or being 'different' as a result of their current illness or injury
- Do not mistake the size of the teenager as a measure of their maturity
- Avoid becoming frustrated or angry if the teenager does not want to communicate or is uncooperative
- Enlist the help of their friends to assist when the teenager is being uncooperative, although keep in mind the teenager's right to confidentiality.

2.4 Primary survey

The primary survey in the infant and child is the same as for adults, except for the general impression component, which should include use of the paediatric assessment triangle (PAT). The PAT is advantageous in children because it can be undertaken without actually touching the child and can be performed 'across the room' to avoid increasing a child's anxiety, by getting too close initially [AAP, 2013].

2.4.1 General impression

It is important to gain a general impression of the health of an infant or child from 'across the room', before your presence has an adverse effect on their level of anxiety or distress. To help you achieve this, use the paediatric assessment triangle (PAT) [Dieckmann, 2010]. As the name suggests, it consists of three key components:
- Appearance
- Work of breathing
- Circulation to skin.

Appearance

The child's general appearance is probably the most significant aspect of the PAT as it provides information about the perfusion of the brain. The parts of this component can be remembered using the mnemonic TICLS [AAP, 2013]:

- **T**one: Is the infant/child moving spontaneously or are they floppy and listless?
- **I**nteractiveness: Does the infant/child respond to people, objects and sounds or are they uninterested in their surroundings?
- **C**onsolability: Can the infant/child be consoled by their parent/carer?
- **L**ook/Gaze: Does the infant/child look at you or do they have a 'glass-eyed' stare into the distance?
- **S**peech/Cry: Is their speech or cry strong or weak, muffled or hoarse?

Work of breathing

In children, it is their work of breathing that provides a better indication as to the adequacy of oxygenation and ventilation, rather than the more traditional respiratory rate and/or auscultation in adults [AAP, 2013]. Look for signs of increased work of breathing as well as listening for abnormal airway sounds:

- Abnormal airway sounds: These include snoring, muffled or hoarse speech, stridor, grunting and wheezing
- Abnormal positioning: Children who can sit up may adopt a 'sniffing the morning air' position, tripod position and/or refuse to lie down
- Recession: Recession of the chest muscles provides an indication of increased work of breathing, as does head bobbing in infants. Beware the child over 5 who has signs of recession, as this is a sign of serious respiratory compromise [Maconochie, 2012]
- Flaring: Look for nasal flaring, an exaggerated opening of the nostrils during laboured inspiration.

Circulation to skin

When cardiac output is not sufficient to meet the body's metabolic demands, the circulation to non-essential organs, such as the skin, reduces. This can manifest in children as [AAP, 2013]:

- Pallor: White or pale skin indicating a reflex shunting of blood away from the skin. This may be the only sign of compensated shock
- Cyanosis: This is blue discolouration of the skin caused by inadequate oxygenation. Note that blue hands and feet in newborns and infants

under the age of 2 months (acrocyanosis) is a normal finding

- Mottling: This is caused by abnormal blood vessel tone in the capillary beds of the skin. There are patchy areas of pallor and cyanosis. This can be normal when the child is exposed to a cold environment.

2.4.2 Airway

Assessment

Obstruction of the airway is common in seriously ill children, causing hypoxia, which can lead to unconsciousness and cardiorespiratory arrest (such as in cases of choking) [Maconochie, 2012]. The lesson on CHOKING IN THE PAEDIATRIC PATIENT (chapter 9) covered the former, so will not be revisited here.

Look for apparent difficulty in breathing or increased work of breathing. In conscious children, they may be in visible distress. Listen for additional noises, such as stridor, a high-pitched (usually) inspiratory sound [Maconochie, 2012].

Management

Children who are conscious should be allowed to adopt a position of comfort, ideally one that they themselves adopt to maximise the efficiency of their airway, and supplemental high-flow oxygen via a non-rebreathe mask should be administered.

For unconscious children, their head needs positioning appropriately to open the airway and prevent the tongue from falling backwards and occluding the airway. This can be achieved in children using a head tilt–chin lift, or jaw thrust manoeuvre as described in the MANAGING THE AIRWAY lesson (chapter 9). Remember that in infants, their head should be placed in the neutral position, with padding under the shoulders to account for their proportionally larger head (Figure 2.1). Care must be taken not to compress the soft tissues under a child's jaw as this can also occlude the airway [Maconochie, 2012].

Suction is useful in children, as in adults, but in infants, suction pressures should not exceed 120 mmHg.

Oropharyngeal airways (OPAs) can be used in children as for adults. For small children and infants, it is generally recommended that the

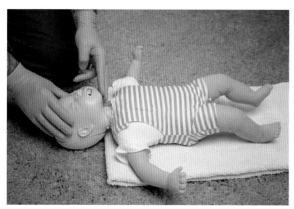

Figure 2.1 An infant, with their airway in neutral alignment

OPA is introduced the 'right way round' and not rotated 180°. This is likely to require a tongue depressor or, if that is not available, a laryngoscope [Gregory, 2010b].

2.4.3 Breathing

Assessment
The most effective way of determining whether the airway is obstructed is to look, listen and feel [Biarent, 2010]:

- Look for chest (and abdominal) movements
- Listen at the child's mouth and nose for breath (plus added) sounds
- Feel for air movement on your cheek.

Note that the chest may move in children, even with an obstruction, making it important to listen and feel.

As part of gaining a general impression, you will already have considered the patient's work of breathing, which includes [AAP, 2013]:

- Abnormal airway sounds
- Abnormal positioning
- Recession
- Flaring.

Other signs of increased work of breathing include elevated respiratory rates and accessory muscle use.

Abnormal airway sounds
Stridor is a high-pitched inspiratory sound, which indicates an upper airway obstruction. This may be an object, or swelling due to infection. In severe cases, it can also occur on expiration. A wheeze, on the other hand, is usually an expiratory sound and is a sign of lower airway obstruction. You may be able to hear it with just your ears, but often it will only be heard on auscultation [AAP, 2013].

Grunting is usually heard in neonates and small infants, although it can occur in small children. It occurs when the infant exhales against a partially closed glottis. This generates a small amount of end-expiratory pressure, keeping the small airways from collapsing at the end of expiration. It is an indication of severe respiratory compromise [Maconochie, 2012].

Abnormal positioning
Children in respiratory distress typically adopt a position that maximises their respiratory efficiency. In upper airway obstruction, this will be a 'sniffing the morning air' position. In lower respiratory problems they may adopt a 'tripod' position, sitting forward with their arms outstretched and resting on their knees Maconochie, 2012].

Recession
Recession can be sternal, subcostal and/or intercostal. Note that significant recession can be seen in infants and young children, even in mild respiratory distress, due to their compliant chest wall (Figure 2.2). However, as previously mentioned, it is a serious sign in children over 5 years of age [AAP, 2013].

Respiratory rate
An increased respiratory rate (tachypnoea) is often the first sign of respiratory problems,

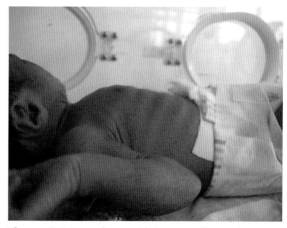

Figure 2.2 A newborn with intercostal recession
By Bobjgalindo (Own work) [CC-BY-SA-3.0-2.5-2.0-1.0], via Wikimedia Commons

although it can be difficult to assess in the crying infant/child (Table 2.1) [Maconochie, 2012].

Table 2.1: Respiratory rate ranges in infants and children

Age (years)	Respiratory rate (breath/min)
< 1	30–40
1–2	26–34
2–5	24–30
5–12	20–24
> 12	12–20

Accessory muscle use

Additional muscles are often recruited when the work of breathing increases. One group is the sternocleidomastoid muscles in the neck. These cause 'head bobbing' in infants, who will nod their head up and down with each breath. However, this is not an efficient method of breathing [Maconochie, 2012].

Pulse oximetry

This can be unreliable when a child has poor peripheral circulation, but if obtainable, a reading of less than 90% on air, or 95% on high-flow oxygen, is a sign of respiratory failure and urgent intervention is required [Biarent, 2010].

Management

All seriously ill children should receive high-flow oxygen via a non-rebreathe mask, unless their ventilation is insufficient. In this case, assistance should be provided with bag-valve-mask ventilation. For children who are conscious, placing a mask over the child may be distressing. In this case, attempt administration using the least-threatening method, for example by asking the parent/carer to hold an oxygen mask close to the patient's mouth and nose [AACE, 2013].

2.4.4 Circulation

Assessment

When assessing circulation, look for signs of blood and other fluid losses, which are causing shock. Children can compensate very well, maintaining their blood pressure until they have significant fluid losses. However, you can spot the child in compensated circulatory failure by examining the following [Maconochie, 2012]:

- Heart rate
- Pulse volume
- Capillary refill time.

Heart rate

Tachycardia is common in children and has a number of causes including pain, anxiety and fever. Bradycardia, however, is a serious sign and you should make your senior clinician aware if you discover an infant's heart rate less than 80 beats/min or a child's heart rate less than 60 beats/min [Maconochie, 2012].

Pulse volume

When a child develops shock, peripheral pulses will become weak and thready. If central pulses (such as a carotid pulse) become weak and thready, the child is in cardiorespiratory failure and arrest is imminent [Maconochie, 2012].

As children become peripherally vasoconstricted in response to shock, their extremities will become cool. Sometimes there is a clear demarcation line between cool skin and warm skin, that will either move towards the torso if shock progresses, or move distally if perfusion and circulation improve [AACE, 2013].

Capillary refill time

Capillary refill time can be a useful indicator of circulatory status, as was covered in the ASSESSMENT OF CIRCULATION lesson (chapter 11).

Management

The principal method of maintaining circulation is to ensure that airway and breathing are adequately addressed and any life-threatening conditions, such as tension pneumothorax, are identified and treated. However, for seriously fluid-depleted children, intravenous access will be required and fluid replacement in 20 ml/kg boluses of normal saline will be required [AACE, 2013].

2.4.5 Disability

Assessment

Often, you will already have an idea about the patient's level of consciousness (LOC) from the general impression. Use the AVPU mnemonic to quickly gauge the child's LOC:

- A : Alert
- V: Responds to voice
- P: Responds to pain
- U: Unresponsive.

Pupils should be checked for dilation, equality and reactivity. Seriously ill children are typically hypotonic and floppy, but in cases of serious brain dysfunction, posturing (particularly in response to pain) such as abnormal flexion and extension may be seen [Maconochie, 2012].

Management

Ensure that airway, breathing and circulation are managed adequately. Don't forget to check blood glucose, and during the history determine whether there is a risk of poisoning or meningococcal septicaemia [AACE, 2013].

2.4.6 Exposure/Environment

In order to complete the primary survey it may be necessary to remove some of the child's clothing, but be mindful that children lose heat rapidly, particularly infants. Use this time to thoroughly examine infants and children who are ill, for rashes [Pilbery, 2013].

Chapter 19: Learning Disabilities

1 Supporting the care of people with learning disabilities

1.1 Learning objectives

By the end of this lesson you will be able to:

- Define the term 'learning disability'
- Explain the needs of a person with a learning disability in emergency care situations
- Describe how you may need to adapt your methods of communication when assisting a person with a learning disability
- Give examples of sources of information, advice and guidance to support the well-being of people with learning disabilities.

1.2 Introduction

A learning disability is a reduced intellectual ability and difficulty with everyday activities – for example household tasks, socialising or managing money – which affects someone for their whole life [Mencap, 2015]. Learning disability includes the presence of [DoH, 2001]:

- a significantly reduced ability to understand new or complex information, to learn new skills (impaired intelligence), with;
- a reduced ability to cope independently (impaired social functioning);
- which started before adulthood, with a lasting effect on development.

It is thought that up to 350,000 people in the UK have severe learning disabilities and this figure is increasing [NHS Choices, 2013].

1.3 Causes of learning disabilities

There are four main causes that are responsible for learning disabilities [Holland, 2011]:

- Genetics
- Events before birth
- Events during birth
- Events after birth.

Genetics

Chromosomal conditions, such as Down's syndrome or Fragile X syndrome, are not in themselves learning disabilities, but they do frequently cause learning disabilities.

Events before birth

Infections that a mother suffers during pregnancy can be transmitted to the fetus, leading to developmental problems and learning disabilities. Other maternal factors, including dietary deficiencies, excessive alcohol consumption during the pregnancy, and endocrine disorders such as phenylketonuria, can also cause learning disabilities.

Events during birth

If during a traumatic or difficult delivery a baby's oxygen supply is interrupted for a significant period of time, brain damage may occur which will cause a learning disability.

Events after birth

In the early years of life, a child is susceptible to many factors which may cause long-term impairment and learning disabilities as a result. Examples of this include infections, particularly meningitis or encephalitis, and traumatic injuries of the brain, sustained by falls, road traffic accidents, or non-accidental injuries.

1.4 Categories of learning disabilities

Learning disabilities are categorised as mild, moderate, severe or profound [Holland, 2011]. As with all conditions, the way in which any individual is challenged by their disability will be unique to them. Many people diagnosed with learning difficulties will be able to lead largely independent lives, whereas others may need more significant help and support.

For people with mild learning difficulties, some occasional support for complex issues may be all that is required, whereas many people with profound and multiple learning disabilities will require more intense help, potentially through to round-the-clock care.

You must always assess any patient with learning difficulties as an individual. Understand how they would normally manage, and what level of support they require on a day-to-day basis. Do not assume, just because a person has a diagnosis of a learning difficulty, that they are incapable of making decisions about their own care needs.

1.5 Communication

As discussed previously, every individual will be affected by their own disability in a unique way, so in order to be able to communicate effectively you need to first understand what is normal for your patient.

For a patient with mild or moderate learning difficulties, you may be able to communicate in a near to normal manner, with maybe just ensuring you use language that is not overly complex or difficult to understand. For patients with more severe or profound learning difficulties it is likely you will need to make more significant adjustments.

Patients with profound, multiple, or severe learning difficulties frequently rely on non-verbal communication, including facial expressions, vocal sounds, body language and behaviour. Some may have a small range of formal communication including words, drawings, gestures or symbols.

For others, they may not have reached any form of intentional communication and you may be relying on feedback from carers as to how changes in behaviour may be indicating pain or distress. In these situations you should seek out the advice of those who know the patient best, as they may be able to better interpret signs the patient is displaying.

You should also consider the use of specialist assessment tools, such as the Abbey pain scale, which is used to assess pain in patients who cannot verbalise, and be mindful that many people with profound learning difficulties also suffer from some degree of visual and/or hearing disability [Mencap, 2008].

1.6 Further support

In the management of an individual incident you should look to friends, family and carers to help support your patient where possible. You may also be able to get further advice and support from:

• Social workers

• Support agencies.

Also consider whether the learning disability makes your patient vulnerable. See the section on safeguarding in chapter 4, LEGAL, ETHICAL AND PROFESSIONAL ISSUES, for more information on this.

Chapter 20: **Older People**

1 Ageing

1.1 Learning objectives

By the end of this lesson you will be able to:

- Describe the anatomical and physiological changes that occur as a person ages.

1.2 Introduction

There are currently around 11 million people in the UK over the age of 65, a figure that is expected to increase by 50% by 2031 [Age UK, 2014]. Although there are no national statistics relating to the number of older people who call the ambulance service, around 45% of the 4,374,611 people who attended an emergency department in 2012/13, and arrived by ambulance, were over the age of 65 [HSCIC, 2014b].

1.3 Anatomy and physiology of ageing

There is no single mechanism of ageing. Instead, there are a range of mechanisms that over time result in the worsening of cell function, causing cellular damage and impairing the body's ability to repair itself. This results in a range of anatomical and physiological changes (Figure 1.1).

1.3.1 Musculoskeletal system

Bones, joints and muscles are all affected by ageing.

Bones

Bone formation is greatest in the period from birth to adolescence, but equalises with bone absorption in a person's twenties, before bone absorption becomes more dominant. This leads to a reduction in body calcium, impairing the body's ability to create bone matrix and increasing the risk of fracture. Cancellous bones, such as those found in the vertebral bodies, wrists and hips, are especially vulnerable. Calcium supplements are often prescribed, as absorption of calcium from the digestive system also declines with age [Farley, 2011].

Joints

The loss of fluid in the fibrocartilage within the intervertebral discs results in kyphosis: the familiar stooped posture of older age, which also reduces the height of the person. With stooping comes a change in the person's centre of gravity and changes to their gait, which becomes slower, shorter and more cautious [Knight, 2008c].

Other joints are affected too, especially synovial joints. The reduction in synovial fluid and articular cartilage leads to bones coming into direct contact with each other. In addition, ligaments are less elastic, shortening and becoming less flexible, all of which contribute to a reduction in the joint's range of movement [Farley, 2011].

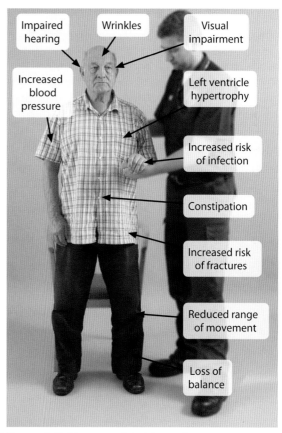

Impaired hearing — Wrinkles — Visual impairment — Increased blood pressure — Left ventricle hypertrophy — Increased risk of infection — Constipation — Increased risk of fractures — Reduced range of movement — Loss of balance

Figure 1.1 Changes related to ageing

Muscles

Muscles atrophy, leading to a reduction in muscle strength and mass, but not endurance. The rate of decline is variable, with some muscles, such as the diaphragm remaining unchanged, whereas the lower limbs can experience noticeable atrophy. Coupled with the decline in nervous system function, movement speed is reduced, and increased muscle rigidity results in limited movement in the neck, shoulders, hips and knees [Farley, 2011].

1.3.2 Respiratory system

The respiratory system is in steady decline from around the age of 25, following a functional peak at 20 years of age. There are a variety of external factors which adversely affect the respiratory system, including poor nutrition, lack of physical exercise and smoking [Farley, 2011]. Changes due to ageing are fairly insignificant compared to the external factors as there is usually sufficient spare capacity in lung function to offset any decline due to older age.

Airway changes

There are a number of changes in the airway itself as we age. Mucus becomes increasingly thick, leading to it lodging in the nasopharynx and causing recurrent coughs. The cilia that line the trachea and smaller airways flatten, reducing the clearance of secretions and other debris, increasing the chance of infection [Knight, 2008].

Ventilatory changes

Respiratory function does deteriorate with age, in tandem with the decline of the musculoskeletal system. Costal cartilages become stiff, decreasing lung compliance and requiring the use of accessory muscles to ventilate. In addition, the strength of the respiratory system declines from around 55 years of age, with intercostal muscle wasting, increasing the work of breathing and making the respiratory system more reliant on the diaphragm [Knight, 2008]. Shortness of breath on exertion (SOBOE) is more common in older people due to [Farley, 2011]:

- Decreasing muscle strength
- Muscles being more prone to fatigue when work of breathing increases
- Muscle wasting
- Decreased blood supply to the muscles of respiration.

A reduction in lung compliance leads to premature airway closing, resulting in areas of poorly ventilated, or unventilated alveoli at resting lung volumes. In addition, reduced elastic recoil of the lungs causes collapse of the small airways at the lung bases, causing secretions to collect, which are difficult to expectorate and become a breeding ground for infections [Farley, 2011].

The loss of lung elasticity also causes a gradual increase in the diameter of the bronchioles and alveolar ducts, increasing the anatomical dead space and adversely affecting gas exchange. The alveolar surface area also declines, further reducing gas exchange.

Most measurements of lung function decline with age, but in healthy patients this is mostly offset by a large reserve capacity of the respiratory system [Farley, 2011].

1.3.3 Cardiovascular system

Blood vessels

As the body ages, blood vessels (particularly the arteries) lose their elasticity and become less compliant. The tunica media of large arteries thicken, due to the increasing number and density of collagen fibres, which makes the arteries more rigid. The inner endothelial layer, normally smooth to encourage blood flow, becomes roughened by muscle fibres that have migrated from the tunica media, which increases the resistance to blood flow [Knight, 2008a].

Systolic blood pressure increases, due to the left ventricular hypertrophy (LVH) and the decrease in elasticity and diameter of the blood vessels. Smaller arteries and arterioles, along with baroreceptors, become less sensitive, leading to a sluggish response to changes in posture, such as from sitting to standing, which can cause postural hypotension [Farley, 2011].

Heart

In order to overcome the increase in systemic vascular resistance, the heart needs to pump with greater force; like all muscles that are exercised, it thickens (hypertrophies), particularly the left ventricle.

There are also changes in the electrical conduction system, with the sino-atrial node losing around 50–75% of pacemaker cells by the age of 50. Progressive fibrosis and cell death in the Bundle of His leads to cardiac conduction problems such as a decrease in maximal heart rate and increase in arrhythmias [Knight, 2008a].

1.3.4 Nervous system

Brain and senses

In healthy people the ageing brain functions normally, and learning, for example, is still able to occur. However, brain weight does decline by approximately 5–10% over a lifetime with little change up to the age of 50 years. Indeed, it is not until 60 years of age and older that there is a significant reduction in weight [Farley, 2011].

An important consequence of this is the separation of the brain from the skull, which allows increased movement and stretching of the bridging veins between the brain and the outer layer of the meninges. During trauma involving the head, this can result in tearing of the veins, with subsequent subdural haemorrhage, bleeding into the subdural space [GEMS, 2015].

About 10% of neurons are lost by the age of 75, but this does not result in significant loss of mental function. However, the loss of sensory neurons leads to impaired hearing, vision, smelling, temperature regulation and appreciation of pain. In addition, as proprioception reduces, older people become increasingly reliant on visual, tactile and auditory cues to stay on their feet, which increases the risk of falling, particularly if any/all of these senses are impaired [Knight, 2008b].

Eyes

The muscles of the eyelids lose tone and elasticity and a reduction in orbital fat makes the eyes become sunken, reducing the upward gaze. The cornea flattens and thickens with age, making it duller and less transparent, increasing the risk of visual blurring. At the same time, there is a reduction in the sensitivity of the cornea, decreasing the awareness of any eye injuries. Pupil diameter declines, resulting in a reduction in light entering the eye, which adversely affects vision, particularly at night. Finally, the lens thickens and stiffens, reducing visual acuity and the ability to focus further [Farley, 2011].

Ears

Hearing loss is common, although not inevitable, with around 50% of people over 75 having hearing difficulties. High-pitched sounds and consonants are particularly affected. This may be especially noticeable for the person when there are high levels of background noise, and it makes identifying the direction of sound tricky.

Spinal cord

As the body ages, reflexes slow and there is a delayed response to stimuli because of a reduction in the numbers of conducting nerve fibres. This in turn causes a reduction in reaction time. The loss of large nerve fibres in the sympathetic nervous system contributes to the problem of postural hypotension and, overall, there is a reduction in the efficiency of the autonomic nervous system. This can result in usually well-tolerated stressors, such as heat, cold and extreme exercise, becoming harmful and even life-threatening [Farley, 2011].

1.3.5 Immune system

From a functional peak around puberty, there is a gradual reduction in immune system capacity over a person's lifetime of between 5% and 30%, but the immune system does continue to function even in very old adults. However, older people are more likely to die of infectious diseases such as pneumonia, influenza and gastroenteritis, for example. In addition, older adults respond differently to infection than younger adults, including [Farley, 2011]:

- Fewer microorganisms are required to cause symptomatic infection
- Confusion prior to a raised temperature is more common
- Symptoms can be masked and/or mistaken for other diseases
- The immune system can be compromised by medication such as steroids and anti-inflammatories
- There is increased risk from chronic diseases such as diabetes and chronic obstructive pulmonary disease.

1.3.6 Integumentary system

The skin is probably the most visible sign of older age and all layers are affected [Farley, 2011]:

- Epidermis: Loss of melanocytes and other skin cells leads to decreased surface contact between the dermis and epidermis, which reduces the exchange of nutrients and other products of metabolism. In addition the epidermis atrophies, causing roughened skin that takes longer to heal and provides less of a barrier

- Dermis: This layer also atrophies, becoming thinner. In addition, there is a reduction in mast cells, which play an important role in the injury and infection responses. The dramatic reduction in dermal blood vessels leads to pallor, decreased temperature and impaired thermoregulation compounded by a loss of sensory nerve endings, increasing the risk of injury
- Hypodermis: A reduction in subcutaneous fat leads to increased conductive heat loss, and the redistribution of the fat leads to bony prominences, which are vulnerable to pressure ulcers and fractures following trauma. Clinically, the skin looks dry, lax and wrinkly. The wrinkles are due to a combination of gravity, decreasing subcutaneous fat and, in the face, repeated traction by facial muscles. In addition photo-ageing caused by ultraviolet radiation from the sun increases the number of skin lesions, which are usually benign, although they can become cancerous later in life.

1.3.7 **Digestive system**
Food intake declines with age, with about a 10% reduction in calorific intake each decade after 50 years of age. Older people may experience altered taste, linked mainly to a decrease in the sense of smell and smell discrimination, as the appeal of foods is based on its smell and taste. In addition, they are more likely to have missing teeth and poorly fitting dentures, all of which contribute to weight loss and malnutrition becoming more common. Increased intake of sugar and salt can contribute to the development of diabetes and high blood pressure [Nigam, 2008].

Muscular contractions that initiate the swallowing reflex also decline with age, leading to dysphagia and increased risk of choking. Lower down the gastrointestinal tract, there is impaired absorption of essential fats and other nutrients, while in the large intestine peristalsis slows, increasing the transit time of bowel contents, which can cause constipation. This in turn can lead to the formation of haemorrhoids due to the increased straining required to defecate [Nigam, 2008].

2 **Dementia**
2.1 **Learning objectives**
By the end of this lesson you will be able to:
- Define dementia
- Explain the differences between dementia and delirium
- Describe a number of strategies that can assist when communicating with a patient with dementia
- Identify a number of causes of challenging behaviour
- Explain how to manage challenging behaviour.

2.2 **Introduction**
Dementia is a set of behaviours or 'symptoms' which suggest difficulties with cognitive function. The most common symptoms include: memory loss, confusion, mood and personality changes, and problems with planning and with doing tasks in the right order. Dementia is diagnosed when the symptoms cause such problems with the everyday tasks of daily life that the person affected can no longer carry on living independently, without care.

Dementia is an 'organic' disorder, meaning there is an associated physical deterioration of the brain tissue, which can be seen via a brain scan or, after death, at autopsy. Dementia is progressive – the damage and symptoms get worse over time. It is therefore not a normal result of ageing, but rather is the result of a disease [SCIE, 2013].

There are over 100 types of dementia, with Alzheimer's disease being the most common single cause in the UK, making up around 66% of cases, and vascular dementia coming in second. However, multiple disease processes are even more common than single disease processes, with Alzheimer's disease and vascular dementia, and Alzheimer's disease and Lewy body dementia being common combinations [NG, 2001].

It is estimated that 7.1% of people over 65 have dementia, which translates into around 850,000 people in the UK in 2015 [Age UK, 2014a].

2.3 **Dementia vs delirium**
If dementia can be thought of as chronic brain failure, then delirium is acute brain failure

[Barrett, 2014]. It is a common and serious condition that is characterised by disruptions in thinking, consciousness, attention, cognition and perception. Unlike dementia, it comes on over a short period of time (typically hours to days). To complicate matters, patients with dementia can also develop delirium and this has been associated with serious complications and poor outcome, including death [Fick, 2002].

Delirium is often divided into three variants [SAS, 2014]:

- Hyperactive: Characterised by anxiety, restlessness, irritability, anger and frustration. Patients may be easily startled and distracted, and unable to sit still. Speech can be loud, but incoherent with frequent topic hopping
- Hypoactive: Patients with hypoactive delirium are typically lethargic, apathetic, slow in movement, withdrawn, drowsy and difficult to wake
- Mixed: A combination of the two other variants, with patients fluctuating between hyperactive and hypoactive delirium throughout the day.

Differentiating between delirium and dementia can be difficult, so if in doubt, it is safer to assume delirium and ensure patients receive prompt medical attention [SAS, 2014]. Table 2.1 lists some of the differences between dementia and delirium to help with identification [GEMS, 2015].

Causes of delirium

Delirium can be the result of virtually any medical condition or drug treatment as well as having a number of other causes, including [SAS, 2014]:

- Infection: Examples include urinary tract infections, pneumonia, or fever from a viral infection
- Medication: Such as anticholinergics, analgesics and corticosteroids
- Serious medical illnesses: For example diseases of the liver, kidneys, lungs and heart
- Sudden alcohol and/or drug withdrawal
- Major surgery
- Acute stress
- Epilepsy
- Brain injury or infection
- Terminal illness
- Constipation

- Urinary catheters
- Immobility.

2.4 Communication

Although the principles of communication have already been covered in chapter 3 on COMMUNICATION, there are some additional points to consider when you are caring for a patient with dementia:

- Get their attention: Approach the patient from the front so they can see you coming. Try to make eye contact and ensure they can see your face and body movements
- Use their name: Using their name can help them understand that you are not a stranger (although this may not be true), which can be reassuring
- Frequently remind them who you are: This can reduce anxiety and avoid the patient becoming alarmed at being treated by a stranger
- Keep ambient noise and activity to a minimum: Reducing distractions, activity and noise will help a patient with dementia (indeed most patients) to concentrate on what you are saying
- Don't rush: Take your time. Slowing your rate of speech can help, but increase the time spent speaking AND listening. It may help if you silently count to seven between short

Table 2.1: The differences between dementia and delirium

Dementia	Delirium
Gradual (chronic) onset	Sudden (acute) onset
Impaired recent memory	Inattention
Regression	Disorganised thinking
At least two of the following:	
Disjointed thinking	Reduced level of consciousness
Poor judgement	Perceptual disturbances e.g. hallucinations
Loss of mental function	Increased/decreased psychomotor activity

sentences, and then give the patient the same time to answer

- Keep calm: Adopt a calm tone and manner to reduce distress and make the patient feel more comfortable with you. Patients with dementia maintain the ability to determine your body language even after their ability to understand speech has been lost
- Keep things simple: Avoid jargon and speak in short and simple to understand sentences. When giving instruction, break down the task into simple stages. Give clear instructions; for example, rather than saying "sit there" you could try saying "sit in this blue chair, please"
- Use the patient's preferred method of communication: Establish this early from the patient and others who know them. This includes speaking to the patient in their first language or using communication aids such as pictures or talking mats.

2.5 Challenging behaviours

Many patients with dementia are placid and sweet-tempered, but over 90% will exhibit some form of challenging behaviour. This includes [Barrett, 2014]:

- Sleeplessness
- Wandering
- Agitation
- Pacing
- Aggression (including spitting)
- Disinhibition
- Jealousy (especially sexual jealousy).

Challenging behaviour needs to be seen as a manifestation of unmet need, which the patient may not be able to express, such as boredom, frustration and/or annoyance.

Managing challenging behaviour

It is important to appreciate that each patient will be slightly different, so the best way of managing challenging behaviour will need to be tailored to them. Advice from carers and/or relatives may help, but general principles include [YAS, 2013]:

- Trying to find out what is the cause of the behaviour
- Reducing the stress and/or demands placed on the patient
- Explaining what is happening using the patient's name and saying who you are. You are likely to have to repeat this process often
- Giving patients time to respond to your requests or questions
- Trying not to show criticism or irritation and avoiding confrontation with patients
- Watching for warning signs that they are becoming more anxious or agitated. Get help if the situation does not calm down quickly
- Including carers and/or relatives who know the patient and who will have experience in managing the patient's challenging behaviour
- Not making sudden movements or using a sharp tone. Instead, remain calm and keep your voice low.

Chapter 21: **Cardiac Arrest**

1 **Adult basic life support**

1.1 **Learning objectives**
By the end of this lesson you will be able to:
- Explain the benefits of the chain of survival to basic life support
- Explain the procedure for providing basic life support to adults.

1.2 **Introduction**
Cardiac arrest is the ultimate medical emergency, but you will have the ability to undertake the two most effective treatments for this: cardiopulmonary resuscitation (more commonly called basic life support in healthcare circles) and defibrillation. However, the role of the ambulance service is just one link in a chain which maximises the patient's chance, not only of a return of spontaneous circulation (ROSC), but also of surviving to hospital discharge neurologically intact (i.e. with normal or near-normal brain function) [Koster, 2010]. That chain is known as the chain of survival [Nolan, 2006].

Chain of survival
The chain of survival encompasses four key principles that are required if a resuscitation is to be successful in adults (Figure 1.1) [Koster, 2010]:
- Early recognition and call for help
- Early bystander cardiopulmonary resuscitation (CPR)
- Early defibrillation
- Post-resuscitation care.

The Chain of Survival

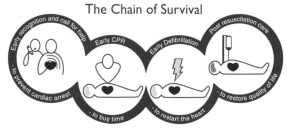

Figure 1.1 The chain of survival
Image reproduced by the kind permission of Laerdal Medical

Early recognition and call for help
This relies on patients and the public calling for help early and can be influenced by the ambulance service with public education and training sessions. Recognition of cardiac chest pain is particularly important as around 21–33% of patients with acute myocardial ischaemia will suffer a cardiac arrest in the first hour following onset [Müller, 2006].

Early CPR
Performing CPR immediately following cardiac arrest can double or triple the chance of the patient surviving [Koster, 2010]. When someone calls 999 they will be given advice on how to perform chest compressions only, as this has been shown to produce higher survival rates in adults than conventional CPR (chest compression and mouth-to-mouth ventilation) [Hüpfl, 2010].

Early defibrillation
Providing good quality CPR and defibrillating in the first 3–5 minutes of a cardiac arrest can produce a survival rate of 50–75%, but, conversely, the chance of surviving to hospital discharge falls by 10–12% for every minute of delay [Koster, 2010].

Post-resuscitation care
Restarting your patient's heart and palpating a pulse (ROSC) is a great feeling, but the patient is not out of the woods yet. The true measure of success is returning the patient to their pre-cardiac-arrest state, with brain function intact so that they can leave hospital. Providing post-resuscitation care on scene, en route and in hospital is crucial if this is to happen [Nolan, 2012].

Children
In stark contrast to adults, children usually suffer a cardiac arrest secondary to hypoxia. The outcomes from these secondary cardiac arrests are very poor and the emphasis with children is to intervene before their heart arrests [Maconochie, 2012].

1.3 **Adult BLS**

Basic life support (BLS) refers to maintenance of airway patency, and supporting breathing and circulation, with artificial ventilation and chest compressions as required [AACE, 2013]. The procedure described is for a single rescuer, but tasks are usually shared when there is more than one rescuer on scene, such as when you are working as a crew.

Procedure

Take the following steps to perform adult BLS: [Koster, 2010; AACE, 2013]

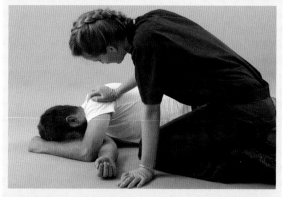

1. Ensure the scene is safe for you, your colleague, the patient and other bystanders. Check the patient to see if they are responsive by gently shaking their shoulders and asking if they are alright

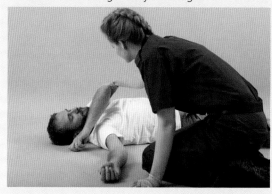

2. If the patient responds, obtain a history and undertake a further patient assessment. If the patient does not respond, inform your colleague so they can assist. Turn the patient onto their back

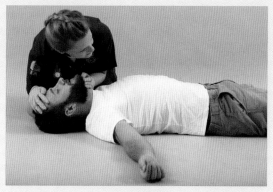

3. Open the patient's airway and look, listen and feel for breathing for no more than 10 seconds. Note that agonal breathing (occasional gasps) is common immediately following cardiac arrest and should not be confused with normal breathing or taken as a sign of life. If the patient is breathing, place them in the recovery position

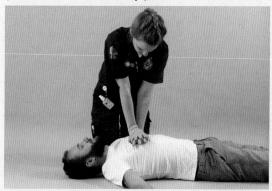

4. If the patient is not breathing or there are no signs of life (not moving, no normal breathing or coughing), start chest compressions:

- Kneel beside the patient
- Place the heel of one hand in the centre of the chest (lower half of the sternum)
- Place the heel of your other hand on top of the first
- Interlock your fingers and ensure that pressure is NOT applied over the patient's ribs
- Keeping your arms straight and with you positioned directly over the patient's chest, apply downward pressure to compress the chest by 5–6 cm
- After each compression release the pressure on the chest, but maintain contact with the patient's skin
- Repeat at a rate of 100–120 compressions/min

Procedure continued →

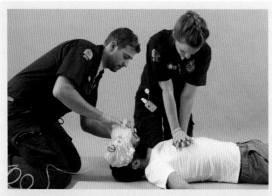

5. After 30 compressions, open the airway (you can insert an oropharyngeal airway if available) and provide two rescue breaths with a pocket mask or bag-valve-mask. If your colleague is available, they may well have already assembled the equipment and be prepared to ventilate. Each ventilation should deliver a tidal volume of 500–600 ml, enough to cause the chest to rise and take about 1 second to deliver. Do not attempt to compress the chest while ventilation is being provided, but keep your hands in the correct position so that chest compressions can immediately resume once the ventilations have been administered

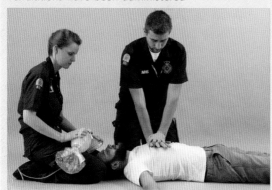

6. Continue with chest compressions and ventilations at a ratio of 30:2. You should alternate chest compressions with your colleague every two minutes, but keep the changeover time to a minimum

2 Paediatric basic life support

2.1 Learning objectives

By the end of this lesson you will be able to:

• Explain the procedure for providing basic life support to paediatric patients.

2.2 Introduction

You will recall from the CHILDREN AND INFANTS lesson (chapter 18) that paediatric patients are not small adults. This is true of cardiac arrest where, unlike adults, who experience a primary cardiac arrest typically due to a cardiac arrhythmia, infants and children usually suffer a secondary cardiac arrest [Maconochie, 2012]. This is not the sudden event experienced by adults, but a progressive worsening of the patient's condition until they cannot continue to compensate. Outcome from secondary cardiac arrest is poor.

Paediatric basic life support (BLS) is different from that of adults, and there are also some differences between infants (paediatric patients under 1 year of age) and children (between 1 year of age and puberty) and so they are presented separately in this lesson.

2.3 Infant BLS

Procedure

Take the following steps to perform basic life support on an infant [Maconochie, 2012; AACE, 2016]:

1. Ensure the scene is safe for you, your colleague, the patient and other bystanders. Check for responsiveness by placing a hand on the infant's forehead to stabilise it and tug their hair while calling their name. If they do not have hair, consider flicking the soles of their feet. Never shake an infant

2. If the patient responds, assess the infant's ABCDE, call for assistance and reassess regularly. If they do not respond, summon additional assistance

3. Open the infant's airway by placing one hand on their forehead and gently tilt it back until it is in a neutral position (Figure 2.1). Perform a chin lift by placing the fingertips of your other hand on the bony part of the lower jaw and lift upwards. Don't compress the soft tissues under the jaw as this will occlude the airway. Placing a towel under the infant's shoulders and upper body can help keep their head in a neutral position

4. If a head tilt–chin lift is not effectively opening the airway, you can use a jaw thrust to open the airway:
   • Position yourself behind the infant
   • Place two fingers under both angles of the jaw
   • Rest your thumbs on the infant's cheeks
   • Lift the jaw upwards

Procedure continued →

5. Look, listen and feel for normal breathing by placing your face close to the infant's face:
   - Look for chest and abdominal movements
   - Listen for airflow at the mouth and nose
   - Feel for airflow at the mouth and nose
6. If the infant is breathing normally, turn them onto their side and monitor their breathing
7. If the infant is not breathing or there are no signs of life (not moving, no normal breathing or coughing), check for, and carefully remove, any airway obstruction and provide 5 rescue breaths:
   - Ensure the head is in a neutral position and apply a chin lift
   - Either place a bag-valve-mask over the infant's mouth and nose (Figure 2.2), or take a breath and place your mouth over the mouth and nose of the infant
   - Ventilate the chest steadily for 1 second, just enough to make the chest rise
   - Maintain head tilt–chin lift and watch the chest fall
   - Repeat this sequence 5 times
8. If the infant's chest is not rising and falling in a similar fashion to normal breathing, open the infant's mouth and check for any visible obstruction. Do not blindly sweep in the infant's mouth. Reposition the head to ensure it is in the neutral position, using a jaw thrust if the head tilt–chin lift manoeuvre is not effective. Make no more than 5 attempts to achieve effective ventilation before moving on to chest compressions
9. Check for signs of life (movement, coughing or normal breathing). If you are confident in checking for a pulse, feel for a brachial pulse in the medial aspect of the infant's arm. Unless you are sure you can feel a pulse, assume it is absent and start chest compressions. If there are signs of circulation, reassess airway and breathing and manage appropriately
10. If there are no signs of life and/or no pulse or a pulse rate of less than 60 beats/min, start chest compressions:
    - If you are on your own, use the tips of two fingers (Figure 2.3), otherwise adopt the encircling technique by placing both thumbs side by side on the lower sternum and spreading the remaining fingers around to the infant's back (Figure 2.4)
    - Avoid compressing the abdomen, by placing your fingers one finger's width above the xiphisternum
    - Compress the sternum at least one-third of the depth of the chest and then fully release the pressure while maintaining contact with the sternum

- Repeat the compressions at a rate of 100–120/min for 15 compressions and then give 2 ventilations
- Continue compressions and ventilations at a ratio of 15:2 unless you are on your own, in which case a ratio of 30:2 may be easier
- Continue until the infant shows signs of life or you become exhausted

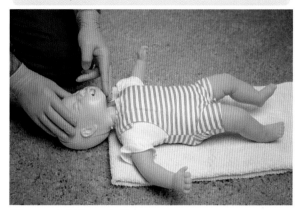

Figure 2.1 Neutral alignment

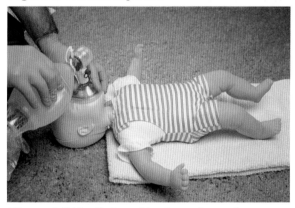

Figure 2.2 Ventilating with a bag-valve-mask

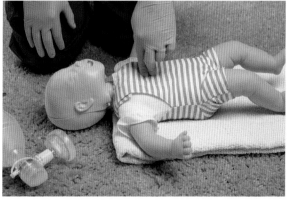

Figure 2.3 Chest compressions using the two-finger technique

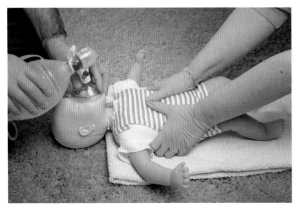

Figure 2.4 Chest compressions using the encircling technique

2.4 Child BLS

Procedure

Take the following steps to perform basic life support on a child [Maconochie, 2012; AACE, 2016]:

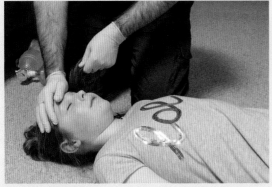

1. Ensure the scene is safe for you, your colleague, the patient and other bystanders. Check for responsiveness by placing a hand on the child's forehead to stabilise it and tug their hair while calling their name or telling them to wake up. Never shake a child

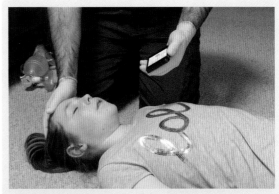

2. If the patient responds, assess the child's ABCDE, call for assistance and reassess regularly. If they do not respond, summon additional assistance

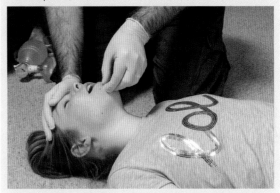

3. Open the child's airway by placing one hand on their forehead and gently tilt it back until it is in a 'sniffing' position. Perform a chin lift by placing the fingertips of your other hand on the bony part of the lower jaw and lift upwards. Don't compress the soft tissues under the jaw as this will occlude the airway. Do not use a head tilt–chin lift technique in children who you suspect have a cervical spine injury: use a jaw thrust instead

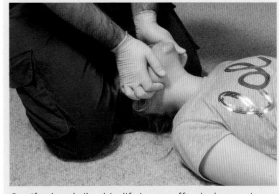

3a. If a head tilt–chin lift is not effectively opening the airway, or you suspect a cervical spine injury, use a jaw thrust to open the airway

Procedure continued →

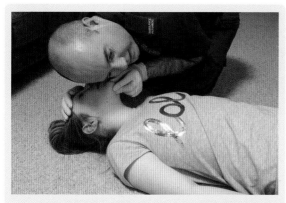

4. Look, listen and feel for normal breathing by placing your face close to the child's face:

- Look for chest and abdominal movements
- Listen for airflow at the mouth and nose
- Feel for airflow at the mouth and nose

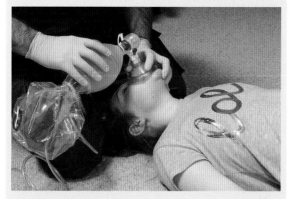

5. If the child is not breathing or there are no signs of life (not moving, no normal breathing or coughing), check for, and carefully remove, any airway obstruction and provide 5 rescue breaths:

- Apply a head tilt–chin lift
- Either place a bag-valve-mask over the child's mouth and nose, or take a breath and place your mouth over the mouth of the child and pinch their nose to prevent air escaping
- Ventilate the chest steadily for 1 second, just enough to make the chest rise
- Maintain head tilt–chin lift and watch the chest fall
- Repeat this sequence 5 times

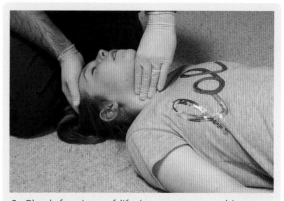

6. Check for signs of life (movement, coughing or normal breathing). If you are confident in checking for a pulse, feel for a carotid pulse at the neck. Unless you are sure you can feel a pulse, assume it is absent and start chest compressions. If there are signs of circulation, reassess airway and breathing and manage appropriately

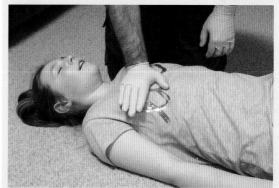

7. If there are no signs of life and/or no pulse or a pulse rate of less than 60 beats/min, start chest compressions:

- Position yourself at the side of the child
- Avoid compressing the abdomen, by locating the xiphisternum and placing the heel of one hand one finger's width above this point
- Lock your elbows and position your body so that your shoulders are directly over the child's chest
- Compress the sternum at least one-third of the depth of the chest (or by 5 cm) and then fully release the pressure while maintaining contact with the sternum. If this is difficult, use the two-handed technique as you would for adults
- Repeat the compressions at a rate of 100–120/min for 15 compressions and then give 2 ventilations
- Continue compressions and ventilations at a ratio of 15:2 unless you are on your own, in which case a ratio of 30:2 may be easier
- Continue until the child shows signs of life or you become exhausted

3 Defibrillation

3.1 Learning objectives

By the end of this lesson you will be able to:

- Describe the types of cardiopulmonary arrest
- Recognise when it is appropriate to use a defibrillator
- Explain the safety considerations when using a defibrillator.

3.2 Introduction

Heart rhythms associated with cardiac arrest are divided into shockable and non-shockable rhythms, depending on whether they should receive an electric current across the myocardium (heart muscle) to depolarise a sufficient amount of the heart muscle simultaneously and allow the normal heart pacemaker (the sino-atrial node) to resume control of the electrical conduction system. Delivering electricity to the heart in this way is known as defibrillation [Nolan, 2012].

In patients who have a shockable rhythm, the sooner they receive defibrillation, the greater the chance it will be successful and the patient will survive. However, it is equally important to ensure that defibrillation minimises the interruption of cardiopulmonary resuscitation (CPR). For each 5-second delay in CPR prior to delivering a shock, the chance of the shock being successful is halved [Nolan, 2012].

3.3 Shockable rhythms

There are two shockable rhythms, ventricular fibrillation and ventricular tachycardia.

Ventricular fibrillation (VF)

VF is a rapid and disorganised ventricular rhythm and is never associated with a palpable pulse. On an electrocardiogram (ECG), you will not see any discernible P, QRS or T waves and complexes and the rate of the undulations is typically between 150 and 500 [Garcia, 2004]. The height (amplitude) of the electrical activity you can see is often referred to as its coarseness (Figure 3.1). This is important, as fine VF, that is VF with an amplitude of less than 0.2 mV (the height of two small squares), should not be defibrillated [Koster, 2005]. As a rule of thumb, if you find it difficult to decide whether the rhythm is VF or asystole (more on this shortly), you should not shock the patient [Deakin, 2010].

Ventricular tachycardia

Ventricular tachycardia (VT) is known as a broad- or wide-complex tachycardia, because the QRS complexes are >0.12 seconds in duration (typically 0.16–0.20 seconds). It usually originates from the ventricles, is monomorphic (has one shape), and has a regular rhythm at a rate of 100–300/min (Figure 3.2) [Nolan, 2012; Garcia, 2004]. Unlike patients with VF, patients with VT may have a pulse and/or signs of life, so always check before defibrillating.

3.4 Non-shockable rhythms

As with shockable rhythms, there are two non-shockable rhythms: asystole and pulseless electrical activity. As the name implies, these are patients who will not benefit from defibrillation.

Asystole

Asystole is the term given to the absence of electrical activity from the heart. On an ECG, you will see a flat (isoelectric) or almost flat line (Figure 3.3) [Garcia, 2004]. A variant of asystole is an agonal rhythm, which is characterised by a slow (a rate of <10/min) broad, sinusoidal complex which interrupts the otherwise isoelectric line on the ECG [SWAST, 2014c].

Pulseless electrical activity (PEA)

PEA is organised electrical activity in the absence of a palpable pulse. Typically, patients in PEA will have some mechanical myocardial activity, but it is not sufficiently strong to produce adequate cardiac output to lead to a detectable pulse or blood pressure [Nolan, 2012]. PEA is associated with a number of reversible causes that are a key component of advanced life support. As with VT, it is important to feel for a pulse and/or look for signs of life prior to determining the need for CPR.

3.5 Defibrillators

There are many brands and types of defibrillator on the market and it is important that you are familiar with the equipment you have in your workplace/ambulance. Broadly, they fall into two types: automated external defibrillators (AEDs) and manual defibrillators.

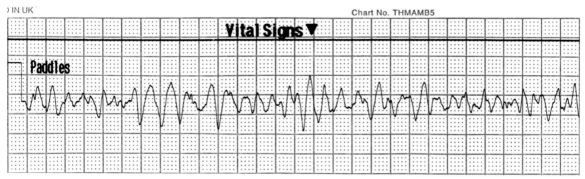

Figure 3.1 Ventricular fibrillation

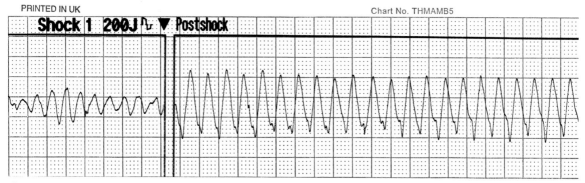

Figure 3.2 Ventricular tachycardia following a 200J shock. The patient was in VF prior to the shock

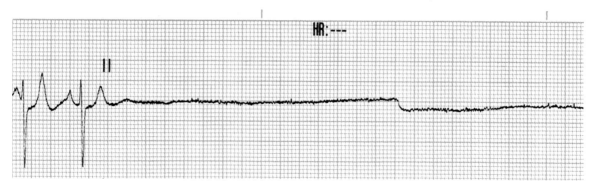

Figure 3.3 Asystole. Note the 2 complexes on the left-hand side of the ECG before the start of asystole. The baseline is not always completely straight in asystole

Automated external defibrillators (AEDs)

These 'shock boxes' are devices that provide voice and visual prompts to guide the public and healthcare professionals to defibrillate safely. AEDs are now widely available in public places such as shopping centres, sports centres, airports and railway stations [BHF, 2013]. Despite their name, some AEDs can be manually overridden by healthcare providers capable of rhythm interpretation, but they are capable of recognising shockable and non-shockable rhythms [Nolan, 2012].

Manual defibrillators

The main advantage with manual defibrillation is the reduction in time for rhythm analysis. This minimises the interruption of chest compressions. In addition, manual defibrillators in the ambulance service are usually capable of other functions such as monitoring vital signs as well as being able to deliver synchronised shocks and external pacing (Figure 3.4).

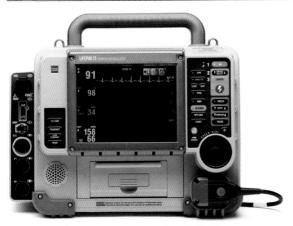

Figure 3.4 A LIFEPAK 15 monitor/defibrillator commonly used by ambulance services

3.5.1 **Safety**

The only person who should receive a shock when a defibrillator is used is the patient. This can be achieved as long as members of the resuscitation team communicate well, so that everyone is well clear of the patient at the time of defibrillation.

Other ways of maximising safety include [Nolan, 2012; EEAST, 2014; Kerber, 2012]:

• Use self-adhesive pads, rather than paddles

• Do not defibrillate patients while they are in water* or near an explosive or combustible environment

• Ensure that the rescuers do not hold intravenous infusion equipment or the ambulance trolley during defibrillation

• Wear gloves

• Shave the patient's chest, if required, to obtain a good skin-to-electrode contact

• Avoid placing the pads over jewellery, piercings, medication patches, wounds and tumours

• Ensure that the pads are well away from pacemaker sites (8 cm in adults and 12 cm in children)

• Remove oxygen from the patient unless the ventilation bag is directly connected to an endotracheal tube or supraglottic airway device.

*Patients who are wet can be defibrillated as long as you dry the patient's chest first.

3.5.2 **Adult defibrillation**

Pad placement

The standard placement for defibrillator pads is to place one just below the right clavicle, to the right of the sternum, and the other in the left mid-axillary line, about level with the V6 ECG electrode or female breast. This should ensure that it is clear of breast tissue [Deakin, 2010].

Alternative positions include:

• Anterior-posterior: One pad is placed over the left precordium, and the other on the back, just under the left scapula (shoulder blade)

• Postero-lateral: One pad placed in the left mid-axillary line, level with the V6 ECG electrode or female breast and the other over the right scapula

• Bi-axillary: One pad placed on either side of the lateral chest wall.

AED procedure

Take the following steps to defibrillate using an AED [Nolan, 2012]:

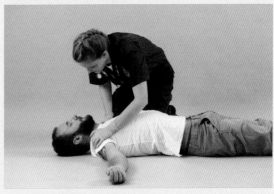

1. Check for danger and ensure that you, your colleagues, the patient and bystanders are safe. Assess the patient's responsiveness

Procedure continued →

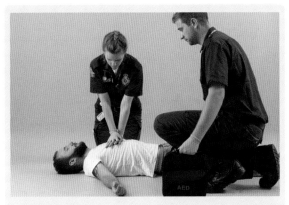

2. If the patient is unresponsive and not breathing normally, start CPR at a ratio of 30 compressions to 2 ventilations (30:2)

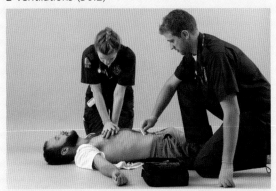

3. Bare the patient's chest and ensure that the pad sites are free from jewellery, piercings, medication patches, pacemakers, wounds and tumours. Shave the chest if required

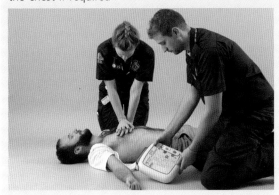

4. Switch on the AED and attach the pads to the patient, ensuring they make a good contact

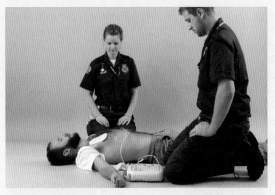

5. Follow visual/voice prompts, ensuring that no-one touches the patient while the AED is analysing the rhythm

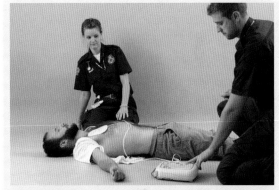

6. Shock?
- If a shock is advised, make sure everyone is clear of the patient and push the shock button. Follow visual/voice prompts
- If a shock is not advised, restart CPR at a ratio of 30:2

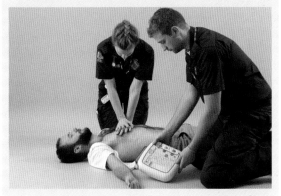

7. Continue until senior help arrives and takes over, the patient shows signs of life or you become exhausted

Manual defibrillation procedure

Take the following steps to manually defibrillate a patient [Nolan, 2012]:

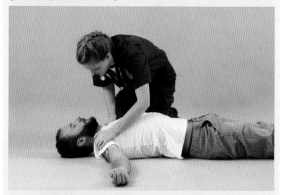

1. Ensure that the scene is safe for you, your colleagues, the patient and other bystanders. Assess the patient's responsiveness

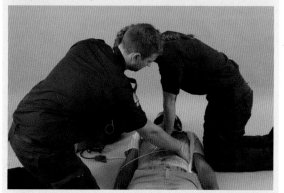

2. Confirm cardiac arrest and start chest compressions. Bare the patient's chest and ensure that the pad sites are free from jewellery, piercings, medication patches, pacemakers, wounds and tumours. Do not interrupt chest compressions while applying the self-adhesive defibrillator pads

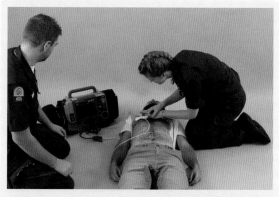

3. Plan actions before pausing chest compressions for rhythm analysis and make sure all team members know their role and the sequence of actions. Stop chest compressions to analyse the rhythm. If not VF or asystole, check for a pulse and/ or signs of life

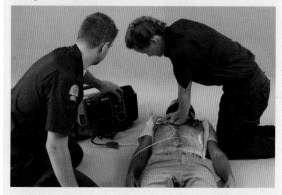

4. If VF/pulseless VT, follow instructions below. If PEA/asystole, skip to step 5

- Immediately resume chest compressions

- The designated person should charge the defibrillator according to the manufacturer's recommendation (typically 120–200J)

- While the defibrillator is charging, everyone except for the chest compressor should stand back and move oxygen away

- Once the defibrillator is charged, the person defibrillating should tell the chest compressor to "stand clear" and deliver the shock as soon as they have done so

Procedure continued →

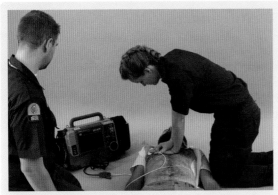

5. Restart CPR immediately at a ratio of 30:2 without checking for a pulse or assessing the rhythm

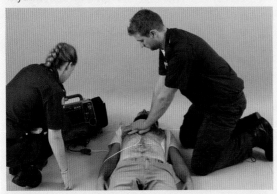

6. Continue for a further 2 minutes and ensure that roles are allocated as the chest compressor should be changed every 2 minutes. Once the two minutes is up, chest compressions should be briefly paused and the rhythm analysed

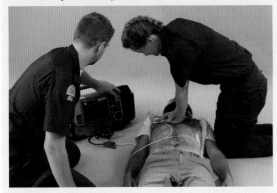

7. Repeat steps 4–6

3.5.3 **Paediatric defibrillation**

Pad placement

The standard placement for defibrillator pads is to place one just below the right clavicle, to the right of the sternum, and the other in the left mid-axillary line. Adult defibrillator pads can be used on children who are >25 kg (about 8 years of age), but they must not touch each other. Use paediatric pads for children under 25 kg (under 8 years of age), if available, but adult pads can be used in smaller children if there is no alternative [Biarent, 2010].

If sufficient gap between the defibrillator pads is not possible due to patient size, use the anterior-posterior pad placement described above.

AED procedure

Take the following steps to defibrillate a child with an AED [Maconochie, 2012]:

1. Check for danger and ensure that you, your colleagues, the patient and bystanders are safe

2. Start basic life support (BLS). If you are on your own, perform one minute of CPR before attaching the AED

3. Bare the patient's chest and ensure that the pad sites are free from jewellery, piercings, medication patches, pacemakers, wounds and tumours

4. Switch on the AED and attach the pads to the patient, ensuring they make a good contact. Use paediatric pads on patients under 25 kg if available

5. Follow visual/voice prompts, ensuring that no-one touches the patient while the AED is analysing the rhythm

6. Shock?
   - If a shock is advised, make sure everyone is clear of the patient and push the shock button. Follow visual/voice prompts
   - If a shock is not advised, restart CPR at a ratio of 15:2 (30:2 if you are on your own)

7. Continue until senior help arrives and takes over, the patient shows signs of life or you become exhausted

Manual defibrillation procedure

Take the following steps to manually defibrillate a child [Maconochie, 2012]:

1. Ensure that the scene is safe for you, your colleague, the patient and other bystanders
2. Start basic life support (BLS)
3. Bare the patient's chest and ensure that the pad sites are free from jewellery, piercings, medication patches, pacemakers, wounds and tumours
4. Plan actions before pausing chest compressions for rhythm analysis and make sure all team members know their role and the sequence of actions
5. Stop chest compressions to analyse the rhythm. If not VF or asystole, check for a pulse and/or signs of life
6. If VF/pulseless VT follow instructions below. If PEA/asystole, skip to step 7
   - Immediately resume chest compressions
   - The designated person should charge the defibrillator by selecting the appropriate energy (4 J/kg)
   - While the defibrillator is charging, everyone except for the chest compressor should stand back and move oxygen away
   - Once the defibrillator is charged, the person defibrillating should tell the chest compressor to "stand clear" and deliver the shock as soon as they have done so
7. Restart CPR immediately at a ratio of 15:2 without checking for a pulse or assessing the rhythm
8. Continue for a further two minutes and ensure that roles are allocated as the chest compressor should be changed every two minutes
9. Once the two minutes is up, chest compressions should be briefly paused and the rhythm analysed
10. Repeat steps 6–9.

4 Cardiac arrest in special circumstances

4.1 Learning objectives

By the end of this lesson you will be able to:

- Explain the considerations for a pregnant patient in cardiac arrest
- Explain the considerations for a hypothermic patient in cardiac arrest
- Explain the management of a drowned patient in cardiac arrest.

4.2 Introduction

In this chapter, you have been introduced to the principles and techniques of resuscitation of a patient in cardiac arrest. However, in some circumstances, the techniques need to be modified and/or alternative techniques used. In this lesson you will be introduced to three groups of patients who require some extra thought when resuscitating them:

- Pregnant patients
- Patients with hypothermia
- Patients who have drowned.

4.3 Cardiac arrest in pregnancy

The general procedure for resuscitating a pregnant patient is the same as for any other patient. However, for patients who are more than 20 weeks pregnant, there is a risk that their fetus-filled uterus can press down on the inferior vena cava and aorta, restricting venous return and leading to a reduction in cardiac output and uterine perfusion [Nolan, 2012].

To prevent this from occurring, the pregnant patient must not lie supine. In the conscious patient, the left lateral position is often used, but this is not practicable in a cardiac arrest when chest compressions need to be provided. Instead, the uterus should be manually displaced to the left, or the patient placed on a spinal board and tilted 15–30° to the left [ALSG, 2010].

During the latter stages of pregnancy, the patient is more likely to regurgitate their stomach contents and aspirate them into the lungs, particularly with over-enthusiastic bag-valve-mask ventilation. Consider using a supraglottic airway device early on in the resuscitation and keep suction close by. Intubation is ideal, if you have a clinician capable, but anatomical changes in pregnancy can make this difficult [ALSG, 2010].

If there is no response to 4 minutes of CPR, the patient should be transferred to the nearest suitable receiving hospital and a pre-alert call made requesting an obstetrician in the emergency department. When initial resuscitation attempts fail, the best chance for successful resuscitation is an emergency Caesarean section [AACE, 2013].

4.4 Cardiac arrest in hypothermic patients

In cases of moderate and severe hypothermia, signs of life can be difficult to identify. You should therefore check for breathing and a pulse for up to 1 minute [AACE, 2013].

In cases where the patient has a core body temperature less than 30°C, some modification of the advanced life support algorithm is required. In these cases, a maximum of three shocks only should be administered if the patient is in VF or pulseless VT, and no intravenous drugs (such as adrenaline and amiodarone) should be given until the patient has been warmed up. Once the core body temperature is over 30°C, but less than 35°C, defibrillation can continue as usual, but when administering intravenous drugs, the time interval between each administration should be doubled (i.e. every 6–10 minutes). Once the patient is over 35°C, they can be resuscitated as normal. Post-resuscitation care is the same as for other cardiac arrest, including the use of therapeutic hypothermia, if appropriate [Soar, 2010].

4.5 Cardiac arrest in drowned patients

Resuscitation is difficult while in the water and should consist of ventilations only. Chest compressions are futile in deep water, so wait until the patient is on a firm surface, such as the shore or the deck of a boat [Szpilman, 2004]. The incidence of spinal injuries is very low (around 0.5%) and immobilising the spine delays effective resuscitation, so only immobilise the spine when there is a clear mechanism of injury that could cause spinal injury (such as diving into shallow water or water ski-ing) [Watson, 2001; Soar, 2010].

Get the victim out of the water as soon as possible and place them supine (on their back), with head and torso at the same level, and check for breathing. If your patient is not breathing, or is breathing abnormally, administer five rescue breaths via a bag-valve-mask connected to high-flow oxygen. Note that this is different from the usual ABC approach that the current resuscitation guidelines advocate for adults, but reflects that correction of hypoxia is the most important aspect in the management of the drowned patient. It can be difficult to differentiate post-arrest gasping from initial respiratory efforts of the drowning patient, so if you are unsure, administer ventilations and start CPR. Pulse checks are unreliable, so try to utilise other diagnostic tests if available, such as electrocardiogram (ECG) and end-tidal carbon dioxide ($EtCO_2$) monitoring. If in doubt, commence chest compressions with ventilations at a ratio of 30:2. Compression-only CPR is not advocated [Soar, 2010].

Regurgitation of stomach contents and inhaled water is common, so consider intubating early. Supraglottic airway devices are not so useful in drowning patients, as pulmonary compliance is likely to be low, requiring the use of high inflation pressures [Soar, 2010].

Advanced life support follows the normal algorithm, unless the patient is hypothermic, in which case follow the guidance for hypothermic patients in cardiac arrest.

Resuscitation efforts should not be stopped unless it is clear that it would be futile to continue (e.g. due to the patient sustaining massive traumatic injuries). There are no completely accurate prognostic indicators in drowning, although duration of submersion is correlated with risk of death or severe neurological impairment [Szpilman, 2012]. In water above 6°C, survival after submersion for more than 30 minutes is unlikely. At 6°C or below, survival time can be extended up to 90 minutes, although this is more likely to apply to children immersed in ice-cold water [Tipton, 2011]. As with hypothermia, the general rule is that your patient is not dead until they are warm and dead [Soar, 2010]. In addition, any patient, irrespective of age, who has been submerged for less than 90 minutes should be resuscitated [AACE, 2013].

5 Post-resuscitation care

5.1 Learning objectives

By the end of this lesson you will be able to:

- Explain the management of the post-resuscitation patient.

5.2 Introduction

A return of spontaneous circulation (ROSC) in a patient who you have resuscitated is a great feeling, but it is just the first step in the path to complete recovery from a cardiac arrest. A complex pathophysiological process occurs as a result of whole body ischaemia during a cardiac arrest and subsequent reperfusion when ROSC is achieved. This is known as post-cardiac arrest syndrome [Deakin, 2010].

5.3 Management

The following steps should be taken once ROSC is achieved [EEAST, 2014; SWAST, 2014c]:

- Minimise patient movement for at least 10 minutes
- Reassess the patient's airway and breathing:
  - A senior clinician may consider intubation
  - Provide ventilation, if required, at a rate of 10–12 breaths/min
  - Oxygen therapy should be titrated to maintain an SpO_2 of 94–98%, except in trauma, where high-flow oxygen should continue to be administered
  - Use capnography if available and adjust ventilation to maintain normocapnia (4.0–5.7 kPa).
- Reassess the patient's circulation:
  - Maintain continuous ECG monitoring and record a 12-lead ECG
  - Perform frequent pulse and blood pressure checks
  - A senior clinician will obtain IV access, if not already achieved.
- Check blood glucose. The target range is over 4 mmol/l but less than 10 mmol/l
- Convulsions can occur following ROSC and will need to be managed promptly with benzodiazepine drugs, such as diazepam
- Transport:
  - Patients should be kept as flat as possible
  - Patients with evidence of ST-segment elevation myocardial infarction (STEMI) should be transported to an appropriate facility as per local guidance
  - A pre-alert call should be made to the receiving facility.

6 Cardiac arrest decisions

6.1 Learning objectives

By the end of this lesson you will be able to:
- Explain when a resuscitation attempt may be stopped or not commenced
- Describe the procedure for the recognition of life extinct (ROLE)
- State the management of a sudden unexpected death in an infant, child or adolescent.

6.2 When to start and stop resuscitation

Whenever there is a chance that a patient may survive from a cardiac arrest, resuscitation should be attempted unless a patient has stated, via an 'advanced decision to refuse treatment' (ADRT), that this should not occur, or there is a valid 'do not attempt cardiopulmonary resuscitation' (DNACPR) order [AACE, 2013].

However, there are certain patients who have an injury or presenting condition that is unequivocally associated with death, irrespective of age [AACE, 2013; SWAST, 2014c]:
- Massive cranial and cerebral destruction
- Hemicorporectomy (complete amputation of the body below the waist) or similar massive injury
- Decomposition/putrefaction: Tissue damage suggests that the patient has been dead for hours, days or even longer
- Incineration: Full thickness burns and charring covering more than 95% of the total body surface area (TBSA)
- Hypostasis: The pooling of blood in the dependent part of the body after death
- Rigor mortis: Stiffness of the body and limbs following death
- Fetal maceration.

Conditions when resuscitation can be discontinued

Even if resuscitation has been commenced, this should be stopped if any of the following are present [AACE, 2013]:
- A DNACPR
- An ADRT clearly states that the patient is not to be resuscitated

- The patient is in the final stages of a terminal illness and the senior clinician determines that CPR would not be successful even if no formal DNACPR decision has been documented
- There is no realistic chance that CPR would be successful because:
  - At least 15 minutes has elapsed since the onset of cardiac arrest
  - No bystander CPR was provided prior to the arrival of the ambulance service
  - There are no exclusion factors such as drowning, hypothermia, poisoning or pregnancy
  - The ECG shows asystole for more than 30 seconds
- The patient has been submerged for more than 90 minutes.

6.3 End of life decisions

Advance care planning

In terminal conditions, death can often be anticipated, which provides patients with the opportunity to consider their wishes and preferences about future care, particularly as they are likely to be unable to do so when close to death. Unfortunately, only 5% of people put these wishes and preferences in writing by means of an advance care plan (ACP, sometimes also called a preferred priorities for care document) [NatCen, 2013]. The contents of an ACP are not legally binding, but any best interests decision about patients must take into account the patient's wishes and preferences [Watson, 2009].

Advanced decisions to refuse treatment (ADRT)

ADRTs (also known as living wills) are documents that outline specific aspects of care that the patient does not wish to receive. This is then typically referred to when the patient is unable to make these wishes clear. Examples of the interventions that a patient may refuse include being ventilated, being tube fed, receiving antibiotics and being admitted to hospital unless they are suffering from a complaint with a treatable cause.

Unlike the ACP, this is a legal document and, as long as the phrase 'even if life is at risk' is present, and the document is signed, dated and witnessed, the contents must be respected by

healthcare staff. Note that treatment can only be declined and not requested, and the ADRT only comes into effect once the patient loses mental capacity [Henry, 2008].

Do not attempt cardiopulmonary resuscitation (DNACPR) decisions

DNACPR decisions are made by a senior clinician, usually with involvement from the patient's clinical team. This will normally be a consultant, GP or suitably experienced nurse [BMA, 2007]. There are four broad situations when a DNACPR decision will be made [Dimond, 2011]:

- A mentally competent patient refuses resuscitative treatment
- A valid advanced directive clearly states that the patient does not want CPR
- CPR is unlikely to be successful
- Successful CPR is possible, but the length and quality of life following resuscitation is not in the patient's best interests.

Ideally, this is written and agreed ahead of time and documentary evidence of the decision will be presented to you before you commence resuscitation. However, even if there is no formal DNACPR in place, the senior clinician can still elect not to start or continue resuscitation if the patient is in the final stages of a terminal illness and they think that CPR would not be successful. Ultimately, if you are unsure about the validity of previously made decisions, then commencing resuscitation is defendable [AACE, 2103].

6.4 Recognition of life extinct (ROLE)

The actions to take following the confirmation of death will be determined by local guidelines and you should ensure that you are familiar with them. The UK Ambulance Services Clinical Practice Guidelines provide a suggested guideline (Figure 6.1) [AACE, 2013].

6.5 Sudden unexpected death in infants, children and adolescents

Sudden unexpected death in infants, children and adolescents (SUDICA) is a collective term covering all deaths in patients under 18 years of age. You may be familiar with the terms 'sudden unexpected death in infants' (SUDI), which

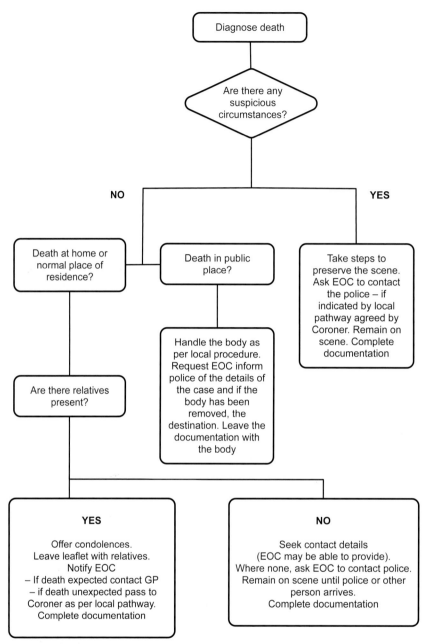

Figure 6.1 Action to be taken after verification of death

incorporates 'sudden infant death syndrome' (SIDS) or cot death [Krous, 2010].

This is likely to be one of the most difficult experiences for you as an SW, particularly as you are likely to be the first on scene. It is also going to be a devastating experience for parents. Although the vast majority of SUDICA will

ultimately be attributable to natural causes, it is important that you are aware of the potential of abuse to be a cause. As such, guidelines have been developed to ensure that specialist paediatric and police involvement occurs in every case.

You should follow your local ambulance service guidelines for these cases, but there are a number of principles that are likely to apply to all services [Lee, 2004; GB, 2013; AACE, 2013]:

- All infants and children should have resuscitation attempted unless there is a presenting condition unequivocally associated with death (excluding hypostasis and rigor mortis)
- All infants and children should be transported to the local emergency department (ED), not a mortuary, unless the police decide that forensic evidence is required first
- Support the family: remember that the vast majority of these cases are due to natural causes and not abuse. Think before you speak and do not criticise the parents/carers

- Use the infant's/child's name whenever you are referring to them
- Avoid placing an infant/child in a body bag
- Parents will need to accompany the infant or child to hospital. If appropriate, offer to take them in the ambulance or ensure that they have alternative means of transport and know where to go. The police may be able to assist with this
- Don't underestimate the effect that an incident like this can have on you. Follow your ambulance service post-critical incident debriefing guidelines and seek support from your colleagues as well as formal counselling, if required.

Glossary

Medical terminology can be rather overwhelming at first. This glossary will provide an explanation of various terms.

Anterior

The front surface of the body, or situated nearer to the front of the body (particularly if comparing the position of one structure to another).

Arrhythmia

A problem with the rate or rhythm of the heartbeat.

Aspiration

Fluid or solid entering the lower respiratory tract (larynx and below).

Aspirin

Aspirin has an anti-platelet action which reduces clot formation and has analgesic (pain-relieving), anti-pyretic (temperature reducing) and anti-inflammatory actions.

Auscultation

The technique of listening to sounds within the body using a stethoscope.

Autoimmune disease

Autoimmune diseases arise from an abnormal immune response of the body against itself, i.e. against substances and tissues that are normally present in the body.

Avulsion

An injury that occurs when a body structure is forcibly detached from its normal point of insertion by a traumatic force.

Battles sign

Bruising behind the ears, which can indicate a skull fracture.

Body mass index

Body mass index (BMI) is defined as a persons weight divided by the square of their height in metres (kg/m^2). This can be adjusted for age and gender, and supplemented with waist circumference measurements, if appropriate. A patient with a BMI of 2529.9 kg/m^2 is considered to be overweight, and if over 30 kg/m^2, obese.

Bradycardia

Slow heart rate.

Brittle asthma

Brittle asthma is a rare form of severe asthma which can result in very serious and often life-threatening attacks.

BVM

Bag-valve-mask.

Care Quality Commission

An independent health and adult social care regulator for England. Their job is to make sure health and social care services provide people with safe, effective, compassionate, high-quality care. They do this by monitoring, inspecting and regulating services to make sure they meet fundamental standards of quality and safety.

Cartilage

Cartilage is a flexible connective tissue found in areas of the body, including the joints between bones, the ribcage, the ear, the nose, the bronchial tubes and the intervertebral discs. It is not as hard and rigid as bone but is stiffer and less flexible than muscle. It does not contain blood vessels, so grows and repairs slowly.

Catastrophic haemorrhage

Bleeding severe enough to cause exsanguination, i.e. blood loss causing death, typically within minutes, or less.

Choking

A mechanical obstruction of the airway occurring anywhere between the mouth and carina.

Circadian rhythms

Circadian rhythms are physical, mental and behavioural changes that follow an approximate 24-hour cycle, responding primarily to light and darkness in a persons environment.

Cognitive function

A persons ability to process thoughts. It encompasses memories, perception, thinking and reasoning.

Connective tissue

Basic tissue type that binds, supports and separates other tissue and organs.

Crepitus

The grating, crackling or popping sounds and sensations experienced under the skin and joints, or a crackling sensation due to the presence of air under the skin. A type of crepitus, bone crepitus, can be heard and felt when two fragments of a fracture are moved against each other.

Distal

Further from the point of attachment of a limb.

Dysphagia

Difficulty swallowing.

Dysphasia

Language disorder marked by a deficiency in the generation of speech, and sometimes also in its comprehension, due to brain disease or damage.

Dyspnoea

Difficulty breathing.

EtCO$_2$

End-tidal carbon dioxide. The measurement of carbon dioxide at the end of expiration.

Focal

Affecting a specific region of the body. For example, a focal neurological deficit may result in a weakness or paralysis of a limb following an impairment of nerve, spinal cord, or brain function.

Glasgow Coma Scale score

The Glasgow Coma Scale (GCS) was developed in 1974 as a way of objectively testing the level of consciousness in brain-injured patients and to improve communication between healthcare professionals. It was originally a 14-point score, but the division of limb flexion into withdrawal and abnormal flexion led to the 15-point score familiar today. Although designed for in-hospital use, it is now routinely used by the ambulance service and is an important marker for the early management of traumatic brain injury (TBI).

Korotkoff sounds

Turbulent blood flow that can be heard when using the manual auscultatory technique to record blood pressure. Named after a Russian surgeon, Nikolai Korotkoff, who first described them in 1905.

Lateral

Of, at, towards, or from the side or sides.

Medial

Towards or at the midline of the body.

METHANE

The mnemonic METHANE is designed to provide the initial communication surrounding details of a major incident. It consists of:

- **M**ajor incident declared or standby. The person making the report should be explicit whether this is a major incident declaration or a standby in anticipation of the occurrence of a major incident
- **E**xact location of the incident. Where possible the grid reference or GPS co-ordinates should be included, along with any landmarks or iconic sites
- **T**ype of incident. What is the exact nature of the incident? For example rail, chemical, road or terrorist
- **H**azards. What hazards are known to be present or could potentially manifest themselves?
- **A**ccess and egress. What are the agreed or best routes to and from the scene?
- **N**umber of casualties. How many casualties are there and, if possible to determine, what are the level and severity of injuries?
- **E**mergency services. Which emergency services are present and which are required? Include specialist resource request if known.

Microorganism

A very small organism that lives outside and inside larger organisms such as the human body.

Multiparity

Having given birth to more than two babies.

Necrosis

Death of body tissue.

OPA

Oropharyngeal airway. A curved plastic tube, with a reinforced flange at one end and designed so that it fits between the tongue and hard palate to help keep the airway open.

OPQRST

- **O** Onset. When did it (the presenting complaint) start?
- **P** Provocation/palliation. What makes it worse/better? Include self-treatment such as taking analgesia
- **Q** Quality. How does the patient describe their symptom, particularly pain? Is it sharp or dull, for example?
- **R** Region/radiation/referral. Where is the symptom located? In the case of pain, does it stay in one place (can the patient point to it with one finger) or does it go elsewhere?
- **S** Severity. On a scale of 0 to 10, where 0 is no pain and 10 is the worst pain imaginable, what score does the patient give it now?
- **T** Time. How long has the patient had it and if it has been relieved, when did this occur? In the case of pain, also consider whether the pain is intermittent (comes and goes).

Palpable

Able to be touched or felt.

Panda eyes

Bruising around both eyes that can be a sign of skull fracture.

Partial pressure

In a mixture of gases, each gas has a partial pressure which is the hypothetical pressure of that gas if it alone occupied the volume of the mixture at the same temperature. The total pressure of the gas mixture is the sum of the partial pressures of each individual gas in the mixture.

Percussion

A method of tapping on a surface to determine the underlying structure. It is used in clinical examinations to assess the condition of the thorax or abdomen.

Pleuritic chest pain

Chest pain that is usually sharp and stabbing, localised to a specific area of the chest (the patient can often point to the pain with a finger) and made worse by coughing and deep inspiration.

Posterior

Further back in position; of or nearer the rear or hind end.

Primary assessment

A swift patient assessment and management process, which can be completed within 60–90 seconds. It is designed to be a stepwise approach, meaning that any abnormalities identified in one step should be addressed before moving on to the next.

Primiparity

Having only given birth once before.

Proprioception

The sense of the relative position of neighbouring parts of the body and strength of effort being employed in movement.

Proximal

Located nearer to the centre of the body or the point of attachment.

Psychomotor

Physical behaviour that is the result of conscious mental processes.

Pulse oximetry

The technique of measuring the oxygen saturation of the haemoglobin in the blood.

Rigors

Shaking or exaggerated shivering which usually occurs in response to a high temperature.

SADs

Supraglottic Airway Devices. Airway devices that sit just above the glottis. The most common SAD is the laryngeal mask airway.

SAMPLE

An acronym for:
- **S** Signs and symptoms of the presenting complaint
- **A** Allergies (particularly to medication but food allergies might be relevant)
- **M** Medications
- **P** Past medical history
- **L** Last oral intake
- **E** Events that led to the current illness or injury

Scope of practice

The area or areas of a persons profession where they have the knowledge, skill and experience to practise safely and effectively.

SOCRATES

- **S** Site
- **O** Onset
- **C** Character. Same as Quality above
- **R** Radiation
- **A** Association. Are there any other signs and symptoms associated with the presenting complaint?
- **T** Timing
- **E** Exacerbating/relieving factors
- **S** Severity

Splanchnic

Referring to organs in the abdominal cavity.

Stridor

High-pitched (usually) inspiratory breath sound, indicating upper airway narrowing.

Superior

Located above or directed upward. In human anatomy, situated nearer to the top of the head (vertex). Opposite of inferior.

Supine

Lying face up, usually referring to a patient who is lying on their back.

Tachycardia

Rapid heart rate.

Tachypnoea

Rapid breathing rate.

TILE

- **T**ask. Consider if the lift:
  - Involves holding the load away from the body
  - Involves long distances
  - Requires strenuous effort or twisting
- **I**ndividual. Consider whether the lift:
  - Requires specialist training
  - Presents a hazard
  - If you and your colleagues are capable of performing the lift
- **L**oad. Is the load:
  - Heavy
  - Difficult to get hold of
  - Unstable
  - Unpredictable
  - Harmful
  - Likely to grab out when alarmed at being carried down the stairs
- **E**nvironment. Determine the presence of:
  - Constraints on posture, e.g. low ceiling, confined spaces
  - Poor, uneven flooring
  - Hot/cold/wet weather
  - Poor lighting
  - Noise
- **E**quipment: Consider what equipment:
  - Is available
  - Will reduce risk to you and the patient
  - Is safe to use
  - You are trained and competent in the use of.

Trendelenburg position

Trolley positioned with the feet-end of the trolley raised, and the head-end lowered.

Trismus

A spasm of the jaw muscles that makes it difficult to open the mouth. Also called lockjaw.

References

A & Ors v East Sussex CC
A & Ors, R (on the application of) v East Sussex County Council & Anor [2003] EWHC 167 (Admin), Available at: http://www.bailii.org/ew/cases/ewhc/admin/2003/167.html [Accessed August 27, 2014].

AACE, 2013
Association of Ambulance Chief Executives, 2013. *UK Ambulance Services Clinical Practice Guidelines 2013.* Bridgwater: Class Professional Publishing.

AAFP, 2012
American Academy of Family Physicians, 2012. *Advanced Life Support in Obstetrics: Provider Manual*, Kansas: AAFP.

AAOS, 2011
American Academy of Orthopaedic Surgeons and American College of Emergency Physicians, 2011. *Critical Care Transport.* Sudbury: Jones and Bartlett Publishers.

AAP, 2006
American Academy of Pediatrics, 2006. The Apgar Score. *Advances in Neonatal Care*, 6(4), 220–223.

AAP, 2013
American Academy of Pediatrics & Pediatric Education for Prehospital Professionals (Program), 2013. *Pediatric Education for Prehospital Professionals* 3rd ed., Burlington: Jones & Bartlett Learning.

Aaronson, 2004
Aaronson PI, 2004. *The Cardiovascular System At A Glance*. 2nd ed. At a glance, Malden, Mass: Blackwell.

Abrassart, 2013
Abrassart S, Stern R and Peter R, 2013. Unstable pelvic ring injury with hemodynamic instability: What seems the best procedure choice and sequence in the initial management? *Orthopaedics and Traumatology: Surgery & Research*, 99(2), 175–182.

Adults with Incapacity (Scotland) Act 2000
The Scottish Government, 2008. Adults with Incapacity (Scotland) Act 2000. Available at: http://www.scotland.gov.uk/publications/2008/06/13114117/0 [Accessed 5 January 2015].

Age UK, 2014
Age UK, 2014. Later Life in the United Kingdom. Available at: http://www.ageuk.org.uk/documents/en-gb/factsheets/later_life_uk_factsheet.pdf?dtrk=true [Accessed 8 January 2015].

Age UK, 2014a
Age UK, 2014. Dementia and cognitive decline: A review of the evidence. Available at: http://www.ageuk.org.uk/documents/en-gb/for-professionals/research/cognitive_decline_and_dementia_evidence_review_age_uk.pdf?dtrk=true [Accessed 15 January 2015].

Age UK, 2014b
Age UK, 2014. Safeguarding older people from abuse. Available at: http://www.ageuk.org.uk/documents/en-gb/factsheets/fs78_safeguarding_older_people_from_abuse_fcs.pdf?epslanguage=en-gb [Accessed 21 January 2015].

ALK-Abello, 2013
ALK-Abello, 2013. Jext 150 and 300 micrograms solution for injection in pre-filled pen: Patient information leaflet. Available at: http://www.medicines.org.uk/emc/pil.23888.latest.pdf [Accessed 5 November 2014].

Allan, 2004
Allan MA and Marsh J, 2004. *History And Examination*. 2nd ed. Mosby's crash course, Edinburgh: Mosby.

Allen, 2007
Allen LA and O'Connor CM, 2007. Management of acute decompensated heart failure. *Canadian Medical Association Journal*, 176(6), 797–805.

Allison, 2004
Allison K and Porter K, 2004. Consensus on the pre-hospital approach to burns patient management. *Accident and Emergency Nursing*, 12(1), 53–57.

ALSG, 2010
Advanced Life Support Group, 2010. *Pre-hospital Obstetric Emergency Training*, Chichester: Wiley-Blackwell.

Althaus, 1982
Althaus, U. et al., 1982. Management of profound accidental hypothermia with cardiorespiratory arrest. *Annals of Surgery*, 195(4), 492.

Ambu, 2011
Ambu, 2011. *Ambu Perfit ACE: Instructions for Use.* Denmark: Ambu D/S.

Angell-James, 1975
Angell-James JE & Daly MB, 1975. Some aspects of upper respiratory tract reflexes. *Acta Oto-laryngologica*, 79(3-4), 242–252.

Anne Kelly, 2004
Anne Kelly C, Upex A and Bateman DN, 2004. Comparison of consciousness level assessment in the poisoned patient using the alert/verbal/painful/unresponsive scale and the Glasgow Coma Scale. *Annals of Emergency Medicine*, 44(2), 108–113.

Apgar, 1953
Apgar V, 1953. A proposal for a new method of evaluation of the newborn infant. *Current Researches in Anesthesia & Analgesia*, 32(4), 260–267.

Ashbury, 2014
Asbury S and Jacobs E, 2014. *Dynamic Risk Assessment: The Practical Guide To Making Risk-based Decisions With The 3-level Risk Management Model.* 1st ed. Abingdon, Oxon: Routledge.

ATLS, 2008
American College of Surgeons and Committee on Trauma, 2008. *ATLS, Advanced Trauma Life Support For Doctors: Student Course Manual.* Chicago: American College of Surgeons.

Austin, 2010
Austin MA, Wills KE, Blizzard L, et al., 2010. Effect of high flow oxygen on mortality in chronic obstructive pulmonary disease patients in prehospital setting: randomised controlled trial. *British Medical Journal*, 341(Oct18 2), c5462.

Band, 2011
Band RA, Gaieski DF, Hylton JH, et al., 2011. Arriving by emergency medical services improves time to treatment endpoints for patients with severe sepsis or septic shock. *Academic Emergency Medicine*, 18(9), 934–940.

Barrett, 2014
Barrett E and Burns A, 2014. Dementia revealed: What Primary Care needs to know. Available at: http://www.england.nhs.uk/wp-content/uploads/2014/09/dementia-revealed-toolkit.pdf [Accessed 15 January 2015].

Bartlett, 2008
Bartlett, N. et al., 2008. Optimal duration of cooling for an acute scald contact burn injury in a porcine model. *Journal of Burn Care & Research: Official Publication of the American Burn Association*, 29(5), 828–834.

Bazarian, 2003
Bazarian JJ, Eirich MA and Salhanick SD, 2003. The relationship between pre-hospital and emergency department Glasgow Coma Scale scores. *Brain Injury*, 17(7), 553.

BCS, 2010
British Cardiovascular Society, 2010. *Recording A Standard 12-lead Electrocardiogram*. Available at: http://www.scst.org.uk/resources/consensus_guideline_for_recording_a_12_lead_ecg_rev_072010b.pdf [Accessed 11 December 2014].

Benger, 2009
Benger J, Nolan J and Clancy M, (eds) 2009. *Emergency Airway Management*. Cambridge; New York: Cambridge University Press.

Berry, 2001
Berry M., Evison D and Roberts AH., 2001. The influence of body mass index on burn surface area estimated from the area of the hand. Burns, 27(6), 591–594.

Betsy, 2012
Betsy T and Keogh JE, 2012. *Microbiology Demystified*. 2nd ed. New York: McGraw-Hill.

BHF, 2013
British Heart Foundation & Resuscitation Council (UK), 2013. A guide to automated external defibrillators (AED). Available at: http://www.resus.org.uk/pages/AED_Guide.pdf [Accessed August 12, 2014].

Biarent, 2010
Biarent D, Bingham R, Eich C, et al., 2010. European Resuscitation Council Guidelines for Resuscitation 2010 section 6. Paediatric life support. *Resuscitation*, 81(10), 1364–1388.

Bickley, 2006
Bickley LS, Szilagyi PG and Bates B, 2006. *Bates' Guide To Physical Examination And History Taking*. 9th ed. Philadelphia: Lippincott Williams and Wilkins.

Blaber, 2008
Blaber A, 2008. *Foundations For Paramedic Practice: A Theoretical Perspective*. 1st ed. Maidenhead: Open University Press.

Bledsoe, 2014
Bledsoe BE, Porter RS and Cherry RA, 2014. *Paramedic Care: Principles And Practice. Vol. 3*. Harlow: Pearson.

BLF, 2007
British Lung Foundation, 2007. Invisible lives: chronic obstructive pulmonary disease (COPD) – finding the missing millions. British Lung Foundation, Available at: http://www.blf.org.uk/files/94ff4ae1-1858-485f-ae85-a06200ded618/invisible-lives-report.pdf [Accessed 29 December 2014].

BMA, 2007
British Medical Association, Resuscitation Council (UK) & Royal College of Nursing, 2007. Decisions relating to cardiopulmonary resuscitation. Available at: http://www.resus.org.uk/pages/dnar.pdf [Accessed March 26, 2014].

BMA, 2014
British Medical Association, 2014. *Safe Handover: Safe Patients*. Available at: http://bma.org.uk/-/media/files/pdfs/practical%20advice%20at%20work/contracts/safe%20handover%20safe%20patients.pdf%20 [Accessed 19 January 2015].

BNF, 2014
British Medical Association and Royal Pharmaceutical Society of Great Britain, 2014. British national formulary. Available at: https://www.medicinescomplete.com/about/publications.htm [Accessed 26 January 2015].

BOC, 2013a
BOC Healthcare, 2013. *Medical Oxygen*. Available at: http://www.bochealthcare.co.uk/internet.lh.lh.gbr/en/images/504370-healthcare%20medical%20oxygen%20integral%20valve%20cylinders%20leaflet%2006409_54069.pdf%20 [Accessed 22 December 2014].

BOC, 2013b
BOC Healthcare, 2013. *ENTONOX® (50% Nitrous Oxide/50% Oxygen)*. Available at: http://www.bochealthcare.co.uk/internet.lh.lh.gbr/en/images/504365-healthcare%20entonox%20integral%20valve%20cylinder%20instructions%20leaflet-04409_57216.pdf [Accessed 22 December 2014].

Body, 2010
Body R, Carley S, Wibberley C, et al., 2010. The value of symptoms and signs in the emergent diagnosis of acute coronary syndromes. *Resuscitation*, 81(3), 281–286.

Bone, 1992
Bone RC, Balk RA, Cerra FB, et al., 1992. Definitions for sepsis and organ failure and guidelines for the use of innovative therapies in sepsis. The ACCP/SCCM Consensus Conference Committee. American College

of Chest Physicians/Society of Critical Care Medicine. *CHEST Journal*, 101(6), 1644–1655.

Bonner, 2011
Bonner TJ, Eardley WGP, Newell N, et al., 2011. Accurate placement of a pelvic binder improves reduction of unstable fractures of the pelvic ring. *Journal of Bone & Joint Surgery, British Volume*, 93-B(11), 1524–1528.

Booker, 2007
Booker R, 2007. Peak expiratory flow measurement. *Nursing Standard*, 21(39), 42–43.

Bose, 2006
Bose P, Regan F and Paterson-Brown S, 2006. Improving the accuracy of estimated blood loss at obstetric haemorrhage using clinical reconstructions. *BJOG: An International Journal of Obstetrics and Gynaecology*, 113(8), 919–924.

Bowers, 2007
Bowers B & Scase C, 2007. Tracheostomy: facilitating successful discharge from hospital to home. *British Journal of Nursing*, 16(8), 476–479.

Boyett, 2009
Boyett MR, 2009. 'And the beat goes on.' The cardiac conduction system: the wiring system of the heart. *Experimental Physiology*, 94(10), 1035–1049.

Briar, 2003
Briar C and Lasserson D, 2003. *Nervous System*. 2nd ed. London: Mosby.

Brophy, 2012
Brophy GM, Bell R, Claassen J, et al., 2012. Guidelines for the evaluation and management of status epilepticus. *Neurocritical Care*, 17(1), 3–23.

BTS, 2008
O'Driscoll BR, Howard LS, Davison AG, et al., 2008. BTS guideline for emergency oxygen use in adult patients. *Thorax*, 63(Supplement 6), vi1–vi68.

BTS, 2010
Levy ML, Le Jeune I, Woodhead MA, et al., 2010. Primary care summary of the British Thoracic Society guidelines for the management of community acquired pneumonia in adults: 2009 update. endorsed by the Royal College of General Practitioners and the Primary Care Respiratory Society UK. *Primary Care Respiratory Journal*, 19(1), 21.

BTS, 2012
British Thoracic Society, 2012. British guidelines on the management of asthma. Available at: https://www.brit-thoracic.org.uk/document-library/clinical-information/asthma/btssign-guideline-on-the-management-of-asthma/%20 [Accessed 29 December 2014].

Burgess, 1990
Burgess AR, Eastridge BJ, Young JW, et al., 1990. Pelvic ring disruptions: effective classification system and treatment protocols. *The Journal of Trauma*, 30(7), 848–856.

Burton, 2006
Burton JH, Harrah JD, Germann CA, et al., 2006. Does end-tidal carbon dioxide monitoring detect respiratory events prior to current sedation monitoring practices?

Academic Emergency Medicine: Official Journal of the Society for Academic Emergency Medicine, 13(5), 500–504.

Buss, 2010
Buss J and Thompson G, (eds) 2010. *Auscultation Skills: Breath & Heart Sounds*. 4th ed. Philadelphia: Wolters Kluwer/Lippincott Williams & Wilkins Health.

Canto, 2012
Canto AJ, Kiefe CI, Goldberg RJ, et al., 2012. Differences in symptom presentation and hospital mortality according to type of acute myocardial infarction. *American Heart Journal*, 163(4), 572–579.

Cantwell, 2011
Cantwell R et al., 2011. Saving Mothers' Lives: Reviewing maternal deaths to make motherhood safer: 2006–2008. The Eighth Report of the Confidential Enquiries into Maternal Deaths in the United Kingdom. *BJOG: An International Journal of Obstetrics and Gynaecology*, 118 Suppl 1, 1–203.

Capps, 2010
Capps JA, Sharma V and Arkwright PD, 2010. Prevalence, outcome and pre-hospital management of anaphylaxis by first aiders and paramedical ambulance staff in Manchester, UK. *Resuscitation*, 81(6), 653–657.

Carley, 1998
Carley S, Mackway-Jones K and Donnan S, 1998. Major incidents in Britain over the past 28 years: the case for the centralised reporting of major incidents. *Journal of Epidemiology and Community Health*, 52(6), 392–398.

CCI, 2011
Clement Clarke International, 2011. Mini-wright peak flow meter instructions for use. Available at: http://www.clement-clarke.com/portals/0/1902169%20mini-wright%20pfm%20instructions-iss6%202011.pdf [Accessed 21 November 2014].

Champion, 1989
Champion HR, Sacco WJ, Copes WS, et al., 1989. A revision of the trauma score. *The Journal of Trauma*, 29(5), 623–629.

Chan, 2003
Chan MM, 2003. What is the effect of fingernail polish on pulse oximetry? *Chest*, 123(6), 2163–2164.

Chapin, 2013
Chapin MM, Rochette LM, Annest JL, et al., 2013. Nonfatal choking on food among children 14 years or younger in the United States, 2001–2009. *Pediatrics*, 132(2), 275–281.

Children Act 2004 Section 11
United Kingdom, 2004. *Children Act 2004. Section 11*. Available at: http://www.legislation.gov.uk/ukpga/2004/31/section/11 [Accessed 7 July 2014].

Chin, 2004
Chin RFM, Neville BGR and Scott RC, 2004. A systematic review of the epidemiology of status epilepticus. *European Journal of Neurology*, 11(12), 800–810.

Civil Contingencies Act 2004
United Kingdom, 2004. *Civil Contingencies Act 2004.* Available at: http://www.legislation.gov.uk/ukpga/2004/36/contents [Accessed 12 November 2012].

Control of Substances Hazardous to Health Regulations 2002
United Kingdom, 2002. The Control of Substances Hazardous to Health Regulations 2002. Available at: http://www.legislation.gov.uk/uksi/2002/2677/regulation/7/made [Accessed 27 December 2014].

Connor, 2013
Connor D, Greaves I, Porter K, et al., 2013. Pre-hospital spinal immobilisation: an initial consensus statement. *Emergency Medicine Journal*, 30(12), 1067–1069.

Cook, 2006
Cook TM and Hommers C, 2006. New airways for resuscitation? *Resuscitation*, 69(3), 371–387.

CoP, 2014
College of Paramedics, 2014. *Paramedic Curriculum Guidance*. 3rd ed. Available at: https://www.collegeofparamedics.co.uk/downloads/curriculum_guidance_2014.pdf [Accessed 5 January 2015].

Corcoran, 2013
Corcoran N, 2013. *Communicating Health: Strategies For Health Promotion,* 2nd ed. Los Angeles: Sage Publications Ltd.

Cox, 2009
Cox ED, Schreiber MA, McManus J, et al., 2009. New hemostatic agents in the combat setting. *Transfusion*, 49, 248S–255S.

Crawford, 2008
Crawford J and Doherty L, 2008. Recording a standard 12-lead ECG: filling in gaps in knowledge. *British Journal of Cardiac Nursing*, 3(12), 572–577.

Crook, 2013
Crook J and Taylor RM, 2013. The agreement of fingertip and sternum capillary refill time in children. *Archives of Disease in Childhood*, 98(4), 265–268.

CSCB, 2014
Coventry Safeguarding Children Board, 2014. Serious case review: Daniel Pelka. Available at: http://www.coventrylscb.org.uk/dpelka.html [Accessed 21 January 2015].

Cure the NHS, 2014
Cure the NHS, 2014. *Cure The NHS Campaign*. Available at: http://www.curethenhs.co.uk/cure-the-nhs-campaign/%20 [Accessed 31 December 2014].

Cuttle, 2008
Cuttle L et al., 2008. The optimal temperature of first aid treatment for partial thickness burn injuries. *Wound Repair and Regeneration: Official Publication of the Wound Healing Society [and] the European Tissue Repair Society*, 16(5), 626–634.

Cuttle, 2009
Cuttle L et al., 2009. A review of first aid treatments for burn injuries. *Burns*, 35(6), 768–775.

Cuttle, 2010
Cuttle, L. et al., 2010. The optimal duration and delay of first aid treatment for deep partial thickness burn injuries. *Burns*, 36(5), 673–679.

Czura, 2011
Czura CJ, 2011. 'Merinoff Symposium 2010: Sepsis' – Speaking with One Voice. *Molecular Medicine*, 17(1–2), 2–3.

Daniels, 2011a
Daniels R, 2011. Surviving the first hours in sepsis: getting the basics right (an intensivist's perspective). *Journal of Antimicrobial Chemotherapy*, 66(Supplement 2), ii11–ii23.

Daniels, 2011b
Daniels R, Nutbeam T, McNamara G, et al., 2011. The sepsis six and the severe sepsis resuscitation bundle: a prospective observational cohort study. *Emergency Medicine Journal*, 28(6), 507–512.

Data Protection Act (1998)
UK Government, 1998. *Data Protection Act 1998*. London: The Stationery Office.

Datta, 2006
Datta A & Tipton M, 2006. Respiratory responses to cold water immersion: neural pathways, interactions, and clinical consequences awake and asleep. *Journal of Applied Physiology*, 100(6), 2057–2064.

Davis, 2003
Davis PD and Kenny GNC, 2003. *Basic Physics And Measurement In Anaesthesia*. Edinburgh: Butterworth-Heinemann.

DCA, 2014
Department for Constitutional Affairs, 2014. Mental Capacity Act Code of Practice. Available at: https://www.gov.uk/government/publications/mental-capacity-act-code-of-practice [Accessed 5 January 2015].

Deakin, 2010
Deakin CD, Nolan JP, Soar J, et al., 2010. European Resuscitation Council guidelines for resuscitation 2010 section 4. Adult advanced life support. *Resuscitation*, 81(10), 1305–1352.

Deary, 1993
Deary IJ, Hepburn DA, MacLeod KM, et al., 1993. Partitioning the symptoms of hypoglycaemia using multi-sample confirmatory factor analysis. *Diabetologia*, 36(8), 771–777.

DfE, 2013
Department for Education, 2013. Working together to safeguard children. Available at: https://www.gov.uk/government/publications/working-together-to-safeguard-children [Accessed 21 January 2015].

Diabetes UK, 2014
Diabetes UK, 2014. Diabetes prevalence 2013. Available at: http://www.diabetes.org.uk/about_us/what-we-say/statistics/diabetes-prevalence-2013/%20 [Accessed 5 November 2014].

Dieckmann, 2010
Dieckmann RA, Brownstein D and Gausche-Hill M, 2010. The pediatric assessment triangle: a novel

approach for the rapid evaluation of children. *Pediatric Emergency Care*, 26(4), 312.

Dimond, 2008
Dimond BC, 2008. *Legal Aspects Of Mental Capacity*. 1st ed. Oxford: Wiley-Blackwell.

Dimond, 2011
Dimond MB, 2011. *Legal Aspects of Nursing* 6th ed. London: Pearson Education.

Dixon, 2009
Dixon M, Carmody N and O'Donnell C, 2009. The effectiveness of supraglottic airway devices in pre hospital basic life support airway management. *Emergency Medicine Journal*, 26(10), 4.

DoH, 2000
Department of Health, 2000. No secrets: guidance on protecting vulnerable adults in care. Available at: https://www.gov.uk/government/publications/no-secrets-guidance-on-protecting-vulnerable-adults-in-care%20 [Accessed 21 January 2015].

DoH, 2001
Department of Health, 2001. Valuing people. Available at: https://www.gov.uk/government/uploads/system/uploads/attachment_data/file/250877/5086.pdf [Accessed 14 June 2015].

DoH, 2003
Department of Health, 2003. Confidentiality: NHS Code of Practice. Available at: https://www.gov.uk/government/publications/confidentiality-nhs-code-of-practice [Accessed 8th December 2014].

DoH, 2005
Department of Health Emergency Preparedness Division, *NHS Emergency Planning Guidance 2005*. Available at: http://www.dh.gov.uk/en/publicationsandstatistics/publications/publicationspolicyandguidance/dh_4121072 [Accessed 15 October 2014].

DoH, 2006a
Department of Health, 2006. *Medical Gases: Health Technical Memorandum 02-01: Medical Gas Pipeline Systems*. London: Stationery Office, Available at: https://www.gov.uk/government/uploads/system/uploads/attachment_data/file/153576/htm_02-01_part_b.pdf [Accessed 22 December 2014].

DoH, 2006b
Department of Health, 2006. A review of services for allergy: The epidemiology, demand for and provision of treatment and effectiveness of clinical interventions. Publication, Available at: http://webarchive.nationalarchives.gov.uk/20130107105354/http://www.dh.gov.uk/en/publicationsandstatistics/publications/publicationspolicyandguidance/dh_4137365 [Accessed 5th November, 2014].

DoH, 2007
Department of Health, 2007. *Mass Casualties Incidents: A Framework For Planning*. Available at: http://webarchive.nationalarchives.gov.uk/20130107105354/http://www.dh.gov.uk/en/publicationsandstatistics/publications/publicationspolicyandguidance/dh_073395%20 [Accessed 15 October 2014].

DoH, 2007a
Department of Health, 2007. Making experiences count: a new approach to responding to complaints – a document for information and comment. Consultation, Available at: http://webarchive.nationalarchives.gov.uk/+/www.dh.gov.uk/en/consultations/liveconsultations/dh_075652%20 [Accessed 31 December 2014].

DoH, 2009
Department of Health and Health Protection Agency, 2009. Pandemic (H1N1) 2009 Influenza. Available at: https://www.gov.uk/government/uploads/system/uploads/attachment_data/file/356986/pandemic_influenza_guidance_for_infection_control_in_ambulance_services.pdf [Accessed 22 December 2014].

DoH, 2009a
Department of Health, 2009. Reference Guide to Consent for Examination or Treatment. Available at: https://www.gov.uk/government/publications/reference-guide-to-consent-for-examination-or-treatment-second-edition [Accessed 5 January 2015].

DoH, 2010
Department of Health, 2010. Confidentiality: NHS Code of Practice – supplementary guidance: public interest disclosures. Available at: https://www.gov.uk/government/publications/confidentiality-nhs-code-of-practice-supplementary-guidance-public-interest-disclosures [Accessed 8th December 2014].

DoH, 2010a
Department of Health, 2010. *Essence Of Care 2010: Benchmarks For The Fundamental Aspects Of Care: Benchmarks For Personal Hygiene*. London: Stationery Office.

DoH, 2010b
Department of Health, 2010. Personal hygiene. Available at: http://www.health.gov.au/internet/publications/publishing.nsf/content/ohp-enhealth-manual-atsi-cnt-l%7Eohp-enhealth-manual-atsi-cnt-l-ch3%7Eohp-enhealth-manual-atsi-cnt-l-ch3.7 [Accessed 21 December 2014].

DoH, 2010c
Department of Health, 2010. Ambulance Guidelines: Reducing Infection Through Effective Practice in the Pre-hospital Environment. Available at: http://webarchive.nationalarchives.gov.uk/20120118164404/hcai.dh.gov.uk/files/2011/03/document_ambulance-_guidelines_reducing_infection_in_prehospital_final_271%e2%80%a6.pdf [Accessed 22 December 2014].

DoH, 2011
Department of Health, 2011. The Health and Social Care Act 2008: Code of Practice on the prevention and control of infections and related guidance. Available at: https://www.gov.uk/government/publications/the-health-and-social-care-act-2008-code-of-practice-on-the-prevention-and-control-of-infections-and-related-guidance [Accessed 24 December 2014].

DoH, 2011a
Department of Health, 2011. Safeguarding adults: the role of health services. Available at: https://www.gov.uk/government/publications/safeguarding-

adults-the-role-of-health-services [Accessed 21 January 2015].

DoH, 2013
Department of Health, 2013. *Managining Healthcare Fire Safely*, Available at: https://www.gov.uk/government/publications/managing-healthcare-fire-safety [Accessed 28th July, 2014].

DoH, 2013a
Department of Health, 2013. Health Technical Memorandum 07-01: Safe management of healthcare waste. Available at: https://www.gov.uk/government/uploads/system/uploads/attachment_data/file/167976/htm_07-01_final.pdf [Accessed 21 December 2014].

DoH, 2013b
Department of Health, 2013. *Berwick Review into Patient Safety*. Available at: https://www.gov.uk/government/publications/berwick-review-into-patient-safety [Accessed 31 December 2014].

DoH, 2013c
Department of Health, 2013. *The Health and Care System Explained*. Available at: https://www.gov.uk/government/publications/the-health-and-care-system-explained/the-health-and-care-system-explained [Accessed 31 December 2014].

DoH, 2013d
Department of Health, 2013. Winterbourne View Hospital: Department of Health review and response. Available at: https://www.gov.uk/government/publications/winterbourne-view-hospital-department-of-health-review-and-response [Accessed 21 January 2015].

Dougherty, 2011
Dougherty L and Lister SE, 2011. *The Royal Marsden Hospital Manual Of Clinical Nursing Procedures*. Chichester: Wiley-Blackwell.

Douglas, 2005
Douglas G, Nicol EF, Robertson C, et al., 2005. *Macleod's Clinical Examination*. 11th ed. Edinburgh: Elsevier Churchill Livingstone.

Drake, 2005
Drake RL, 2005. *Gray's Anatomy For Students*. Edinburgh: Churchill Livingstone.

Dunn, 2005
Dunn L, 2005. Pneumonia: classification, diagnosis and nursing management. *Nursing Standard*, 19(42), 50–54.

Durrer, 2003
Durrer B, Brugger H, Syme D, et al., 2003. The medical on-site treatment of hypothermia: ICAR-MEDCOM recommendation. *High Altitude Medicine & Biology*, 4(1), 99–103.

Durrington, 2005
Durrington HJ, Flubacher M, Ramsay CF, et al., 2005. Initial oxygen management in patients with an exacerbation of chronic obstructive pulmonary disease. *QJM*, 98(7), 499–504.

DWI, 2012
Drinking Water Inspectorate, 2012. Legislation. Available at: http://dwi.defra.gov.uk/stakeholders/legislation/ [Accessed 27 December 2014].

Dykes, 2002
Dykes M, 2002. *Crash Course: Anatomy*. 2nd ed. London: Mosby.

Eastridge, 2007
Eastridge BJ, Salinas J, McManus JG, et al., 2007. Hypotension begins at 110 mmHg: redefining 'hypotension' with data: *The Journal of Trauma: Injury, Infection, and Critical Care*, 63(2), 291–299.

EC, 2013
European Commission, 2013. *Chemicals At Work – A New Labelling System*. Available at: http://ec.europa.eu/social/blobservlet?docid=10450&langid=en [Accessed 15 December 2014].

ECA, 2011
European Chemicals Agency, 2011. Guidance on Labelling and Packaging in accordance with Regulation (EC) No 1272/2008. Available at: http://echa.europa.eu/documents/10162/13562/clp_labelling_en.pdf [Accessed 15 December 2014].

EEAST, 2013
East of England Ambulance Service NHS Trust, 2013. Major Incident Plan. Available at: http://www.eastamb.nhs.uk/board%20papers/2013/november%202013/27%2011%2013%20trust%20brd%20pub%20sess%20agenda%20item%2019%20civil%20cont%20act%20compliance%20b%20-%20major%20incident%20plan.pdf%20 [Accessed June 28, 2014].

EEAST, 2014
East of England Ambulance Service, 2014. *Clinical Manual 2014*. Bridgwater: Class Professional Publishing.

Enoch, 2009
Enoch S, Roshan A and Shah M, 2009. Emergency and early management of burns and scalds. BMJ, 338(apr08 1), b1037–b1037.

Epstein, 1980
Epstein RA, Reznik AM and Epstein MA, 1980. Determinants of distortions in CO2 catheter sampling systems: a mathematical model. *Respiration Physiology*, 41(1), 127–136.

Equality Act 2010
United Kingdom. Equality Act 2010. Available at: http://www.legislation.gov.uk/ukpga/2010/15/contents [Accessed 11 January 2015].

EROS, 2009
The European Registers of Stroke (EROS) Investigators, 2009. Incidence of stroke in Europe at the beginning of the 21st century. *Stroke*, 40(5), 1557–1563.

Evans, 2012
Evans JDW and Sutton P, 2012. *Cardiovascular System*. Edinburgh: Mosby/Elsevier.

Falk, 2003
Falk E and Thuesen L, 2003. Pathology of coronary microembolisation and no reflow. *Heart*, 89(9), 983–985.

Farley, 2011
Farley A and Hendry C, 2011. *The Physiological Effects Of Ageing*. 1st ed. Chichester: Wiley-Blackwell.

Feber, 2006
Feber T, 2006. Tracheostomy care for community nurses: basic principles. *British Journal of Community Nursing*, 11(5), 186.

Ferno, 2001
Ferno-Washington, 2001. *Model 125 KED User Manual*. Wilmington: Ferno-Washington.

Ferno, 2006
Ferno-Washington, 2006. *Scoop EXL Stretcher Series User Manual*, Wilmington: Ferno-Washington.

Ferreira, 2005
Ferreira, J. et al., 2005. *Evaluation of Manual Handling Tasks Involving the Use of Carry Chairs by UK Ambulance Personnel*, Sudbury: HSE Books.

Fick, 2002
Fick DM, Agostini JV and Inouye SK, 2002. Delirium Superimposed on Dementia: A Systematic Review. *Journal of the American Geriatrics Society*, 50(10), 1723–1732.

Food Safety Act 1990
United Kingdom, 1990. Food Safety Act 1990. Available at: http://www.legislation.gov.uk/ukpga/1990/16/contents [Accessed 27 December 2014].

Francis, 2013
Francis R, 2013. *Final report – Mid Staffordshire NHS Foundation Trust Public Inquiry*. Available at: http://www.midstaffspublicinquiry.com/report [Accessed 31 December 2014].

Francis, 2015
Francis R, 2015. *Freedom To Speak Up Review*. Available at: https://freedomtospeakup.org.uk/wp-content/uploads/2014/07/f2su_web.pdf [Accessed 15 February 2015].

Frank, 2010
Frank M, Schmucker U, Stengel D, et al., 2010. Proper estimation of blood loss on scene of trauma: tool or tale? *The Journal of Trauma: Injury, Infection, and Critical Care*, 69(5), 1191–1195.

Freyenhagen, 2009
Freyenhagen F, 2009. Personal autonomy and mental capacity. *Psychiatry*, 8(12), 465–467.

Frykberg, 1988
Frykberg ER & Tepas JJ, 1988. Terrorist bombings. Sections learned from Belfast to Beirut. *Annals of Surgery*, 208(5), 569–576.

Fuchs, 2012
Fuchs S, Yamamoto L, American Academy of Pediatrics, et al., 2012. *APLS: The Pediatric Emergency Medicine Resource*. Burlington: Jones & Bartlett Learning.

Gabbe, 2011
Gabbe BJ, de Steiger R, Esser M, et al., 2011. Predictors of mortality following severe pelvic ring fracture: results of a population-based study. *Injury*, 42(10), 985–991.

Garcia, 2004
Garcia TB and Miller GT, 2004. *Arrhythmia Recognition: The Art Of Interpretation*. Sudbury: Jones and Bartlett Publishers.

Garcia, 2015
Garcia TB, 2015. *12-lead ECG: The Art Of Interpretation*. 2nd ed. Burlington, MA: Jones & Bartlett Learning.

Garlapati, 2012
Garlapati AK and Ashwood N, 2012. An overview of pelvic ring disruption. *Trauma*, 14(2), 169–178.

Geerts, 2012
Geerts BF, van den Bergh L, Stijnen T, et al., 2012. Comprehensive review: is it better to use the Trendelenburg position or passive leg raising for the initial treatment of hypovolemia? *Journal of Clinical Anesthesia*, 24(8), 688–674.

GEMS, 2015
Snyder DR, American Geriatrics Society and National Association of Emergency Medical Technicians (U.S.), 2015. *Geriatric Education For Emergency Medical Services: (GEMS)*. 2nd ed. Burlington, MA: Jones & Bartlett Learning.

Gibbs, 1988
Gibbs G, 1988. *Learning By Doing: A Guide To Teaching And Learning Methods*. London: FEU.

Ginsberg, 2004
Ginsberg L, 2004. *Lecture Notes: Neurology*. 8th ed. Oxford: Wiley-Blackwell.

Gitelman, 2008
Gitelman A, Hishmeh S, Morelli BN, et al., 2008. Cauda equina syndrome: a comprehensive review. *American Journal of Orthopedics*, 37(11), 556–562.

GMC, 2009
General Medical Council, 2009. Confidentiality guidance: Disclosure after a patient's death. Available at: http://www.gmc-uk.org/guidance/ethical_guidance/confidentiality_70_72_disclosure_after_patient_death.asp [Accessed 8th December 2014].

Goldberg, 2007
Goldberg A, Southern DA, Galbraith PD, et al., 2007. Coronary dominance and prognosis of patients with acute coronary syndrome. *American Heart Journal*, 154(6), 1116–1122.

Golden, 1997
Golden FSC et al., 1997. *Review of Rescue and Immediate Post-immersion Problems: A Medical/Ergonomic Viewpoint*, Sudbury: HSE Books.

Granville-Chapman, 2011
Granville-Chapman J, Jacobs N and Midwinter MJ, 2011. Pre-hospital haemostatic dressings: a systematic review. *Injury*, 42(5), 447–459.

Gray, 2013
Gray A, Ward K, Lees F, et al., 2013. The epidemiology of adults with severe sepsis and septic shock in Scottish emergency departments. *Emergency Medicine Journal*, 30(5), 397–401.

Greaves, 2008
Greaves I, Porter K, Ryan J, et al., 2008. *Trauma Care Manual*. 2nd ed. London: Hodder Arnold.

Greaves, 2010
Greaves I, Porter Keith and Smith J, 2010. *Practical Prehospital Care: The Principles And Practice Of Immediate Care*. 1st ed. London: Churchill Livingstone.

Gregory, 2010a
Gregory P, Ward A and Sanders MJ, 2010. *Sanders' Paramedic Textbook*. Edinburgh: Mosby.

Gregory, 2010b
Gregory P, 2010. *Manual Of Clinical Paramedic Procedures*. Chichester: Wiley-Blackwell.

Guly, 2010
Guly HR, Bouamra O, Little R, et al., 2010. Testing the validity of the atls classification of hypovolaemic shock. *Resuscitation*, 81(9), 1142–1147.

Gupta, 2009
Gupta A, Taly AB, Srivastava A, et al., 2009. Non-traumatic spinal cord lesions: epidemiology, complications, neurological and functional outcome of rehabilitation. *Spinal Cord*, 47(4), 307–311.

Hammell, 2009
Hammell CL and Henning JD, 2009. Prehospital management of severe traumatic brain injury. *BMJ*, 338, b1683.

Harbison, 2003
Harbison J, Hossain O, Jenkinson D, et al., 2003. Diagnostic accuracy of stroke referrals from primary care, emergency room physicians, and ambulance staff using the face arm speech test. *Stroke*, 34(1), 71–76.

Harrison, 2007
Harrison P, 2007. *Managing Spinal Cord Injury: The First 48 Hours*. Milton Keynes: Spinal Injuries Association.

Hart, 2006
Hart CA and Thomson APJ, 2006. Meningococcal disease and its management in children. *BMJ*, 333(7570), 685–690.

Hartley, 1999
Hartley P, 1999. *Interpersonal Communication*. 2nd ed. London: Routledge.

Hasler, 2011
Hasler RM, Nüesch E, Jüni P, et al., 2011. Systolic blood pressure below 110 mmHg is associated with increased mortality in blunt major trauma patients: multicentre cohort study. *Resuscitation*, 82(9), 1202–1207.

Hasler, 2011a
Hasler RM, Exadaktylos AK, Bouamra O, et al., 2011. Epidemiology and predictors of spinal injury in adult major trauma patients: European cohort study. *European Spine Journal*, 20(12), 2174–2180.

Hasler, 2012
Hasler RM, Nüesch E, Jüni P, et al., 2012. Systolic blood pressure below 110 mmHg is associated with increased mortality in penetrating major trauma patients: multicentre cohort study. *Resuscitation*, 83(4), 476–481.

Hazardous Waste Regulations 2005
United Kingdom, 2005. The Hazardous Waste (England and Wales) Regulations 2005. Available at: http://www.legislation.gov.uk/uksi/2005/894/contents/made [Accessed 27 December 2014].

HC, 2009
The Healthcare Commission, 2009. *Investigation Into Mid Staffordshire NHS Foundation Trust*. London: Healthcare Commission. Available at: http://webarchive.nationalarchives.gov.uk/20110504135228/http://www.cqc.org.uk/_db/_documents/investigation_into_mid_staffordshire_nhs_foundation_trust.pdf [Accessed 31 December 2014].

HCPC, 2012
Health and Care Professions Council, 2012. Standards of Conduct, Performance and Ethics. Available at: http://www.hpc-uk.org/aboutregistration/standards/standardsofconductperformanceandethics/ [Accessed 31 December 2014].

HCPC, 2014
Health and Care Professions Council, 2014. Standards of Proficiency – Paramedics. Available at: http://www.hcpc-uk.org.uk/publications/standards/index.asp?id=48%20 [Accessed 8 December 2014].

Health and Safety at Work etc. Act 1974
United Kingdom, 1974. Health and Safety at Work etc. Act 1974. Available at: http://www.legislation.gov.uk/ukpga/1974/37 [Accessed 27 December 2014].

Health and Social Care Act 2008
United Kingdom, 2008. Health and Social Care Act 2008. Available at: http://www.legislation.gov.uk/ukpga/2008/14/contents [Accessed 27 December 2014].

Helm, 2003
Helm M, Schuster R, Hauke J, et al., 2003. Tight control of prehospital ventilation by capnography in major trauma victims. *British Journal of Anaesthesia*, 90(3), 327–332.

Henry, 2008
Henry C & Seymour J, 2008. Advanced Care Planning: A Guide for Health and Social Care Staff. Available at: http://www.ncpc.org.uk/sites/default/files/advancecareplanning.pdf [Accessed 14 August, 2014].

Hettiaratchy, 2004
Hettiaratchy S and Papini R, 2004. Initial management of a major burn: II – assessment and resuscitation. *BMJ*, 329(7457), 101–103.

Hinkelbein, 2007
Hinkelbein J, Genzwuerker HV, Sogl R, et al., 2007. Effect of nail polish on oxygen saturation determined by pulse oximetry in critically ill patients. *Resuscitation*, 72(1), 82–91.

HMFSIPS, 1998
HM Fire Service Inspectorate Publications Section, 1998. *Fire Service Manual. Vol. 1, No. 1*. London: Stationery Office.

HMG, 2006
HM Government, 2006. *Making Your Premises Safe*, Available at: https://www.gov.uk/government/publications/making-your-premises-safe-from-fire [Accessed 28 July, 2014].

Hodgetts, 2006
Hodgetts TJ, Mahoney PF, Russell MQ, et al., 2006. Abc to <c>abc: redefining the military trauma paradigm. *Emergency Medicine Journal*, 23(10), 745–746.

Holland, 2011
Holland K, 2011. Factsheet: learning disabilities. Available at: http://www.bild.org.uk/EasySiteWeb/GatewayLink.aspx?alId=2522 [Accessed 14 June 2015].

Holt, 2010
Holt TA, 2010. *ABC Of Diabetes*. 6th ed. ABC series, Chichester: Wiley-Blackwell/BMJ.

Howlett, 2011
Howlett JG, 2011. Acute heart failure: sections learned so far. *Canadian Journal of Cardiology*, 27(3), 284–295.

HPA, 2009
Health Protection Agency, 2009. *Generic Incident Management*. Available at: http://webarchive.nationalarchives.gov.uk/20140714084352/http://www.hpa.org.uk/webc/hpawebfile/hpaweb_c/1194947395416 [Accessed 5 January 2015].

HPA, 2009a
Health Protection Agency, 2009. ORCHIDS project: Optimisation through Research of Chemical Incident Decontamination Systems. Available from: http://www.orchidsproject.eu/index.html [Accessed 6 June 2015].

HSCIC, 2013
Health and Social Care Information Centre, 2013. NHS written complaints data released. Available at: http://www.hscic.gov.uk/article/3414/nhs-written-complaints-data-released [Accessed 19 January 2015].

HSCIC, 2014
Health and Social Care Information Centre, 2014. Caldicott Guardians. Available at:http://systems.hscic.gov.uk/infogov/caldicott [Accessed 8 December 2014].

HSCIC, 2014a
Health and Social Care Information Centre, 2014. NHS Pathways. Available at: http://systems.hscic.gov.uk/pathways [Accessed 6 January 2015].

HSCIC, 2014b
Health and Social Care Information Centre, 2014. *Accident And Emergency Attendances In England – 2012–13*. Available at: http://www.hscic.gov.uk/catalogue/pub13464/acci-emer-atte-eng-2012-13-data.xls [Accessed 23 December 2014].

HSE, 1998
Health and Safety Commission, 1998. *Safe Use Of Lifting Equipment: Lifting Operations And Lifting Equipment Regulations 1998*. Available at: http://www.hse.gov.uk/pubns/indg290.pdf [Accessed 29 December 2014].

HSE, 2003
Health and Safety Executive, 2003. The principles of good manual handling: Achieving a consensus. Available at: http://www.hse.gov.uk/research/rrpdf/rr097.pdf [Accessed 21 August, 2014].

HSE, 2004
Health and Safety Executive, 2004. Manual Handling Operations Regulations 1992 (as amended): Guidance on Regulations. Available at: http://www.hse.gov.uk/pubns/priced/l23.pdf [Accessed 21 August, 2014].

HSE, 2004a
Health and Safety Executive, 2004. *Manual Handling: Manual Handling Operations Regulations 1992, Guidance On Regulations L23*. Available at: http://www.hse.gov.uk/pubns/priced/l23.pdf [Accessed 29 December 2014].

HSE, 2006
Health and Safety Executive, 2006. *Essentials of Health and Safety at Work*. Sudbury: HSE Books.

HSE, 2007
Health and Safety Executive, 2007. *Managing The Causes Of Work-related Stress: A Step-by-step Approach Using The Management Standards*. Suffolk: HSE.

HSE, 2008
Health and Safety Executive, 2008. *Working Together To Reduce Stress At Work*. Available at: http://www.hse.gov.uk/pubns/indg424.pdf [Accessed 12 August 2014].

HSE, 2009
Health and Safety Executive, 2009. *Health and Safety Law*. Available at: http://www.hse.gov.uk/pubns/law.pdf [Accessed 29 December 2014].

HSE, 2011
Health and Safety Executive, 2011. Risk factors associated with pushing and pulling loads. Available at: http://www.hse.gov.uk/msd/pushpull/risks.htm [Accessed 21 August, 2014].

HSE, 2012
Health and Safety Executive, 2012. Manual handling at work. Available at: http://www.hse.gov.uk/pubns/indg143.pdf [Accessed 21 August, 2014].

HSE, 2013
Health and Safety Executive, 2013. Handling injuries in Great Britain, 2013. Available at: http://www.hse.gov.uk/statistics/causinj/handling-injuries.pdf [Accessed 21 August, 2014].

HSE, 2013a
Health and Safety Executive, 2013. *Managing For Health And Safety*. Available at: http://www.hse.gov.uk/pubns/priced/hsg65.pdf [Accessed 29 December 2014].

HSE, 2013b
Health and Safety Executive, 2013. *Control Of Substances Hazardous To Health: Approved Code Of Practice*. Available at: http://www.hse.gov.uk/pubns/priced/l5.pdf [Accessed 29 December 2014].

HSE, 2013c
Health and Safety Executive, 2013. *Personal Protective Equipment (PPE) At Work*. Available at: http://www.hse.gov.uk/pubns/indg174.pdf [Accessed 29 December 2014].

HSE, 2014
Health and Safety Executive, 2014. Work Related Stress: Signs and Symptoms. Available at: http://www.hse.gov.uk/stress/furtheradvice/signsandsymptoms.htm [Accessed 8 December 2014].

HSE, 2014a
Health and Safety Executive, 2014. Risk management. Available at: http://www.hse.gov.uk/risk/controlling-risks.htm [Accessed 9 December 2014].

HSE, 2014b
Health and Safety Executive, 2014. Risk assessment – A brief guide to controlling risks in the workplace. Available at: http://www.hse.gov.uk/pubns/indg163.htm [Accessed 9 December 2014].

HSE, 2014c
Health and Safety Executive, 2014. *Safe Use Of Work Equipment*. Available at: http://www.hse.gov.uk/pubns/priced/l22.pdf [Accessed 29 December 2014].

HSE, 2014d
Health and Safety Executive, 2014. *Carriage Of Dangerous Goods Manual*. Available at: http://www.hse.gov.uk/cdg/manual/index.htm [Accessed 15 December 2014].

Hüpfl, 2010
Hüpfl M, Selig HF and Nagele P, 2010. Chest-compression-only versus standard cardiopulmonary resuscitation: a meta-analysis. *The Lancet*, 376(9752), 1552–1557.

Iacono, 2005
Iacono L and Lyons K, 2005. Making GCS as easy as 1, 2, 3, 4, 5, 6. *Journal of Trauma Nursing*, 12(3), 77–81.

Iankova, 2006
Iankova A, 2006. The Glasgow Coma Scale. *Emergency Nurse*, 14(8), 30–35.

Idris, 2003
Idris AH et al., 2003. Recommended guidelines for uniform reporting of data from drowning. *Circulation*, 108(20), 2565–2574.

ILAE, 1993
International League Against Epilepsy, 1993. Guidelines for Epidemiologic Studies on Epilepsy. *Epilepsia*, 34(4), 592–596.

Ireland, 2011
Ireland S, Endacott R, Cameron P, et al., 2011. The incidence and significance of accidental hypothermia in major trauma – A prospective observational study. *Resuscitation*, 82(3), 300–306.

James, 2004
James CY, Riemann BL, Munkasy BA, et al., 2004. Comparison of cervical spine motion during application among 4 rigid immobilization collars. *Journal of Athletic Training*, 39(2), 138–145.

James, 2011
James B, 2011. *Lecture Notes: Ophthalmology*. 11th ed. Chichester, West Sussex: Wiley-Blackwell.

Jasper, 2003
Jasper M, 2003. *Beginning Reflective Practice*. Cheltenham: Nelson Thornes.

JCO, 2010a
Judicial Communications Office, 2010. *Coroner's Inquests into the London Bombings of the 7 July 2005*, Available at: http://webarchive.nationalarchives.gov.uk/20120216072438/http:/7julyinquests.independent.gov.uk/ [Accessed 15 January 2015].

JCO, 2010b
Judicial Communications Office, 2010. *Coroner's Inquests into the London Bombings of 7 July 2005: Hearing Transcripts*. Available at: http://webarchive.nationalarchives.gov.uk/20120216072438/http://7julyinquests.independent.gov.uk/hearing_transcripts/09122010am.htm [Accessed 28 June 2014].

Jenkins, 2008
Jenkins JL, McCarthy M, Sauer L, et al., 2008. Mass-casualty triage: time for an evidence-based approach. *Prehospital Disaster Medicine*, 23(1), 3–8.

JESIP, 2013
Joint Emergency Services Interoperability Programme, 2013. Joint doctrine: the interoperability framework. Available at: http://www.jesip.org.uk/wp-content/uploads/2013/07/jesip-joint-doctrine.pdf [Accessed 10 February 2015].

Johnson, 2004
Johnson S and Henderson SO, 2004. Myth: the Trendelenburg position improves circulation in cases of shock. *CJEM*, 6(1), 48.

Johnson, 2012
Johnson G, Hill-Smith, Ian, 2012. *The Minor Illness Manual*. London: Radcliffe Publishing.

JRCALC, 2008
Joint Royal Colleges Ambulance Liaison Committee, 2008. A Critical Reassessment of Ambulance Service Airway Management in Pre-Hospital Care. Available at: http://www.jrcalc.org.uk/airway17.6.8.pdf [Accessed June 19, 2014].

Kaeser, 2010
Kaeser P-F and Kawasaki A, 2010. Disorders of pupillary structure and function. *Neurologic Clinics*, 28(3), 657–677.

Kalson, 2012
Kalson NS et al., 2012. Burns represent a significant proportion of the total serious trauma workload in England and Wales. *Burns: Journal of the International Society for Burn Injuries*, 38(3), 330–339.

Kapit, 2000
Kapit W, Macey RI and Meisami E, 2000. *The Physiology Coloring Book*. San Francisco: Addison Wesley Longman.

Kapit, 2001
Kapit W and Elson LM, 2001. *The Anatomy Coloring Book*. 3rd ed. London: Benjamin Cummings.

Kauffman, 2014
Kauffman M, 2014. *History And Physical Examination: A Common Sense Approach*. Burlington, MA: Jones & Bartlett Learning.

Kerber, 2012
Kerber RE, 2012. Hands-on defibrillation – the end of 'I'm clear, you're clear, we're all clear'? *Journal of the American Heart Association*, 1(5), e005496.

Kilner, 2002
Kilner T, 2002. Triage decisions of prehospital emergency health care providers, using a multiple casualty scenario paper exercise. *Emergency Medicine Journal*, 19(4), 348–353.

Kimmel, 1999
Kimmel EC and Still KR, 1999. Acute lung injury, acute respiratory distress syndrome and inhalation injury: an overview. *Drug and Chemical Toxicology*, 22(1), 91–128.

King, 2014
King D, Morton R and Bevan C, 2014. How to use capillary refill time. *Archives of Disease in Childhood – Education & Practice Edition*, 99(3), 111–116.

Kligfield, 2007
Kligfield P, Gettes LS, Bailey JJ, et al., 2007. Recommendations for the standardization and interpretation of the electrocardiogram Part I: the electrocardiogram and its technology. A scientific statement from the American Heart Association Electrocardiography and Arrhythmias Committee, Council on Clinical Cardiology; the American College of Cardiology Foundation; and the Heart Rhythm Society, endorsed by the International Society for Computerized Electrocardiology. *Journal of the American College of Cardiology*, 49(10), 1109–1127.

Knight, 2008
Knight J and Nigam Y, 2008. Exploring the anatomy and physiology of ageing. Part 2 – the respiratory system. *Nursing Times*, 104(32), 24–25.

Knight, 2008a
Knight J and Nigam Y, 2008. Exploring the anatomy and physiology of ageing. Part 1 – the cardiovascular system. *Nursing Times*, 104(31), 26–27.

Knight, 2008b
Knight J and Nigam Y, 2008. Exploring the anatomy and physiology of ageing. Part 5 – the nervous system. *Nursing Times*, 104(35), 18–19.

Knight, 2008c
Knight J and Nigam Y, 2008. Exploring the anatomy and physiology of ageing. Part 10 – muscles and bone. *Nursing Times*, 104(48), 22–23.

Knops, 2011
Knops SP, 2011. Comparison of three different pelvic circumferential compression devices: a biomechanical cadaver study. *The Journal of Bone and Joint Surgery (American)*, 93(3), 230.

Kodali, 2013
Kodali BS, 2013. Capnography Outside the Operating Rooms. *Anesthesiology*, 118(1), 192–201.

Koster, 2005
Koster R, 2005. Vf waveform characteristics predict defibrillation success. Available at: http://www.escardio.org/congresses/esc_congress_2005/documents/koster-fp1294-slides-congress05.pdf [Accessed 11 August 2014].

Koster, 2010
Koster RW, Baubin MA, Bossaert LL, et al., 2010. European Resuscitation Council Guidelines for Resuscitation 2010 Section 2. Adult basic life support and use of automated external defibrillators. *Resuscitation*, 81(10), 1277–1292.

Krassioukov, 2009
Krassioukov A, Warburton DE, Teasell R, et al., 2009. A systematic review of the management of autonomic dysreflexia after spinal cord injury. *Archives of Physical Medicine and Rehabilitation*, 90(4), 682–695.

Krassioukov, 2012
Krassioukov A, 2012. Autonomic dysreflexia. *Clinical Journal of Sport Medicine*, 22(1), 39–45.

Krell, 2006
Krell J, McCoy M, Sparto P, et al., 2006. Comparison of the ferno scoop stretcher with the long backboard for spinal immobilization. *Prehospital Emergency Care*, 10(1), 46–51.

Krous, 2010
Krous H, 2010. Sudden unexpected death in infancy and the dilemma of defining the sudden infant death syndrome. *Current Pediatric Reviews*, 6(1), 5–12.

Lange, 2010
Lange RT, Iverson GL, Brubacher JR, et al., 2010. Effect of blood alcohol level on Glasgow Coma Scale scores following traumatic brain injury. *Brain Injury*, 24(7/8), 919–927.

Layon, 2009
Layon AJ and Modell JH, 2009. Drowning: update 2009. *Anesthesiology*, 110(6), 1390–1401.

Lee, 2004
Lee JA, 2004. Sudden unexpected death in infancy. Available at: http://www.rcpath.org/resources/rcpath/migrated%20resources/documents/s/sudi%20report%20for%20web.pdf [Accessed 17 August 2014].

Lee, 2007a
Lee C, Revell M, Porter K, et al., 2007. The prehospital management of chest injuries: a consensus statement. faculty of pre-hospital care, Royal College of Surgeons of Edinburgh. *Emergency Medicine Journal: EMJ*, 24(3), 220–224.

Lee, 2007b
Lee C, Porter KM and Hodgetts TJ, 2007. Tourniquet use in the civilian prehospital setting. *Emergency Medicine Journal*, 24(8), 584–587.

Lee, 2011
Lee JK and Vadas P, 2011. Anaphylaxis: mechanisms and management. *Clinical & Experimental Allergy*, 41(7), 923–938.

Leigh-Smith, 2005
Leigh-Smith S and Harris T, 2005. Tension pneumothorax – time for a re-think? *Emergency Medicine Journal*, 22(1), 8–16.

LESLP, 2012
London Emergency Services Liaison Panel, 2012. Major Incident Procedure Manual. Available at: http://www.leslp.gov.uk/docs/major_incident_procedure_manual_8th_ed.pdf [Accessed June 28, 2014].

Levy, 2010
Levy M, Dellinger R, Townsend S, et al., 2010. The Surviving Sepsis Campaign: results of an international guideline-based performance improvement program targeting severe sepsis. *Intensive Care Medicine*, 36(2), 222–231.

Lewin, 2008
Lewin J and Maconochie I, 2008. Capillary refill time in adults. *Emergency Medicine Journal*, 25(6), 325–326.

Lifting Operations and Lifting Equipment Regulations 1998
United Kingdom, 1998. The Lifting Operations and Lifting Equipment Regulations 1998. Available at: http://www.legislation.gov.uk/uksi/1998/2307/contents/made [Accessed 29 December 2014].

Lipman, 2013
Lipman GS, Eifling KP, Ellis MA, et al., 2013. Wilderness Medical Society practice guidelines for the prevention and treatment of heat-related illness. *Wilderness & Environmental Medicine*, 24(4), 351–361.

Lissauer, 2007
Lissauer T and Clayden G, 2007. *Illustrated Textbook Of Paediatrics*. 3rd ed. Edinburgh: Mosby.

LOLER, 1998
United Kingdom, 1998. The Lifting Operations and Lifting Equipment Regulations. Available at: http://www.legislation.gov.uk/uksi/1998/2307/contents/made [Accessed August 21, 2014].

Lonnecker, 2001
Lonnecker S and Schoder V, 2001. Hypothermia after burn injury – influence of pre-hospital management. *Der Chirurg*, 72(2), 164–167.

Lord, 2005
Lord SR and Davis PR, 2005. Drowning, near drowning and immersion syndrome. *Journal of the Royal Army Medical Corps*, 151(4), 250.

Luke, 2010
Leenen L, 2010. Pelvic fractures: soft tissue trauma. *European Journal of Trauma and Emergency Surgery*, 36(2), 117–123.

MacDuff, 2010
MacDuff A, Arnold A and Harvey J, 2010. Management of spontaneous pneumothorax: British Thoracic Society pleural disease guideline 2010. *Thorax*, 65(Suppl 2), ii18–ii31.

Mackway-Jones, 2012
Mackway-Jones K, Carley S and Advanced Life Support Group, 2012. *Major Incident Medical Management And Support: The Practical Approach At The Scene*. Chichester: Wiley-Blackwell.

Macleod, 2005
Douglas G, Nicol EF, Robertson C, et al., 2005. *Macleod's Clinical Examination*. 11th ed. Edinburgh: Elsevier Churchill Livingstone.

Maconochie, 2012
Maconochie I, Bingham R and Mitchell S, 2012. *European Paediatric Life Support Manual*. 3rd ed. London: Resuscitation Council (UK).

Magill-Cuerden, 2011
Magill-Cuerden J and MacDonald S, 2011. *Mayes' Midwifery: A Textbook for Midwives*, Edinburgh: Bailliere-Tindall.

Magner, 2004
Magner JJ, 2004. Heart failure. *British Journal of Anaesthesia*, 93(1), 74–85.

Management of Health and Safety at Work Regulations 1999
United Kingdom, 1999. The Management of Health and Safety at Work Regulations 1999. Available at: http://www.legislation.gov.uk/uksi/1999/3242/contents/made [Accessed 29 December 2014].

Mancia, 2013
Mancia G et al., 2013. 2013 ESH/ESC Guidelines for the management of arterial hypertension The Task Force for the management of arterial hypertension of the European Society of Hypertension (ESH) and of the European Society of Cardiology (ESC). *European Heart Journal*, 34(28), 2159–2219.

Mangar International, 2012
Mangar International, 2012. *ELK user instructions and warranty*, Available at: http://mangar.co.uk/wp-content/uploads/2013/07/me0117-3_elk_multi_language_user_instructions.pdf [Accessed August 20, 2014].

Marieb, 2013
Marieb E and Hoehn K, 2013. *Human Anatomy And Physiology*. New York: Pearson.

Manual Handling Operations Regulations 1992
United Kingdom, 1992. The Manual Handling Operations Regulations 1992. Available at: http://www.hse.gov.uk/pubns/priced/l23.pdf [Accessed 29 December 2014].

Martineau, 2006
Martineau L and Shek PN, 2006. Evaluation of a bi-layer wound dressing for burn care: I. Cooling and wound healing properties. *Burns*, 32(1), 70–76.

Matis, 2008
Matis G and Birbilis T, 2008. The Glasgow Coma Scale – a brief review. Past, present, future. *Acta Neurologica Belgica*, 108(3), 75–89.

McCormack, 2010
McCormack R, Strauss EJ, Alwattar BJ, et al., 2010. Diagnosis and management of pelvic fractures. *Bulletin of the NYU hospital for joint diseases*, 68(4), 281.

McGrath, 2012
McGrath BA et al., 2012. Multidisciplinary guidelines for the management of tracheostomy and laryngectomy airway emergencies: Tracheostomy management guidelines. *Anaesthesia*, 67(9), 1025–1041.

McMurray, 2012
McMurray JJV et al., 2012. ESC guidelines for the diagnosis and treatment of acute and chronic heart failure 2012: The Task Force for the Diagnosis and Treatment of Acute and Chronic Heart Failure 2012 of the European Society of Cardiology. Developed in collaboration with the Heart Failure Association (HFA) of the ESC. *European Heart Journal*, 33(14), 1787–1847.

Mears, 1986
Mears DC, 1986. *Pelvic And Acetabular Fractures*. Thorofare: Slack.

Medicines Act 1968
United Kingdom, 1968. Medicines Act 1968. Available at: http://www.legislation.gov.uk/ukpga/1968/67 [Accessed 13 June 2015].

Meldrum, 1973
Meldrum BS and Horton RW, 1973. Physiology of status epilepticus in primates. *Archives of Neurology*, 28(1), 1.

Mencap, 2008
Mencap, 2008. About profound and multiple learning disabilities. Available at: https://www.mencap.org.uk/ [Accessed 14 June 2015].

Mencap, 2015
Mencap, 2015. About learning disability. Available at: https://www.mencap.org.uk/about-learning-disability/about-learning-disability [Accessed 14 June 2015].

Mental Capacity Act 2005
United Kingdom, 2005. Mental Capacity Act 2005. Available at: http://www.legislation.gov.uk/ukpga/2005/9/contents [Accessed January 5 2015].

Middleton, 2012
Middleton PM, 2012. Practical use of the Glasgow Coma Scale: A comprehensive narrative review of GCS methodology. *Australasian Emergency Nursing Journal*, 15(3), 170–183.

Misuse of Drugs Act 1971
United Kingdom, 1971. Misuse of Drugs Act 1971. Available at: http://www.legislation.gov.uk/ukpga/1971/38/contents [Accessed 13 June 2015].

Misuse of Drugs Regulations 2001
United Kingdom, 2001. The Misuse of Drugs Regulations 2001. Available at: http://www.legislation.gov.uk/uksi/2001/3998/contents/made [Accessed 13 June 2015].

Mittal, 2009
Mittal R, Vermani E, Tweedie I, et al., 2009. Critical care in the emergency department: traumatic brain injury. *Emergency Medicine Journal*, 26(7), 513–517.

MOD, 2008
Ministry of Defence, 2008. Health and safety risk assessment. Available at: https://www.gov.uk/government/uploads/system/uploads/attachment_data/file/28827/leaf_39.pdf [Accessed 12th December 2014].

Modell, 1999
Modell JH et al., 1999. Drowning without aspiration: is this an appropriate diagnosis? *Journal of Forensic Sciences*, 44, 1119–1123.

Montalescot, 2013
Montalescot G, Sechtem U, Achenbach S, et al., 2013. 2013 ESC guidelines on the management of stable coronary artery disease: the task force on the management of stable coronary artery disease of the European Society of Cardiology. *European Heart Journal*, 34(38), 2949–3003.

Moorhouse, 2007
Moorhouse I et al., 2007. A realistic model for catastrophic external haemorrhage training. *Journal of the Royal Army Medical Corps*, 153(2), 99–101.

Moppett, 2007
Moppett IK, 2007. Traumatic brain injury: assessment, resuscitation and early management. *British Journal of Anaesthesia*, 99(1), 18–31.

Moritz, 1947
Moritz AR and Henriques FC, 1947. Studies of Thermal Injury. *The American Journal of Pathology*, 23(5), 695–720.

Moscati, 1999
Moscati R, Billittier AJ, Marshall B et al., 1999. Blood loss estimation by out-of-hospital emergency care providers. *Prehospital Emergency Care: official journal of the National Association of EMS Physicians and the National Association of State EMS Directors*, 3(3), 239–242.

Moye, 2007
Moye J and Marson DC, 2007. Assessment of decision-making capacity in older adults: an emerging area of practice and research. *The Journals of Gerontology. Series B, Psychological Sciences and Social Sciences*, 62(1), 3–11.

Muehlberger, 2010
Muehlberger T et al., 2010. Emergency pre-hospital care of burn patients. *The Surgeon*, 8(2), 101–104.

Mukherjee, 2008
Mukherjee S and Bhide A, 2008. Antepartum haemorrhage. *Obstetrics, Gynaecology & Reproductive Medicine*, 18(12), 335–339.

Müller, 2006
Müller D, Agrawal R and Arntz H-R, 2006. How sudden is sudden cardiac death? *Circulation*, 114(11), 1146–1150.

Munden, 2002
Munden J and Thorn Barrows S, 2002. *Pathophysiology Made Incredibly Easy*. Philadelphia: Lippincott Williams & Wilkins.

Murakami, 2003
Murakami K and Traber DL, 2003. Pathophysiological basis of smoke inhalation injury. *Physiology*, 18(3), 125–129.

Mutschler, 2013
Mutschler M, Nienaber U, Brockamp T, et al., 2013. A critical reappraisal of the ATLS classification of hypovolaemic shock: does it really reflect clinical reality? *Resuscitation*, 84(3), 309–313.

Mutschler, 2014
Mutschler M, Nienaber U, Müntzberg M, et al., 2014. Assessment of hypovolaemic shock at scene: is the PHTLS classification of hypovolaemic shock really valid? *Emergency Medicine Journal*, 31(1), 35–40.

NAEMT, 2011
National Association of Emergency Medical Technicians, 2011. *Advanced Medical Life Support*. St. Louis, MO: Jones and Bartlett.

NAEMT, 2014
National Association of Emergency Medical Technicians (U.S.) and American College of Surgeons, 2014. *PHTLS: Prehospital Trauma Life Support*. 8th ed. Burlington, MA: Jones & Bartlett Learning.

NAO, 2002
National Audit Office, 2002. Facing the Challenge: NHS Emergency Planning in England. Available at: http://www.nao.org.uk/report/facing-the-challenge-nhs-emergency-planning-in-england/ [Accessed June 28, 2014].

NAO, 2005
National Audit Office, 2005. *Reducing Brain Damage: Faster Access To Better Stroke Care*. London: Stationery Office Books.

NAO, 2010
National Audit Office, 2010. *Progress In Improving Stroke Care: Department Of Health*. London: Stationery Office.

NARU, 2012
National Ambulance Resilience Unit, 2012. *National Ambulance Service Command and Control Guidance*. London: Association of Ambulance Chief Executives.

NASMeD, 2013
National Ambulance Service Medical Directors Group, 2013. Triage Sieve. Available at: http://naru.org.uk/wp-content/uploads/2014/02/naru-triage-sieve-ju5a304d.pdf%20 [Accessed July 7, 2014].

NatCen, 2013
NatCen Social Research, 2013. British Social Attitudes research for Dying Matters. Available at: http://www.dyingmatters.org/sites/default/files/bsa30_full_report.pdf [Accessed March 25, 2014].

NBCG, 2008
National Burn Care Group, 2008. *UK Burn Injury Data 1986-2007*, Available at: http://www.ibidb.org/

downloads/doc_download/4-2008-first-ibid-report[Accessed July 16, 2014].

NBCRC, 2001
National Burn Care Review Committee, 2001. *National Burn Care Review*, Available at: http://www.britishburnassociation.org/downloads/nbcr2001.pdf [Accessed Jul 16, 2014].

NCEC, 2013
National Chemical Emergency Centre, 2013. Dangerous Good Emergency Action Code List. Available at: http://the-ncec.com/assets/resources/eac-dangerous-goods-list-2013.pdf [Accessed 15 December 2014].

NEAS, 2010
North East Ambulance Service NHS Trust, 2010. Infection Prevention and Control Policy and Strategy. Available at: https://www.neas.nhs.uk/media/15946/11%20-%20infection%20prevention%20and%20control%20policy.pdf [Accessed 22 December 2014].

NEAS, 2011
North East Ambulance Service NHS Trust, 2011. Ambulance Response Categories Explained. Available at: https://www.neas.nhs.uk/our-services/accident-emergency/ambulance-response-categories-explained.aspx [Accessed 6 January 2015].

NEAS, 2014
North East Ambulance Service NHS Trust, 2014. *Clinical handbook 2014*, Bridgwater: Class Professional Publishing.

Neligan, 2010
Neligan A and Shorvon SD, 2010. Frequency and prognosis of convulsive status epilepticus of different causes: a systematic review. *Archives of Neurology*, 67(8), 931–940.

NG, 2001
Neuropathology Group of the Medical Research Council Cognitive Function and Ageing Study, 2001. Pathological correlates of late-onset dementia in a multicentre, community-based population in England and Wales. Neuropathology Group of the Medical Research Council Cognitive Function and Ageing Study (MRC CFAS). *Lancet*, 357(9251), 169–175.

NHS Choices, 2011
NHS Choices, 2011. Authorities and Trusts. Available at: http://www.nhs.uk/servicedirectories/pages/ambulancetrustlisting.aspx [Accessed 8 January 2014].

NHS Choices, 2013
NHS Choices, 2013. What is a learning disability? Available at: http://www.nhs.uk/Livewell/Childrenwithalearningdisability/Pages/Whatislearningdisability.aspx [Accessed 14 June 2015].

NHS Choices, 2014
NHS Choices, 2014. Ten stress busters. Available at: http://www.nhs.uk/conditions/stress-anxiety-depression/pages/reduce-stress.aspx [Accessed 8th December 2014].

NHS Choices, 2014a
NHS Choices, 2014. Raising low self-esteem. Available at:http://www.nhs.uk/livewell/mentalhealth/pages/

dealingwithlowself-esteem.aspx [Accessed 11 January 2015].

NHS Choices, 2015
NHS Choices, 2015. Abuse and neglect of vulnerable adults. Available at: http://www.nhs.uk/conditions/social-care-and-support-guide/pages/vulnerable-people-abuse-safeguarding.aspx [Accessed 21 January 2015].

NHS England, 2013
NHS England, 2013. A guide to the FFP3 respirator. Available at: http://www.england.nhs.uk/wp-content/uploads/2013/12/guide-ffp3-leaflet-v2.pdf [Accessed 22 December 2014].

NHS England, 2014
NHS England, 2014. Confidentiality Policy. Available at: http://www.england.nhs.uk/wp-content/uploads/2013/06/conf-policy-1.pdf [Accessed 8th December 2014].

NHS England, 2014a
NHS England, 2014. Transforming Urgent and Emergency Care Services in England. Available at: http://www.nhs.uk/nhsengland/keogh-review/documents/uecreviewupdate.fv.pdf [Accessed 5 January 2015].

NHS England, 2015
NHS England, 2015. Ambulance Quality Indicators Data 2014–15. Available at: http://www.england.nhs.uk/statistics/statistical-work-areas/ambulance-quality-indicators/ambulance-quality-indicators-data-2014-15/ [Accessed 6 January 2015].

NHS England, 2015a
NHS England, 2015. Equality and diversity. Available at: http://www.england.nhs.uk/about/equality/ [Accessed 11 January 2015].

NICE, 2004
National Institute for Health and Care Excellence, 2004. Type 1 diabetes. Available at: http://www.nice.org.uk/guidance/cg15 [Accessed 6 November 2014].

NICE, 2009
National Institute for Health and Care Excellence, 2009. When to suspect child maltreatment. Available at: http://www.nice.org.uk/guidance/cg89 [Accessed 21 January 2015].

NICE, 2010
National Institute for Health and Care Excellence, 2010. Chronic obstructive pulmonary disease: management of chronic obstructive pulmonary disease in adults in primary and secondary care. National Clinical Guideline Centre, Available at: http://guidance.nice.org.uk/cg101/guidance/pdf/english%20 [Accessed 24 November 2014].

NICE, 2010a
National Institute for Health and Care Excellence, 2010. Bacterial meningitis and meningococcal septicaemia. Available at: http://www.nice.org.uk/guidance/cg102%20 [Accessed 16 November 2014].

NICE, 2011
National Institute for Health and Care Excellence, 2011. Hypertension in pregnancy: The management of hypertensive disorders during pregnancy. Available at:

http://www.nice.org.uk/guidance/cg107 [Accessed August 1, 2014].

NICE, 2012
National Institute for Health and Care Excellence, 2012. Infection: Prevention and Control of Healthcare-associated Infections in Primary and Community Care. Available at: http://www.nice.org.uk/guidance/cg139 [Accessed 21 December 2014].

NICE, 2013
National Institute for Health and Care Excellence, 2013. Unstable angina and NSTEMI. *NICE*. Available at: http://www.nice.org.uk/ [Accessed June 11, 2014].

NICE, 2014
National Institute for Health and Care Excellence, 2014. Head injury. Available at: http://www.nice.org.uk/guidance/cg176/ [Accessed 5 December 2014].

Nigam, 2008
Nigam Y and Knight J, 2008. Exploring the anatomy and physiology of ageing. Part 3 – the digestive system. *Nursing Times*, 104(33), 22–23.

NIHR, 2012
National Institute for Health Research, 2012. Diversity and inclusion: what's it about and why is it important for public involvement in research? Available at: http://www.invo.org.uk/wp-content/uploads/2012/10/involvediversityandinclusionoct2012.pdf [Accessed 11 January 2015].

Ninis, 2010
Ninis N, Nadel S and Glennie L, 2010. *Sections From Research For Doctors In Training*. 3rd ed. Bristol: Meningitis Research Foundation.

NNBC, 2012
National Network for Burn Care, 2012. *National Burn Care Referral Guidelines*, NNBC. Available at: http://www.britishburnassociation.org/downloads/national_burn_care_referral_guidance_-_5.2.12.pdf [Accessed July 18, 2014].

Nolan, 2006
Nolan J, Soar J and Eikeland H, 2006. The chain of survival. *Resuscitation*, 71(3), 270–271.

Nolan, 2010
Nolan JP, Soar J, Zideman DA, et al., 2010. European Resuscitation Council guidelines for resuscitation 2010 section 1. Executive summary. *Resuscitation*, 81(10), 1219–1276.

Nolan, 2012
Nolan J, Soar J, Lockey A, et al., 2012. *Advanced Life Support*. 6th ed. London: Resuscitation Council (UK).

Noppen, 2010
Noppen M, 2010. Spontaneous pneumothorax: epidemiology, pathophysiology and cause. *European Respiratory Review*, 19(117), 217–219.

NPSA, 2007
National Patient Safety Agency, 2007. Healthcare risk assessment made easy. Available at: http://www.nrls.npsa.nhs.uk/resources/?entryid45=59825 [Accessed 9th December 2014].

NPSA, 2008
National Patient Safety Agency, 2008. Risk matrix for risk managers. Available at: http://www.npsa.nhs.uk/nrls/improvingpatientsafety/patient-safety-tools-and-guidance/risk-assessment-guides/risk-matrix-for-risk-managers/ [Accessed 9th December 2014].

NTSP, 2014
National Tracheostomy Safety Project (Great Britain), 2014. *Comprehensive Tracheostomy Care: The National Tracheostomy Safety Project Manual*. McGrath BA (ed.), Chichester, West Sussex: John Wiley & Sons

Nutbeam, 2013
Nutbeam T and Boylan M, 2013. *ABC Of Prehospital Emergency Medicine*. Chichester: John Wiley & Sons.

NWSF, 2012
National Water Safety Forum, 2012. *UK water related fatalities 2010 WAID database report*, Available at: http://www.nationalwatersafety.org.uk/waid/info/waid_fatalincindentreport_2010.pdf [Accessed August 10, 2014].

NZGG, 2007
New Zealand Guidelines Group, 2007. *Management of Burns and Scalds in Primary Care*, Wellington: Accident Compensation Corporation.

O'Brien, 2003
O'Brien E, Asmar R, Beilin L, et al., 2003. European society of hypertension recommendations for conventional, ambulatory and home blood pressure measurement. *Journal of Hypertension*, 21(5), 821–848.

O'Donnell, 2010
O'Donnell MJ, Xavier D, Liu L, et al., 2010. Risk factors for ischaemic and intracerebral haemorrhagic stroke in 22 countries (the INTERSTROKE study): a case-control study. *The Lancet*, 376(9735), 112–123.

O'Driscoll, 2008
O'Driscoll BR, Howard LS, Davison AG, et al., 2008. British Thoracic Society guideline for emergency oxygen use in adult patients. *Thorax*, 63(Supplement 6), vi1–vi68.

ONS, 2013
Office for National Statistics, 2013. Deaths registered in England and Wales 2012. Available at: http://www.ons.gov.uk/ons/rel/vsob1/mortality-statistics--deaths-registered-in-england-and-wales--series-dr-/2012/dr-tables-2012.xls [Accessed April 20, 2014].

ONS, 2013a
Office for National Statistics, 2013. Births in England and Wales by Characteristics of Birth 2, 2012. *Office for National Statistics*. Available at: http://www.ons.gov.uk/ons/rel/vsob1/characteristics-of-birth-2--england-and-wales/2012/sb-characteristics-of-birth-2.html?format=print [Accessed August 3, 2014].

Orlowski, 1989
Orlowski JP, Abulleil MM and Phillips JM, 1989. The hemodynamic and cardiovascular effects of near-drowning in hypotonic, isotonic, or hypertonic solutions. *Annals of Emergency Medicine*, 18(10), 1044–1049.

Osler, 2012
Osler W, 2012. Pneumonia part 1: pathology, presentation and prevention. *British Journal of Nursing*, 21(2), 103.

Oyetunji, 2011
Oyetunji TA, Chang DC, Crompton JG, et al., 2011. Redefining hypotension in the elderly: normotension is not reassuring. *Archives of Surgery*, 146(7), 865–869.

Pante, 2010
Pante MD and American Academy of Orthopaedic Surgeons, 2010. *Advanced Assessment And Treatment Of Trauma*. Sudbury: Jones and Bartlett Publishers.

Papadopoulos, 2006
Papadopoulos IN, Kanakaris N, Bonovas S, et al., 2006. Auditing 655 fatalities with pelvic fractures by autopsy as a basis to evaluate trauma care. *Journal of the American College of Surgeons*, 203(1), 30–43.

Patel, 2008
Patel H, 2008. *Crash Course: Respiratory System*. 3rd ed. London: Elsevier Health Sciences.

Paul, 1998
Paul A, 1998. *Where Bias Begins: The Truth About Stereotypes*. Available at: http://www.psychologytoday.com/articles/199805/where-bias-begins-the-truth-about-stereotypes [Accessed 31 December 2014].

Peña, 2012
Peña SB & Larrard AR, 2012. Does the Trendelenburg position affect hemodynamics? A systematic review. *Emergencias*, 24, 143–150.

Personal Protective Equipment at Work Regulations 1992
United Kingdom, 1992. The Personal Protective Equipment at Work Regulations 1992. Available at: http://www.legislation.gov.uk/uksi/1992/2966/regulation/4/made [Accessed 29 December 2014].

PHE, 2014a
Public Health England, 2014. Meningococcal: the green book. Available at: https://www.gov.uk/government/publications/meningococcal-the-green-book-chapter-22%20 [Accessed 16 November 2014].

PHE, 2014b
Public Health England, 2014. Meningococcal disease: guidance, data and analysis. Available at: https://www.gov.uk/government/collections/meningococcal-disease-guidance-data-and-analysis [Accessed 16 November 2014].

Physio-Control, 2009
Physio-Control, 2009. *LifePak 15 Monitor/defibrillator Operating Instructions*. Available at: http://moodle.999cpd.com/%20http:/www.physio-control.com/uploadedfiles/physio85/contents/emergency_medical_care/products/operating_instructions/lifepak15_operatinginstructions_3306222-002.pdf [Accessed 11 December 2014].

Pickard, 2011
Pickard A, Karlen W, Ansermino JM. Capillary Refill Time: Is It Still a Useful Clinical Sign? *Anesthesia & Analgesia*. 2011 Jul;113(1):120–3.

PIE, 2014
Picker Institue Europe, 2014. NHS staff surveys – 2013 results. Available at: http://www.nhsstaffsurveys.com/page/1006/latest-results/2013-results/ [Accessed 8 December 2014].

Piette, 2006
Piette MHA and De Letter EA, 2006. Drowning: Still a difficult autopsy diagnosis. *Forensic Science International*, 163(1-2), 1–9.

Piirilä, 1995
Piirilä P and Sovijärvi ARA, 1995. Crackles: recording, analysis and clinical significance. *European Respiratory Journal*, 8(12), 2139–2148.

Pilbery, 2013
Pilbery R, Caroline NL, American Academy of Orthopaedic Surgeons, et al., 2013. *Nancy Caroline's Emergency Care In The Streets*. United Kingdom 7th ed. Burlington: Jones and Bartlett Learning.

PML, 2014
Prometheus Medical Ltd, 2014. Prometheus pelvic splint: instruction sheet.

Pokorná, 2010
Pokorná M, Nečas E, Kratochvíl J, et al., 2010. A sudden increase in partial pressure end-tidal carbon dioxide (PETCO2) at the moment of return of spontaneous circulation. *The Journal of Emergency Medicine*, 38(5), 614–621.

Porth, 2003
Porth CM, 2003. *Essentials Of Pathophysiology: Concepts Of Altered Health States*. London: Lippincott Williams & Wilkins.

Preston, 2004
Preston ST and Hegadoren K, 2004. Glass contamination in parenterally administered medication. *Journal of Advanced Nursing*, 48(3), 266–270.

Prien, 1988
Prien T and Traber DL, 1988. Toxic smoke compounds and inhalation injury – a review. *Burns, Including Thermal Injury*, 14(6), 451–460.

PROMPT, 2012
Prompt Maternity Foundation, 2012. *PROMPT Course Manual*, Cambridge: Cambridge University Press.

Provision and Use of Work Equipment Regulations 1998
United Kingdom, 1998. The Provision and Use of Work Equipment Regulations 1998. Available at: http://www.legislation.gov.uk/uksi/1998/2306/contents/made [Accessed 29 December 2014].

Pumphrey, 2000
Pumphrey R, 2000. Sections for management of anaphylaxis from a study of fatal reactions. *Clinical & Experimental Allergy*, 30(8), 1144–1150.

Purcell, 2010
Purcell D, 2010. *Minor Injuries: A Clinical Guide*. Edinburgh; New York: Elsevier Churchill Livingstone.

Randle, 2009
Randle J, Coffey F and Bradbury M, 2009. *Oxford Handbook Of Clinical Skills In Adult Nursing*. Oxford; New York: Oxford University Press.

RCOG, 2012
Royal College of Obstetricians and Gynaecologists, 2012. Shoulder dystocia (Green-top Guideline 42). Available at: http://www.rcog.org.uk/womens-health/clinical-guidance/shoulder-dystocia-green-top-42 [Accessed August 3, 2014].

Resuscitation Council UK, 2015
Resuscitation Council UK, 2015. Resuscitation Guidelines. Available at: https://www.resus.org.uk/resuscitation-guidelines [Accessed 26 Oct, 2015]

Roberts, 2014
Roberts JR, Custalow, Thomsen, et al., 2014. *Roberts And Hedges' Clinical Procedures In Emergency Medicine*. 6th edn. New York: Elsevier.

Rodgers, 2004
Rodgers H, Greenaway J, Davies T, et al., 2004. Risk factors for first-ever stroke in older people in the North East of England: a population-based study. *Stroke*, 35(1), 7–11.

Roguin, 2006
Roguin A, 2006. Rene Theophile Hyacinthe Laennec (1781–1826): the man behind the stethoscope. *Clinical Medicine & Research*, 4(3), 230–235.

Ross, 2014
Ross S, 2014. *Rapid Infection Control Nursing*. Rapid series, Chichester, West Sussex: Wiley-Blackwell.

Rossaint, 2010
Rossaint R, Bouillon B, Cerny V, et al., 2010. Management of bleeding following major trauma: an updated European guideline. *Critical Care*, 14(2), R52.

Ryland, 2014
Ryland B and Roy TM, 2014. Pneumothorax. Available at: http://bestpractice.bmj.com/best-practice/monograph/504/highlights/summary.html [Accessed 4 November 2014].

Sampson, 2006
Sampson HA, Muñoz-Furlong A, Campbell RL, et al., 2006. Second symposium on the definition and management of anaphylaxis: summary report – second National Institute of Allergy and Infectious Disease/Food Allergy and Anaphylaxis Network Symposium. *Annals of Emergency Medicine*, 47(4), 373–380.

SAS, 2014
Scottish Ambulance Service, 2014. Dementia Learning Resource. Publication, Available at: http://www.nes.scot.nhs.uk/education-and-training/by-theme-initiative/mental-health-and-learning-disabilities/publications-and-resources/publications-repository/scottish-ambulance-service-dementia-learning-resource.aspx [Accessed 15 January 2015].

Saver, 2006
Saver JL, 2006. Time is brain – quantified. *Stroke*, 37(1), 263–266.

SCAS, 2010
South Central Ambulance Service NHS Trust, 2010. *Major Incident Plan*. Available at: http://www.southcentralambulance.nhs.uk/_assets/documents/scas%20mip%202010%20%20v1.51%20june%202010.pdf [Accessed June 28, 2014].

SCAS, 2013
South Central Ambulance Service NHS Trust, 2013. *Fire Policy and Procedure*, Available at: http://www.southcentralambulance.nhs.uk/_assets/

documents/policies/corporate/cpp%20no.%2022%20 scas%20fire%20policy%202013.pdf [Accessed July 26, 2014].

SCIE, 2013
Social Care Institute for Excellence, 2013. Dementia Gateway. Available at: http://www.scie.org.uk/ publications/dementia/index.asp [Accessed 15 January 2015].

SECAmb, 2011
South East Coast Ambulance Service NHS Foundation Trust, 2011. Resourcing Escalatory Action Plan. Available at: http://www.secamb.nhs.uk/about_us/ news/2013/idoc.ashx?docid=eb9d79c5-5452-485a-818a-7ccf6b004d5f&version=-1 [Accessed 12th December 2014].

SG, 2009
Scottish Government, 2009. Review of Allergy Services in Scotland: A Report by a Working Group of the Scottish Medical and Scientific Advisory Committee. Publication, Available at: http://www.scotland.gov.uk/ publications/2009/06/17135245/0 [Accessed 5 November 2014]).

Sharma, 2008
Sharma A and Jindal P, 2008. Principles of diagnosis and management of traumatic pneumothorax. *Journal of Emergencies, Trauma and Shock*, 1(1), 34–41.

Shattock, 2012
Shattock MJ and Tipton MJ, 2012. 'Autonomic conflict': a different way to die during cold water immersion? *The Journal of Physiology*, 590(14), 3219–3230.

Sheridan, 2012
Sheridan R, 2012. *Burns: A Practical Approach To Immediate Treatment And Long-term Care*. London: Manson Publishing.

Simon, 2010
Simon C, 2010. *Oxford Handbook Of General Practice*. 3rd ed. Oxford Handbooks, Oxford: Oxford University Press.

Simons, 2001
Simons FER, Gu X and Simons KJ, 2001. Epinephrine absorption in adults: Intramuscular versus subcutaneous injection. *Journal of Allergy and Clinical Immunology*, 108(5), 871–873.

Simpson, 2002
Simpson T, Krieg JC, Heuer F, et al., 2002. Stabilization of pelvic ring disruptions with a circumferential sheet. *The Journal of Trauma and Acute Care Surgery*, 52(1), 158–161.

Singer, 2006
Singer AJ, Freidman B, Modi P, et al., 2006. The effect of a commercially available burn-cooling blanket on core body temperatures in volunteers. *Academic Emergency Medicine*, 13(6), 686–690.

Singer, 2010
Singer AJ, Taira BR, Thode Jr HC, et al., 2010. The association between hypothermia, prehospital cooling, and mortality in burn victims. *Academic Emergency Medicine*, 17(4), 456–459.

SJA, SAA, BRC, 2014
St. John Ambulance, St. Andrew's Ambulance Association and British Red Cross, 2014. *First Aid Manual*. 10th ed. London: Dorling Kindersley.

Smith, 2011a
Smith I, Mackay J, Fahrid N, et al., 2011. Respiratory rate measurement: a comparison of methods. *British Journal of Healthcare Assistants*, 5(1), 18–23.

Smith, 2011b
Smith J (ed), 2011. *The Guide to the Handling of People: A Systems Approach*, Teddington, Middlesex: BackCare.

Smith, 2013
Smith LA et al., 2013. Incidence of and risk factors for perineal trauma: a prospective observational study. *BMC Pregnancy and Childbirth*, 13(1), 59.

Smithson, 2012
Smithson H and Walker MC, 2012. *ABC Of Epilepsy*. 1st ed. ABC series, Chichester: John Wiley & Sons.

Smithuis, 2008
Smithuis, R. & Willems, T., 2008. Coronary anatomy and anomalies. *The Radiology Assistant*. Available at: http://www.radiologyassistant.nl/en/ 48275120e2ed5%20 [Accessed June 4, 2014].

Soar, 2008
Soar J, Pumphrey R, Cant A, et al., 2008. Emergency treatment of anaphylactic reactions – guidelines for healthcare providers. *Resuscitation*, 77(2), 157–169.

Soar, 2010
Soar J, Perkins GD, Abbas G, et al., 2010. European Resuscitation Council guidelines for resuscitation 2010 section 8. cardiac arrest in special circumstances: electrolyte abnormalities, poisoning, drowning, accidental hypothermia, hyperthermia, asthma, anaphylaxis, cardiac surgery, trauma, pregnancy, electrocution. *Resuscitation*, 81(10), 1400–1433.

Spiteri, 1988
Spiteri MA, Cook DG and Clarke SW, 1988. Reliability of eliciting physical signs in examination of the chest. *Lancet*, 1(8590), 873–875.

Steg, 2012
Steg G, James SK, Atar D, et al., 2012. ESC guidelines for the management of acute myocardial infarction in patients presenting with ST-segment elevation the task force on the management of ST-segment elevation acute myocardial infarction of the European Society of Cardiology (ESC). *European Heart Journal*, 33(20), 2569–2619.

Stewart, 2013
Stewart M, 2013. Bet 3: pelvic circumferential compression devices for haemorrhage control: panacea or myth? *Emergency Medicine Journal*, 30(5), 425–426.

Studnek, 2012
Studnek JR, Artho MR, Garner Jr CL, et al., 2012. The impact of emergency medical services on the ED care of severe sepsis. *The American Journal of Emergency Medicine*, 30(1), 51–56.

Stuke, 2007
Stuke L, Diaz-Arrastia R, Gentilello LM, et al., 2007. Effect of alcohol on Glasgow Coma Scale in head-injured patients. *Annals of Surgery*, 245(4), 651–655.

SWAST, 2013
South Western Ambulance Service NHS Foundation Trust, 2013. Major haemorrhage. Available at: http://www.swast.nhs.uk/Downloads/Clinical%20 Guidelines%20SWASFT%20staff/CG14_Major_ Haemorrhage.pdf [Accessed 15 June 2016].

SWAST, 2014
South Western Ambulance Service NHS Foundation Trust, 2014. Major Incident Plan. Available at: http:// www.swast.nhs.uk/downloads/swasft%20policies/ swasft_mip.pdf [Accessed June 28, 2014].

SWAST, 2014a
South Western Ambulance Service NHS Foundation Trust, 2014. Risk management strategy. Available at: http://www.swast.nhs.uk/downloads/swasft%20 policies/riskstrategy.pdf [Accessed 5 January 2015].

SWAST, 2014b
South Western Ambulance Service NHS Foundation Trust, 2014. Community first responders. Available at: http://www.swast.nhs.uk/working%20with%20us/ community-first-responders.htm [Accessed 31 December 2014].

SWAST, 2014c
South Western Ambulance Service NHS Foundation Trust, 2013. Cardiac Arrest. Available at: http:// www.swast.nhs.uk/downloads/clinical%20 guidelines%20swasft%20staff/cg07_cardiac_arrest.pdf [Accessed August 11, 2014].

Szpilman, 2004
Szpilman, D. & Soares, M., 2004. In-water resuscitation – is it worthwhile? *Resuscitation*, 63(1), 25–31.

Szpilman, 2012
Szpilman D et al., 2012. Drowning. *Journal of Medicine,* 366(22), 2102–2110.

Tall, 2003
Tall G, Wise D, Grove P, et al., 2003. The accuracy of external blood loss estimation by ambulance and hospital personnel. *Emergency Medicine*, 15(4), 318–321.

Talley, 2006
Talley NJ and O'Connor S, 2006. *Clinical Examination: A Systematic Guide To Physical Diagnosis*. 5th ed. London: Elsevier.

Tapson, 2008
Tapson VF, 2008. Acute pulmonary embolism. *The New England Journal of Medicine*, 358(10), 1037–1052.

Teasdale, 1974
Teasdale G and Jennett B, 1974. Assessment of coma and impaired consciousness. *The Lancet*, 304(7872), 81–84.

Teasdale, 1976
Teasdale G and Jennett B, 1976. Assessment and prognosis of coma after head injury. *Acta neurochirurgica*, 34(1-4), 45–55.

Thadepalli, 2002
Thadepalli H, 2002. Women gave birth to the stethoscope: Laennec's introduction of the art of auscultation of the lung. *Clinical infectious diseases*, 35(5), 587–588.

Thompson, 2006
Thompson MJ, Ninis N, Perera R, et al., 2006. Clinical recognition of meningococcal disease in children and adolescents. *The Lancet*, 367(9508), 397–403.

Thompson, 2006a
Thompson N, 2006. *Anti-Discriminatory Practice*. 4th ed. Basingstoke: Palgrave Macmillan.

Thompson, 2008
Thompson G and Sciarra J (eds), 2008. *Wound Care Made Incredibly Visual*. Ambler: Lippincott Williams and Wilkins.

Tipton, 2011
Tipton MJ and Golden FSC, 2011. A proposed decision-making guide for the search, rescue and resuscitation of submersion (head under) victims based on expert opinion. *Resuscitation*, 82(7), 819–824.

Toon, 2010
Toon MH et al., 2010. Management of acute smoke inhalation injury. *Critical Care and Resuscitation: Journal of the Australasian Academy of Critical Care Medicine*, 12(1), 53–61.

Torbicki, 2008
Torbicki A, Perrier A, Konstantinides S, et al., 2008. Guidelines on the diagnosis and management of acute pulmonary embolism. *European Heart Journal*, 29(18), 2276–2315.

Tortora, 2008
Tortora GJ and Derrickson BH, 2008. *Principles Of Anatomy And Physiology*. 12th ed. Hoboken: John Wiley & Sons.

Tortora, 2013
Tortora GJ, 2013. *Microbiology: An Introduction*. Harlow: Pearson.

Toth, 2012
Toth L, King KL, McGrath B, et al., 2012. Efficacy and safety of emergency non-invasive pelvic ring stabilisation. *Injury*, 43(8), 1330–1334.

US Navy, 2009
United States Navy, 2009. Time Critical Risk Management. Available at: http://www.public.navy.mil/ comnavsafecentest/documents/orm_data/tcrm_jpa/ tcrm_facilitator_notes_v2-aug09_dlt.pdf [Accessed 19 December 2014].

Vacanti, 2011
Vacanti CA, 2011. *Essential Clinical Anesthesia*. Cambridge: Cambridge University Press.

Valensi, 2011
Valensi P, Lorgis L and Cottin Y, 2011. Prevalence, incidence, predictive factors and prognosis of silent myocardial infarction: a review of the literature. *Archives of Cardiovascular Diseases*, 104(3), 178–188.

Vause, 2005
Vause S and Saroya DK, 2005. Functions of the placenta. *Anaesthesia & Intensive Care Medicine*, 6(3), 77–80.

Venema, 2010
Venema AM, Groothoff JW and Bierens JJLM, 2010. The role of bystanders during rescue and resuscitation of drowning victims. *Resuscitation*, 81(4), 434–439.

Vincent, 2006
Vincent J-L, Sakr Y, Sprung CL, et al., 2006. Sepsis in European intensive care units: results of the SOAP study. *Critical Care Medicine*, 34(2), 344–353.

Walfish, 2009
Walfish M, Neuman A and Wlody D, 2009. Maternal haemorrhage. *British Journal of Anaesthesia*, 103(Supplement 1), i47–i56.

Wallis, 2006
Wallis LA and Carley S, 2006. Comparison of paediatric major incident primary triage tools. *Emergency Medicine Journal*, 23(6), 475–478.

Walls, 2012
Walls RM and Murphy MF (eds), 2012. *Manual Of Emergency Airway Management*. 4th ed. Philadelphia: Wolters Kluwer/Lippincott Williams & Wilkins Heath.

Walters, 2005
Walters TJ and Mabry RL, 2005. Issues related to the use of tourniquets on the battlefield. *Military Medicine*, 170(9), 770–775.

Ward, 1998
Ward KR and Yealy DM, 1998. End-tidal carbon dioxide monitoring in emergency medicine, part 1: basic principles. *Academic Emergency Medicine: Official Journal of the Society for Academic Emergency Medicine*, 5(6), 628–636.

Wardrope, 2008
Wardrope J et al., 2008. *Community Emergency Medicine* 1st ed., London: Churchill Livingstone.

Waterhouse, 2005
Waterhouse C, 2005. The Glasgow Coma Scale and other neurological observations. *Nursing Standard*, 19(33), 56.

Waterhouse, 2009
Waterhouse C, 2009. The use of painful stimulus in relation to Glasgow Coma Scale observations. *British Journal of Neuroscience Nursing*, 5(5), 209–215.

Watson, 2001
Watson RS, Cummings P, Quan L, et al., 2001. Cervical spine injuries among submersion victims. *The Journal of Trauma*, 51(4), 658–662.

Watson, 2009
Watson MS ed., 2009. *Oxford Handbook of Palliative Care* 2nd ed., Oxford: Oxford University Press.

Wells, 2001
Wells LC, Smith JC, Weston VC, et al., 2001. The child with a non-blanching rash: How likely is meningococcal disease? *Archives of Disease in Childhood*, 85(3), 218.

Weston, 2014
Weston D, 2014. *Fundamentals Of Infection Prevention And Control: Theory And Practice*. 2nd ed. Chichester, West Sussex: John Wiley & Sons.

Whitaker, 2011
Whitaker DK, 2011. Time for capnography – everywhere. *Anaesthesia*, 66(7), 544–549.

WHO, 1999
World Health Organization, 1999. *Definition, Diagnosis And Classification Of Diabetes Mellitus And Its Complications*. WHO, Available at: http://whqlibdoc.who.int/hq/1999/who_ncd_ncs_99.2.pdf?ua=1 [Accessed 6 November 2014].

WHO, 2009
World Health Organization, 2009. *WHO Guidelines On Hand Hygiene In Health Care: First Global Patient Safety Challenge: Clean Care Is Safer Care*. Geneva: World Health Organization, Patient Safety.

WHO, 2009a
World Health Organization, 2009. *WHO Guidelines For Safe Surgery 2009: Safe Surgery Saves Lives*. Available at: http://whqlibdoc.who.int/publications/2009/9789241598552_eng.pdf?ua=1 [Accessed 19 January 2015].

WHO, 2011
World Health Organization, 2011. Pulse Oximetry Training Manual. Available at: http://www.who.int/patientsafety/safesurgery/pulse_oximetry/who_ps_pulse_oximetry_training_manual_en.pdf [Accessed May 22, 2014].

WHO, 2012
World Health Organization, 2012. *WHO Recommendations For The Prevention And Treatment Of Postpartum Haemorrhage*. Geneva: World Health Organization, Available at: http://apps.who.int/iris/bitstream/10665/75411/1/9789241548502_eng.pdf?ua=1 [Accessed 3 August 2014].

Wijdicks, 2010
Wijdicks EFM, 2010. The Bare Essentials: Coma. *Practical Neurology*, 10(1), 51–60.

Wood, 2002
Wood KE, 2002. Major pulmonary embolism. *Chest*, 121(3), 877 –905.

YAS, 2013
Yorkshire Ambulance Service NHS Trust, 2013. Dementia Learning Resource for Ambulance Staff. Available at: http://www.yas.nhs.uk/calling999/docs/dementia%20learning%20resource%20for%20ambulance%20staff.pdf [Accessed 15 January 2015].

Young, 2014
Young GB, 2014. Assessment of coma. Available at: http://bestpractice.bmj.com/best-practice/monograph/417/overview/summary.html [Accessed 18 November 2014].

Zabir, 2008
Zabir AF, Choy CY and Rushdan R, 2008. Glass particle contamination of parenteral preparations of intravenous drugs in anaesthetic practice: original research. *Southern African Journal of Anaesthesia and Analgesia*, 14(3), 17–19.

Zuercher, 2009
Zuercher M, Ummenhofer W, Baltussen A, et al., 2009. The use of Glasgow Coma Scale in injury assessment: A critical review. *Brain Injury*, 23(5), 371–384.

Index

D

N

O

NOTES

NOTES

NOTES

NOTES